BUCHENWALD: HELL ON A HILLTOP

Murder, Torture & Medical Experiments in the Nazis' Worst Concentration Camp

BUCHENWALD: HELL ON A HILLTOP

Murder, Torture & Medical Experiments in the Nazis' Worst Concentration Camp

Flint Whitlock

CABLE PUBLISHING

Brule, Wisconsin

BUCHENWALD: HELL ON A HILLTOP
Murder, Torture & Medical Experiments in the Nazis' Worst Concentration Camp

First Edition

Published by:
Cable Publishing
14090 E Keinenen Rd
Brule, WI 54820
www.cablepublishing.com
E-mail: nan@cablepublishing.com

Hardcover: 978-1-934980-72-9
Soft cover: 978-1-934980-71-2

Library of Congress Control Number: 2013945438

Excerpts from *War Against the Weak: Eugenics and America's Campaign to Create a Master Race*, by Edwin Black, 2012, expanded edition by Dialog Press, reprinted by permission of the author.

Excerpts from *From the Holocaust to Hogan's Heroes: The Autobiography of Robert Clary*, by Robert Clary, 2001, reprinted by permission of the author.

Excerpts from *Survivor of Buchenwald: My Personal Odyssey Through Hell*, by Louis Gros, 2012, reprinted by permission of Cable Publishing, Inc.

Excerpts from *The Liberators: America's Witnesses to the Holocaust*, by Michael Hirsh, 2010, reprinted by permission of the author.

Excerpts from *168 Jump Into Hell*, by Arthur Kinnis, 1999, reprinted by permission of the author.

Excerpts from *Inhumanity: Death March to Buchenwald and The Last Jews of Bendzin*, by John Ranz, 2007, reprinted by permission of the author.

Excerpts from *Saving Children: Diary of a Buchenwald Survivor and Rescuer*, by Jack Werber, 1996, reprinted by permission of Transaction Publishers.

Cover photo: A composite of two images, Heinrich Himmler with Adolf Hitler and an interior view of a barracks at Buchenwald Concentration Camp, both courtesy of the National Archives.

Printed in the United States of America

TODAY, BUCHENWALD IS ONLY A SYMBOL

Some things never change, and one is evil. It is always with us – lurking right around the corner. It always has been – waiting for its chance. It always will be. Edmund Burke saw the danger clearly:

The only thing necessary for the triumph
of evil is for good men to do nothing.

If anybody doubts the truth of Burke's maxim, the proof of it sits on a hill in Germany near the peaceful town of Weimar, once the capital of that country's first try at real democracy. It is the ultimate in tragic irony: What remains of Nazi Germany's worst camp overlooks the remains of the bright promise of real representative government.

Today, Buchenwald is only a symbol. Like Dachau, where this writer has been, Buchenwald is quiet now, open for people to see where some of the worst atrocities in all of history were committed. But unless the visitor has read and thought deeply about the filthy things that were done within that camp, he or she cannot understand the horror of what happened there…and can happen again. Here.

Few historians know more, or write better, about the horror that was Buchenwald than Flint Whitlock…and the horror that can be again if we, as good people, do nothing and let down our guard. For our world is full of "isms," causes, and radical philosophies. Many of them sound wonderful – they are fair of skin but foul inside.

And our world is full of people ready to perpetrate any horror in the name of their pet fair-sounding philosophy. In their surreal philosophy they are right, of course, and everybody who disagrees with them is therefore wrong. In their eyes, whatever it is their scheme requires, however vicious, however bizarre, it has to be done…for the greater good of everybody, of course.

We cannot convince such fanatics that they are wrong; nobody can. What we *can* do is read this book, and the other two in the Buchenwald series, and tell our kids and grandkids about the horror that was…and can be again.

For if we let it happen again, it is they who will suffer, and that is inexcusable.

— Col. Robert Barr Smith (ret.),
author of *The Robbers*

FLINT WHITLOCK BOOKS

The Buchenwald Trilogy: Volume I
The Beasts of Buchenwald
Karl & Ilse Koch, Human-skin Lampshades, & the War-Crimes Trial of the Century
by Flint Whitlock

The Buchenwald Trilogy: Volume II
Survivor of Buchenwald
My Personal Odyssey through Hell
by Louis Gros with Flint Whitlock

Fight On
A GI's Odyssey Back to Nazi Germany
by Bernard L. Kahn
with Neil Kahn and Flint Whitlock

Turbulence before Takeoff
The Life & Times of Aviation Pioneer Marlon DeWitt Green
by Flint Whitlock

Internal Conflicts
a novel
by Flint Whitlock

Capt. Jepp and the Little Black Book
How Barnstormer & Aviation Pioneer Elrey B. Jeppesen Made the Skies Safer for Everyone
by Flint Whitlock and Terry Barnhart

CONTENTS

Prologue 1
Introduction 6
Chapter 1 Hell under Construction 13
Chapter 2 The Beasts of Buchenwald 25
Chapter 3 Chamber of Horrors 42
Chapter 4 Turning Men into Monsters 51
Chapter 5 What the World Knew 63
Chapter 6 The Devil's Doctors 82
Chapter 7 The Demented Doctor 99
Chapter 8 Super Weapons 104
Chapter 9 Official Indifference 122
Chapter 10 Buchenwald, Inc. 128
Chapter 11 The Little Children Suffer 143
Chapter 12 The End Nears 148
Chapter 13 No Place for a Princess 154
Chapter 14 Fallen to Earth 158
Chapter 15 Mission 132 165
Chapter 16 Life in the Ruins 178
Chapter 17 The Beginning of the End 185
Chapter 18 Third Army to the Rescue 203
Chapter 19 Ordeal at Ohrdruf 211
Chapter 20 Evacuating Buchenwald 229
Chapter 21 Overrunning Ohrdruf 237
Chapter 22 The Liberation of Buchenwald 248
Chapter 23 The Surrender of Weimar 259
Chapter 24 Ike at Ohrdruf 267
Chapter 25 Patton at Buchenwald 275
Chapter 26 Tourist Destination 296
Chapter 27 Unprepared 308
Chapter 28 Marching to Oblivion 319
Chapter 29 Justice? 328
Epilogue 343
Acknowledgments 345
Source Notes 346
Bibliography 357
Index 365

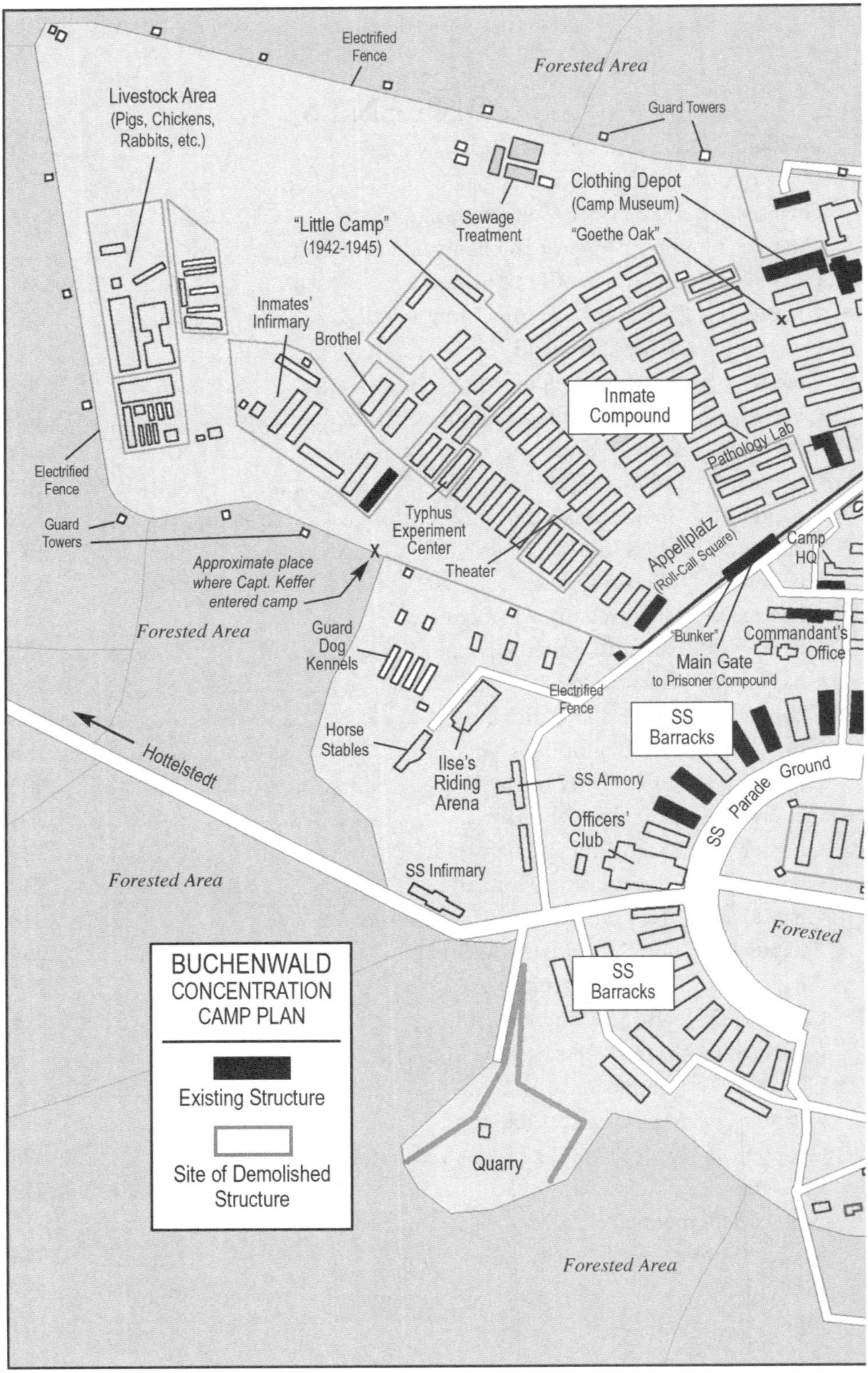
Electrified Fence
Forested Area
Guard Towers
Livestock Area
(Pigs, Chickens, Rabbits, etc.)
Sewage Treatment
Clothing Depot
(Camp Museum)
"Little Camp"
(1942-1945)
"Goethe Oak"
Inmates' Infirmary
Brothel
Inmate Compound
Pathology Lab
Electrified Fence
Guard Towers
Typhus Experiment Center
Theater
Appellplatz
(Roll-Call Square)
Camp HQ
Approximate place where Capt. Keffer entered camp
Forested Area
Guard Dog Kennels
"Bunker"
Commandant's Office
Main Gate
to Prisoner Compound
Electrified Fence
SS Barracks
Horse Stables
Ilse's Riding Arena
SS Armory
Hottelstedt
Officers' Club
SS Parade Ground
SS Infirmary
Forested Area
Forested
SS Barracks
Quarry
Forested Area
BUCHENWALD CONCENTRATION CAMP PLAN
Existing Structure
Site of Demolished Structure

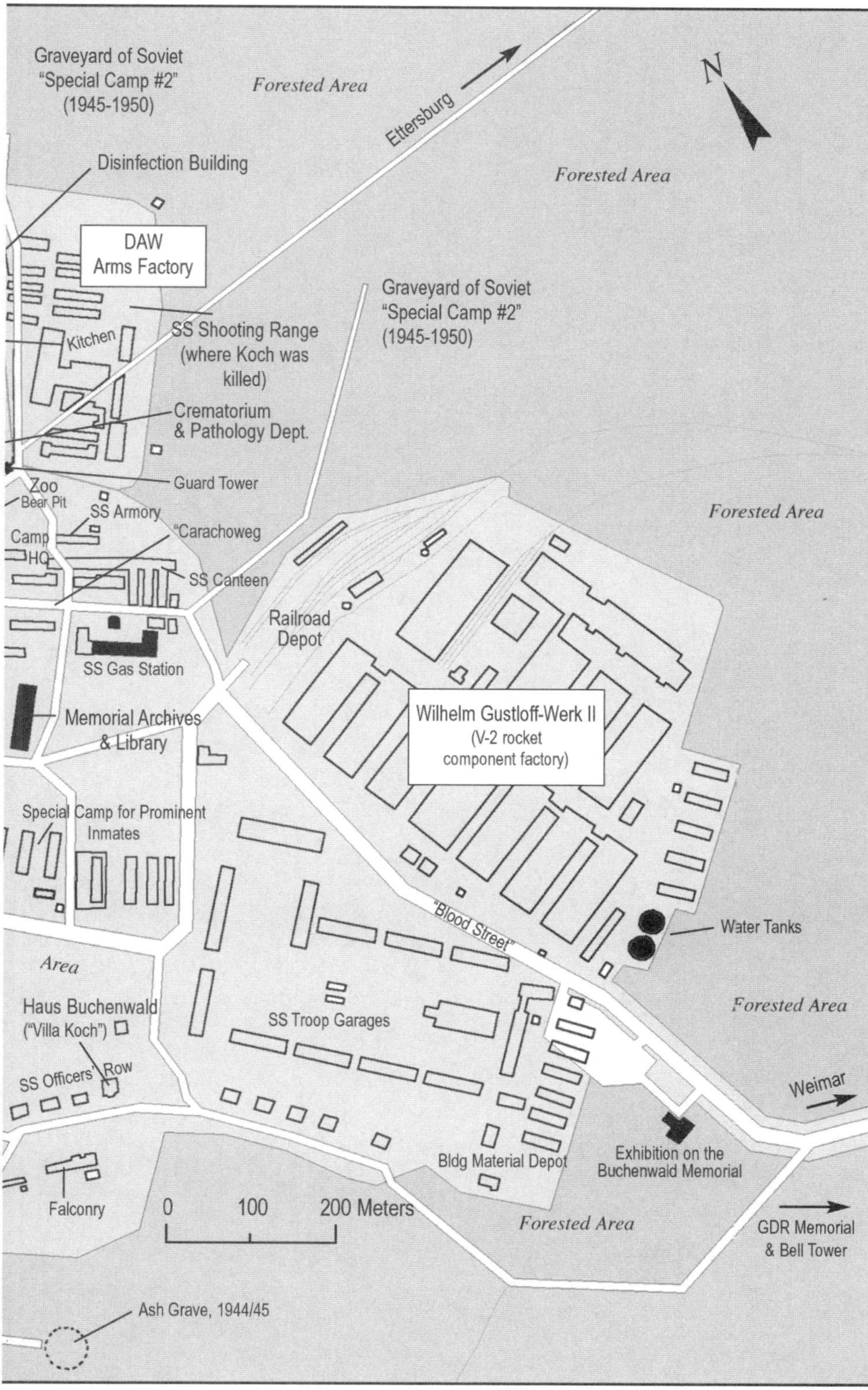

Graveyard of Soviet "Special Camp #2" (1945-1950)
Forested Area
Ettersburg
N
Forested Area
Disinfection Building
DAW Arms Factory
Kitchen
SS Shooting Range (where Koch was killed)
Graveyard of Soviet "Special Camp #2" (1945-1950)
Crematorium & Pathology Dept.
Guard Tower
Zoo
Bear Pit
SS Armory
Camp HQ
"Carachoweg
SS Canteen
Forested Area
Railroad Depot
SS Gas Station
Memorial Archives & Library
Wilhelm Gustloff-Werk II (V-2 rocket component factory)
Special Camp for Prominent Inmates
"Blood Street"
Water Tanks
Area
Haus Buchenwald ("Villa Koch")
SS Troop Garages
Forested Area
SS Officers' Row
Weimar
Exhibition on the Buchenwald Memorial
Bldg Material Depot
Falconry
0 100 200 Meters
Forested Area
GDR Memorial & Bell Tower
Ash Grave, 1944/45

PROLOGUE

THE DAY—MONDAY, April 16, 1945—was a warm, beautiful spring day. Along the paved, tree-lined road leading up the Ettersberg hill from the bomb-damaged German city of Weimar trudged a long line of civilians, many dressed in their best clothing: suits, hats, dresses, polished shoes. The road was steep and the sun was high; the few white, puffy clouds offered no relief from the heat or the strenuous walk. Some of the men removed their suit jackets and slung them over their shoulders. Occasionally a man would stop and mop his brow with a handkerchief before being encouraged by an American soldier with a rifle to continue the upward climb.

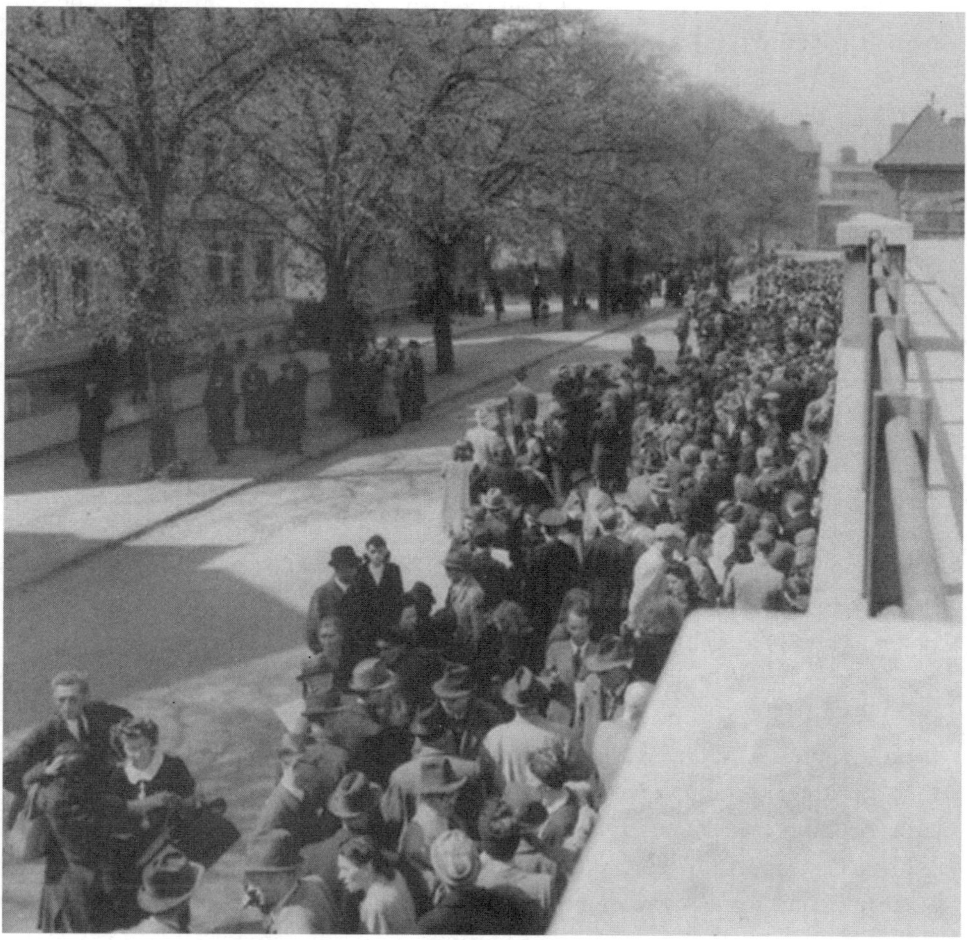

A thousand Weimar citizens, following the orders of General Patton, line up at the main train station and wait to be escorted up the Ettersberg hill for their first visit to the Buchenwald concentration camp, April 16, 1945. What they discovered would shock them. (U.S. National Archives)

Up the road they walked, more than a thousand men and women, speaking little, wondering silently what they were about to be forced to see against their will. There had been rumors, of course, that atop the Ettersberg hill—the only geographic feature that relieved the otherwise gently rolling terrain around Weimar—their now-tottering Nazi regime had been operating a concentration camp since 1937.

The camp with the bucolic name "Buchenwald," meaning Beech Forest, was more than a rumor to most of Weimar's citizens; in 1937 the *Thüringer Gauzeitung*, the regional Nazi Party newspaper, had been full of stories about the new prison camp being built atop the hill—a camp that would provide an economic boost to the community. Many of the citizens talked about how this was the *quid pro quo*—the payoff for all the years that so many of them had been Nazi Party loyalists.

Plenty of SS guards had frequented the taverns of Weimar over the years and, with their lips loosened by *Bier* and *Schnapps*, often talked a little too freely about the camp on top of the hill. Scores of filthy, emaciated prisoners in striped uniforms had also been seen cleaning up the rubble after that terrible day of February 9, 1945, when the American aerial bombing raid had reduced much of the city's historic core to ruins. Anyone who lived near the main train station or the rail line leading up the hill surely had, for quite some time, been aware of the scores of trains packed with prisoners heading either to or from the hilltop camp.

And, of course, there had been the ever-present wispy gray smoke that drifted over the city, carrying with it the unmistakable, unforgettable stench of burning human flesh.

It had not been wise for ordinary citizens to ask too many questions of the Nazi regime that had begun a dozen years earlier. Even if some of them had been opposed to Adolf Hitler and the Nazis (although the Weimar area had been a particularly enthusiastic Nazi hotbed long before Hitler became chancellor), it was well understood that those who dissented, opposed, or otherwise questioned what was taking place under the hypnotic symbol of the swastika soon disappeared, along with, in many cases, their families. It was simply better (and healthier) to shut their eyes and ears and minds, and pretend not to see, hear, or know what was going on atop the Ettersberg.

But the American army was now in the rubble of Weimar with their guns and tanks and hordes of soldiers looking and acting like the conquering heroes they were. And, just yesterday, an American general—someone said his name was Patton—had notified the new, acting mayor of Weimar that he must have a thousand citizens ready on the morning of April 16 to be marched up to the hilltop camp to view the atrocious handiwork of their fellow countrymen. That was why they were on this march.

ONWARD AND UPWARD the well-dressed crowd of sweating marchers continued. As they neared the crest of the hill, they passed the familiar, 140-foot-tall crenellated observation tower known as the Bismarckturm—an imposing stone edifice dedicated to the beloved late Prussian emperor, Otto von Bismarck, and his Second Reich—which overlooked the city and had been a place of happy gatherings, weddings, and picnicking since it opened forty-four years earlier.

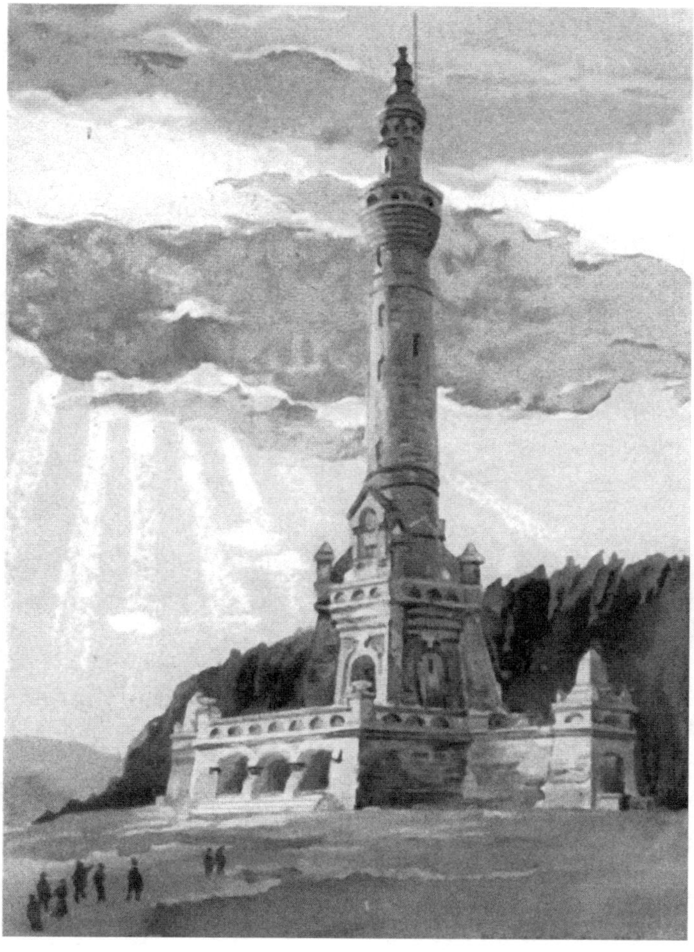

Watercolor sketch on a 1902 postcard showing the Bismarckturm on the Ettersberg hill (Author collection)

After trudging a few hundred yards farther up the road, the group reached the crest of the hill and saw what had been kept from them for the past eight years. On their left was a complex of garages and maintenance facilities that had been used by the SS regiment permanently stationed at the camp. Across the road, to the marchers' right, were the blackened, still-shattered remains of the Wilhelm Gustloff-Werk II factory that once had made components for some secret German weapon (none of the civilians knew exactly what) and which had been destroyed in a precise American bombing raid eight months earlier.

A little farther on, past an assemblage of offices and other low buildings that had been used by the SS, stood the two-story gatehouse and formal entrance to the camp, the words *Jedem das Seine* welded to the wrought-iron gate. Outside the gate, waiting for them, were more American soldiers along with gaunt men in ragged, striped uniforms.

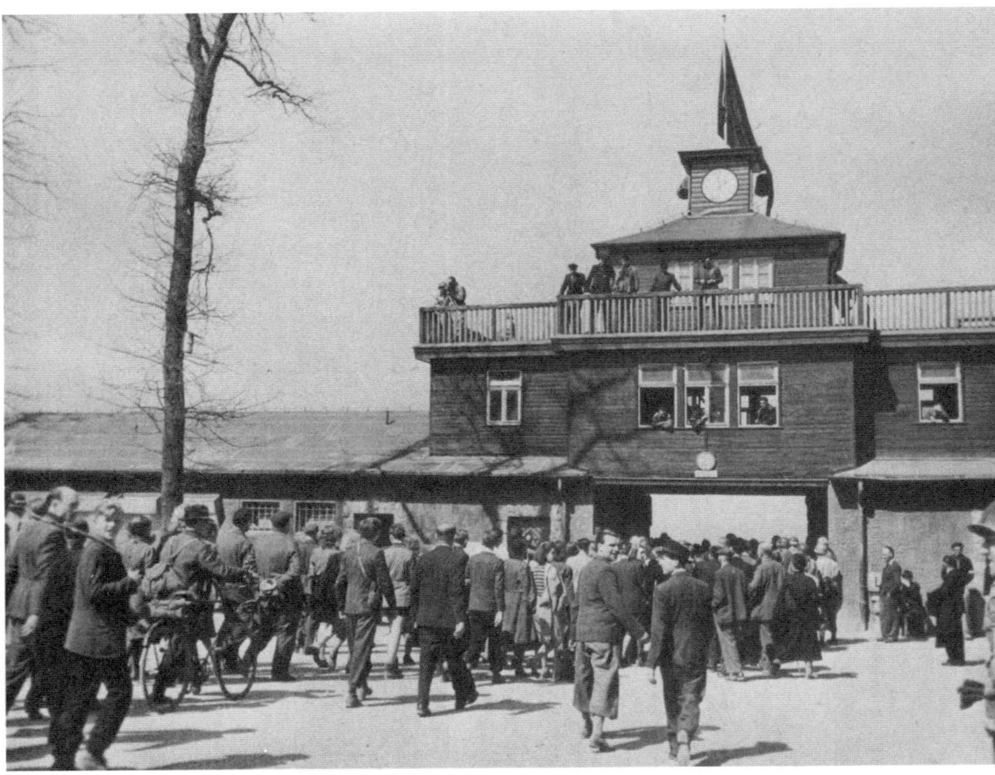

Weimar citizens stream through the camp's main gate as they begin their forced guided tour of Buchenwald, April 16, 1945. Barely visible on the lintel above the gate is an inscription: *Mein Vaterland, Recht Oder Unrecht*—"My Country, Right or Wrong." (U.S. National Archives)

To these thousand burghers of Weimar, the gate was wide open, inviting them inside. Patton's aide, Colonel Charles Codman, had written to his wife: "If you didn't know what it was, you might take it for the entrance to a third-rate amusement park."

The new American proprietors of the camp—a camp about which the Weimarers had heard so many whispered tales since it had opened eight years earlier, in 1937—were about to throw an open house just for them. But there would be no cookies and fruit punch and bouquets of flowers, nor smiling hostesses and a string quartet. The grim-faced American soldiers and a select group of frightfully thin former prisoners would be their hosts and would make sure their "guests" were exposed to everything the camp administrators had once kept hidden.

The unmistakable stench of death was in the air, and the noses of the German civilians were about to be rubbed in it.

The horror show was about to begin.

INTRODUCTION

HIGH ON THE hill overlooking the baroque German city of Weimar there exists to this day an ugly scar that mars an otherwise bucolic scene. This hill, some 1,568 feet (478 meters) high, is called the Ettersberg. Before 1937, it was crowned by a magnificent, untouched forest of beech and oak and fir trees. Birds sang here, and animals in the royal hunting preserve bounded through the underbrush in great profusion. A royal summer palace still stands nears its summit. It was to this hill that Johann Wolfgang Goethe—one of the world's great playwrights and philosophers—came for respite, reflection, and inspiration.

Then, in the warm and sunny summer of 1937, something happened that changed the landscape forever. On July 15, a convoy of trucks carrying inmates from the Sachsenburg concentration camp, southeast of Weimar and near the Czech border, crawled slowly and noisily up the winding road from Weimar to the top of the Ettersberg. Accompanied by shouted threats and orders from armed guards and the barks and snarls of guard dogs straining at their leashes, the frightened, bewildered prisoners jumped down from the trucks. They were handed hammers and saws and buckets full of nails and told to get to work—*Schnell*! What they were building would soon become their new home—a concentration camp that, as yet, had no name.

But soon, perhaps in deference to the leafy setting, it acquired the name Beech Forest Concentration Camp, or, as it is better known in German, *Konzentrationslager* (or *KL*) *Buchenwald*. As if to mock its lovely setting, the camp became one of the ugliest places in *Deutschland das Schöne*—Germany the Beautiful—and not just because of the electric barbed-wire fence that surrounded its 480 acres (194 hectares), nor the sinister guard towers with their spotlights and machine guns and guards who kept constant watch over the inmates like unblinking eyeballs, nor the assortment of dispiriting, shoddily constructed barracks, nor the tall, square chimney of the crematorium that belched flames and smoke and ash composed of the corpses it consumed like some mythological, fire-breathing monster. No, KL Buchenwald was ugly because of the depths of depravity which it represented, of how it debased and destroyed the human spirit.

The questions about KL Buchenwald are many: How did this once-lovely place become a place of unspeakable horror? Who operated it? What terrible secret activities took place there? Most importantly, how were citizens of one of the most civilized nations on earth able to do what they did there?

This book will attempt to answer these and many other questions. But first, a little history lesson. One need only glance through the tremendous time capsule of newspapers and magazines of the period to realize that the decade 1930-1940 was arguably the most pivotal in recent human history. Across the world, much of humanity was struggling to survive the depths of a global financial collapse (the "Great Depression") while, at the same time, freedom and democracy were under assault by the forces of totalitarianism. Widespread unrest was causing millions of people to either embrace or battle against dictators devoted to imposing on others political doctrines such as fascism and communism. Hatred and fear gripped whole populations, and confidence in the future was at low ebb.

The decade was also a period of increasingly violent military action and blatant violations of sovereignty by countries against their neighbors. In 1931, worried that they would not have the natural resources to power their expanding economy and accommodate their burgeoning population, the militants in Japan decided to invade Manchuria, followed by an invasion of China. In Italy, Dictator Benito Mussolini, known to his fervent fascist followers as *Il Duce* ("The Leader"), sought to restore the martial glory of the ancient Roman Empire by invading in 1935 the weakest country he could find: Ethiopia. In Germany, once it became obvious that he probably could not overthrow the democratically elected "Weimar government" by force, Adolf Hitler used legitimate means to obtain power and was appointed that country's chancellor in January 1933; both Hitler and Mussolini would, in 1936, provide material assistance to a renegade Spanish army colonel named Francisco Franco in his efforts to defeat the leftist Spanish monarchy and establish a fascist state—with Franco as *El Supremo* ("Supreme Leader").

And so it went, with one nation after another using the force of arms to impose its will on others. In America, Britain, France, and elsewhere, isolationists and appeasers chose to turn a blind eye to this aggression, hoping that another world war could be averted simply by ignoring the growing problem.

As Adolf Hitler and his Nazi minions soon discovered after ascending to unimagined heights of control in 1933, there was widespread, but not unanimous, support for the new regime, accompanied by a sense that a majority of the German people were willing to grant the Nazis *carte blanche* for anything they wished to do that might restore Germany's former position of power and prestige after the humiliations of the Treaty of Versailles.

Nazi culture quickly infiltrated all aspects of German life. Red, white, and black Nazi Party banners emblazoned with hypnotic swastikas hung in great profusion from public buildings, company offices, department stores, small shops, and private homes. Many homes had a framed portrait of Hitler hanging on the walls, as did offices and school classrooms. Band concerts and symphony productions usually began with the playing of the German national anthem ("*Deutschland über alles*"—"Germany Above All"), followed by the Nazi Party anthem, "The Horst Wessel Song."

When greeting business colleagues at the shop, office, or factory, friends on the street, ministers in church, or government officials in their domain, the expected greeting was a stiff-armed salute and a hearty "*Heil, Hitler!*" Even students—from college down to kindergarten—were required to greet their teachers in such a manner. In 1934, members of the German military were required to swear an oath of allegiance, not to the nation, but to Adolf Hitler personally.

Even those who silently harbored reservations about the Austrian immigrant with the Charlie Chaplain moustache grudgingly admitted that Hitler had brought about an amazing transformation of Germany in a surprisingly short time: the end of ruinous inflation; a renewed faith in the currency; a restoration of nearly full employment; an unprecedented public-works program (which included a nationwide *Autobahn* highway system and modernistic urban-renewal schemes); the International Olympic Committee's awarding of both the 1936 Summer and Winter Olympic Games to the nation; the suppression of communist agitators who wanted to spark a Bolshevik revolution; the expansion of the military in spite of Treaty of Versailles prohibitions; and a regenerated pride in the Fatherland and its armed forces. Uniforms were revered and German men in a wide variety of professions—from garbage collectors to railroad workers—soon appeared in uniforms that closely resembled those of the army or navy.

The Nazis' grand goal was to completely transform German life, to make the state the ultimate arbiter of how the people should live, work, and think—and to make them regard Adolf Hitler, who had christened himself *der Führer* ("The Leader"), as their nation's beloved savior. He was, after all, the man who had rescued the nation from the brink of the abyss of complete social, financial, and economic collapse.

And so, their spirits soaring, the ordinary German people went along with the program, many hoping against hope that all the crazy things Hitler had written in his venom-filled autobiography and political manifesto *Mein Kampf* were only rhetoric, a way to get attention and stand out from all the other political candidates.

To be sure, there were large numbers of opponents to *die Bewegung* ("the Nazi Movement") and Hitler's takeover of power—millions of Germans who refused to goose-step along with the Nazis. A few courageous clergymen spoke out from their pulpits; a few brave editors occasionally wrote scathingly in their newspapers; a handful of professors denounced the "police state" in their classrooms; politicians with the temerity to do so railed against the Nazis; ordinary people grumbled their misgivings in coffee houses, beer halls, work places, and on street corners.

But Germans suddenly realized, after noting that friends and neighbors who expressed any disapproval of Hitler and the Nazis were vanishing at a rapid clip, that it was far healthier to support the new regime and not voice or write anything critical about it. They also realized that they would be regarded as "good citizens" if they turned in their less-than-enthusiastic neighbors to the authorities. Nazi Party spies, too, were everywhere, making notes as to the identity of the agitators and dissidents. Soon carloads of trench-coated Gestapo—the dreaded *Geheime Stattspolizei* (Secret State Police)—came swooping down in the middle of the night to arrest those who had dared to speak against their beloved *Führer*. It did not take long for the jails to become overcrowded, so special detention facilities called *Konzentrationslager* ⋆ (concentration camps) began springing up in old castles, abandoned factories, and disused military bases all over Germany; these proved to be inadequate. In order to house the growing number of opponents being arrested every day, larger, purpose-built facilities were needed.[1]

Thus was the policy of *Schutzhaft* (protective custody) instituted, but the name is ironic. It was not those in custody (*Häftlingen*) who were being protected but rather the state being protected from its opponents. By forcing the *Häftlingen* to endure a harsh, Spartan existence, a rigid discipline, and the performance of hard labor, the concentration camps were also seen as places where the offenders could be "re-educated" so that they might be released and returned to society and lead a productive, pro-Nazi existence.[2]

To shape and control all aspects of German and, ultimately, European life, Hitler and the Nazis came down hard on anyone who did not fit their mold of the perfect Aryan model—particularly criminals, communists, socialists, Jews, Gypsies, the clergy, the mentally feeble, the physically infirm, and anyone who dared to speak out against Hitler's self-proclaimed "Third Reich."

⋆ In German, they were called *Konzentrationslager*, or *KL*, for short. (Later, for unknown reasons, the alternate abbreviation "KZ" became popular; it remains so today. In some German documents, the abbreviation "KZL" appears.)

Besides isolating from society those people whom the Reich felt posed a danger to its rule and order, the main purpose of the concentration camp (as opposed to the death camp) was to break the spirit of dissenters and strike fear into the hearts of those who might even consider opposing Hitler's reign—not slaughter them in huge numbers.

With the coming of the camps, order—the quality many Germans seem to prize most—had been restored. True, order came with a trade-off: a little loss of freedom here, a little more persecution there. It all seemed such a small trade-off at the time but, as the world would soon discover, give the Nazis an inch and they'll take a continent. Sensing this, the Nazis realized that this same program of jailing those whom they didn't like or didn't trust could, in time, be expanded—all the way to the systematic mass slaughter of whole populations.

WHILE THE GROWING armed might of Germany and the increasingly harsh persecutions of certain segments of its citizenry struck fear in the hearts of many, it should be remembered that Nazi Germany was itself a nation ruled by fear. Hitler and his followers were astonishingly fearful.

It is said that we humans hate what we fear, and it is my opinion that probably no nation was ever governed more by fear—and, consequentially, hatred—than Nazi Germany. The Nazis hated the communists for fear that their political rivals would gain power and impose their ideology on Germany. They hated—and feared—the so-called Weimar Republic because its democratic principles were antithetical to its own doctrine of a single strong ruler. They hated—and feared—conventional religion because religion placed a belief in God above a belief in State; religion urged people to be loving and compassionate, not cruel and sadistic. They hated—and feared—Jehovah's Witnesses and Seventh-Day Adventists and Masons because they would not swear oaths of loyalty to them. Mostly they hated—and feared—the Jews because they were convinced that a Jewish cabal was poised to take over Germany—not to mention the even greater, all-consuming fear they had that Jews would mix with the "Aryan" population and thus "pollute" pure German/Aryan/Nordic blood.

Ruled as they were by fear, the Nazis increasingly began to target Jews by imposing laws that greatly restricted their rights and, after the pogroms of 1938, the concentration camps took on the role of becoming massive holding pens for Jews while the Nazis decided their fate. Later, once the war had begun, the inmates of the concentration camps—whether Jew or Gentile—were used as slave laborers (*Sklavenarbeiter*) to serve the economic interests of the Third Reich, especially when German armed forces began suffering heavy losses on the battlefronts and able-bodied men were drafted out of the war industries to serve in the armed forces.

While the vast majority of the camps were not death camps, hundreds of thousands of prisoners died in them, mostly from disease, starvation, beatings, work-site accidents, and small-scale executions. The camps also became handy laboratories for doctors and scientists eager to carry out medical experiments on human subjects rather than on animals. Nor were the concentration camps considered "prisoner-of-war" camps, although, on occasion, captured enemy soldiers—especially Soviet troops—were incarcerated in them. KL Buchenwald, too, became a place where Soviet, British, American, and Canadian soldiers and airmen were held; some never emerged alive.[3]

It should also be noted that Adolf Hitler was not the only German or Austrian (or even Frenchman or Pole) to harbor a deep-seated fear and hatred of Jews and Judaism. As Daniel J. Goldhagen points out so forcefully in *Hitler's Willing Executioners: Ordinary Germans and the Holocaust* (and as does Donald McKale in *Hitler's Shadow War*), much of Europe had for centuries made a career out of despising and persecuting Jews, a phenomenon as normal and natural to them as eating, sleeping, and breathing. Jews were long regarded as wicked, unscrupulous, and Satan incarnate—hence, people to be feared. Virtually all of German society was anti-Semitic; the Holocaust was simply the logical, if tragic, extension of that fear and hatred. When the Nazis came to power and issued orders to their countrymen to mistreat, incarcerate, and eventually murder their Jewish countrymen, their executioners willingly obeyed those orders because they, too, held a deep-seated fear and hatred toward Jews and wanted them expunged from German life, much as a pest exterminator might honor a homeowner's request to eliminate vermin from his home.

KL BUCHENWALD WAS the epitome of cruelty for the way those unfortunate enough to have been warehoused here were treated: the round-the-clock brutality, the non-stop degradation, the palpable fear that drove men mad, the exhausting, never-ending work, the soul-robbing starvation, the unimaginable filth, the rampant disease, and the hideous medical experiments. For nearly eight years, the people who ruled this hilltop domain of evil enjoyed absolute power over their hapless victims. Few places on earth have ever so dramatically showcased the depths of ugliness to which humankind can sink as did Buchenwald.

And, while one might wish to dismiss Buchenwald as some sort of aberration, it was all part of a larger, well-thought-out plan devised by one of the most malevolent, criminal governments ever to rule a nation.

This, then, is the story of Buchenwald. It is not a pretty story, and readers with sensitive dispositions are advised to journey into the following pages with caution. But it is a necessary story so that the world will better understand what happens when power is left unchecked and how, as 18th century Irish statesman Edmund Burke once said, "The only thing necessary for evil to flourish is for good men to do nothing."

1
HELL UNDER CONSTRUCTION

"Tolerance means weakness. In the light of this concept, punishment will be mercilessly handed out whenever the interests of the Fatherland warrant it."

—Theodor Eicke
Supervisor of the Nazi concentration camp system

KL BUCHENWALD was the third in the long line of major concentration camps built by the Nazis. Preceded by Dachau near Munich (1933) and Sachsenhausen north of Berlin (1936), Buchenwald began its infamous existence in the summer of 1937, although without the name it is known by today. Eventually, according to a new study by the U.S. Holocaust Memorial Museum published in March 2013, there were some 42,500 camps of various sizes—everything from tiny, slave-labor work camps to ghettos to medical facilities performing pseudo-scientific experiments to sprawling extermination facilities.[1]

As it was the SS (*Schutzstaffel*, or "Protection Detachment") that provided the personnel to run the camps, a brief history of the SS—and its most notorious leaders—is in order here. Begun in April 1925 as a small, private bodyguard designed to protect Hitler from his communist opponents (and others), the Schutzstaffel grew into a formidable force that became infamous for instilling fear in the Nazis' enemies, both foreign and domestic. In 1929, a former chicken farmer and Hitler loyalist named Heinrich Luitpold Himmler was appointed *Reichsführer-SS*, or "National Leader" of the SS.

On the surface, Himmler seemed like an odd choice for such an exalted position where image was so important. Born to a Munich schoolmaster and his wife on October 7, 1900, little Heinrich was the second of three sons. Heinrich was a serious and studious lad, more interested in German history and mythology than in rugged outdoors or athletic pursuits. He also seemed to be frail and more susceptible to illnesses than other boys his age. In today's parlance, Heinrich would have been called a "wimp," and no doubt was teased and bullied unmercifully by his classmates.

The outbreak of the Great War in 1914 excited in Heinrich a desire for martial glory, and he volunteered for the Kaiser's army a few months before he turned seventeen. He was called up and trained with the 11th Bavarian Infantry

Regiment but never saw combat; he was discharged a month after the armistice in 1918 and, with few prospects in the post-war period, decided to go into farming, attending the University of Munich as an agriculture student. Shy and socially awkward, Himmler forced himself to make friends and even push himself into athletic endeavors, such as swimming, skating, and fencing, while continuing his modest, carefully circumscribed lifestyle and Catholic-churchgoing habits. He also joined a Bavarian military unit as a reservist, but his smallish frame, owlish pince-nez glasses, and a prim and proper outlook on life gave him the appearance and manner of a meek, detail-oriented bank clerk—certainly not the image of the future leader of one of the most powerful and dreaded organizations in history.

Himmler was also anti-Semitic—a not-uncommon trait for Bavarian Catholics. Fiercely nationalistic, and anti-communistic as well, he was appalled at the left-leaning Bavarian government and gladly joined the Nazi Party in 1923 in hopes of ousting the Reds. He even summoned up the courage to play a minor role in Hitler's November 1923 *Putsch*—the attempt to take over the government in Munich. Following the violent police suppression of the Putsch, Himmler became obsessed with politics and slavishly devoted himself to Hitler, who saw in the young man a bright flame in the torch of National Socialism. Like his idol, Himmler discovered a gift for oratory, and soon he attracted his boss's eye after speaking at numerous rallies throughout Bavaria. In 1926 Himmler was made deputy to Party propagandist Josef Goebbels, followed by an appointment to be deputy commander of the black-uniformed SS.

In July 1928, Himmler married Margarete "Marga" Concerzowo, a nurse seven years his senior whom he had met in Berlin. They bought a small chicken farm outside of Munich; the sale of chickens and eggs helped augment his Nazi Party salary of 200 marks a month, but his fortunes were about to take an upward turn. In January 1929, Hitler appointed Himmler to command the SS. In spite of his protégé's decidedly un-Aryan appearance, it was a fateful appointment that would do much to change the Nazi Party, the German nation and, indeed, the world.

In August 1929, the couple had their only child, a pretty little girl named Gudrun*; they would also become foster parents to the son of an SS officer who died before the war. Himmler later had two children by his mistress, Hedwig Potthast.[2]

* After the war, far from being apologetic about the sins of her father, Gudrun Himmler Burwitz remained an ardent neo-Nazi for the rest of her life. (Fabian Leber, "*Gudrun Burwitz und die 'Stille Hilfe': Die schillernde Nazi-Prinzessin*," *Der Tagespiel*, June 10, 2001)

THREE MAIN BRANCHES of the SS eventually were formed: the first was Hitler's personal bodyguard, the *SS-Leibstandarte Adolf Hitler*, or LAH, made up mostly of tall, blond, blue-eyed specimens of the Aryan ideal. A second branch, created in 1934, was the *SS-Verfügungstruppe*, or SS-VT—the Combat Support Force (which would become known as the *Waffen-SS* in July 1940), a hard-core group of "shock troops" that fought alongside the Wehrmacht, the "regular" army. When the first concentration camps were created in 1933, a force of tough, pitiless men was recruited to become the guards and administrators, a branch known as the *SS-Totenkopfverbände*, or "Death's Head" units.

In February 1934, Himmler appointed *SS-Standartenführer* (Colonel) Oswald Pohl, a former naval officer and long-time member of the paramilitary organization known as the *Sturmabteilung*, or SA or Brown Shirts,* to head the

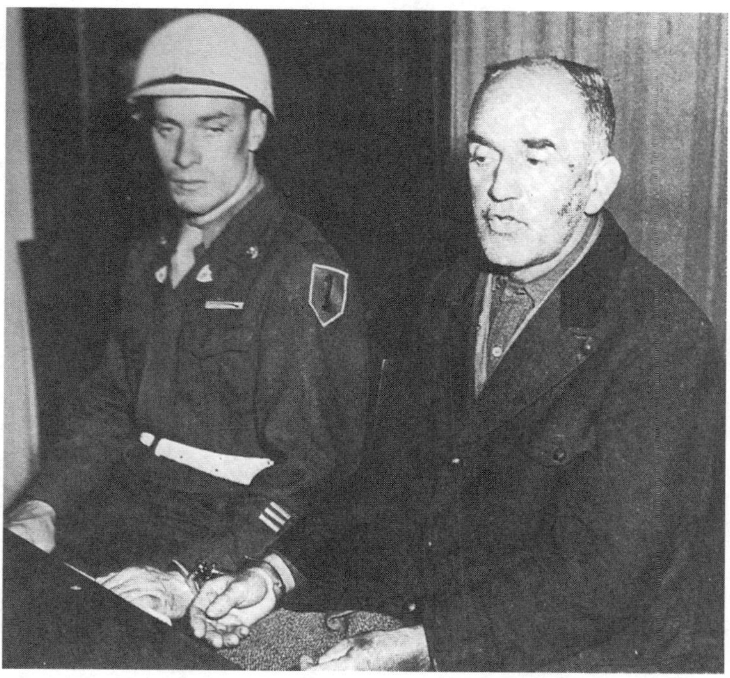

Oswald Pohl shown during his war-crimes trial at Nurnberg, November 1947. Pohl was found guilty and hanged on June 7, 1951. (U.S. National Archives)

* In the words of historian Paul Garson, "Characterized by a solid working-class sense of *gemutlichkeit* or warm comradeship, the SA was composed of many ex-World War I servicemen and a variety of malcontents. They considered themselves 'rough and ready' revolutionary soldiers, preferring beer over the champagne tastes of the SS." (Garson, *New Images of Nazi Germany*, p. 92)

SS Administrative and Economic Department. In that position, Pohl oversaw the fledgling concentration camp system and did much to foster its growth and development.

MEMBERS OF THE *SS-Totenkopfverbände* camp guards and administrators were trained at the SS school at Dachau (dubbed the "School of Violence") and were generally held to a higher standard of conduct and discipline than ordinary German Wehrmacht soldiers. This higher standard included unquestioning obedience to orders, even if the orders involved the torture and murder of human beings.[3]

The first concentration camp to open was at Nohra, created in early March 1933 on the grounds of a military airfield, a farming village five miles west-southwest of Weimar; the guards at the camp were students from an *SS-Führerschule*, a

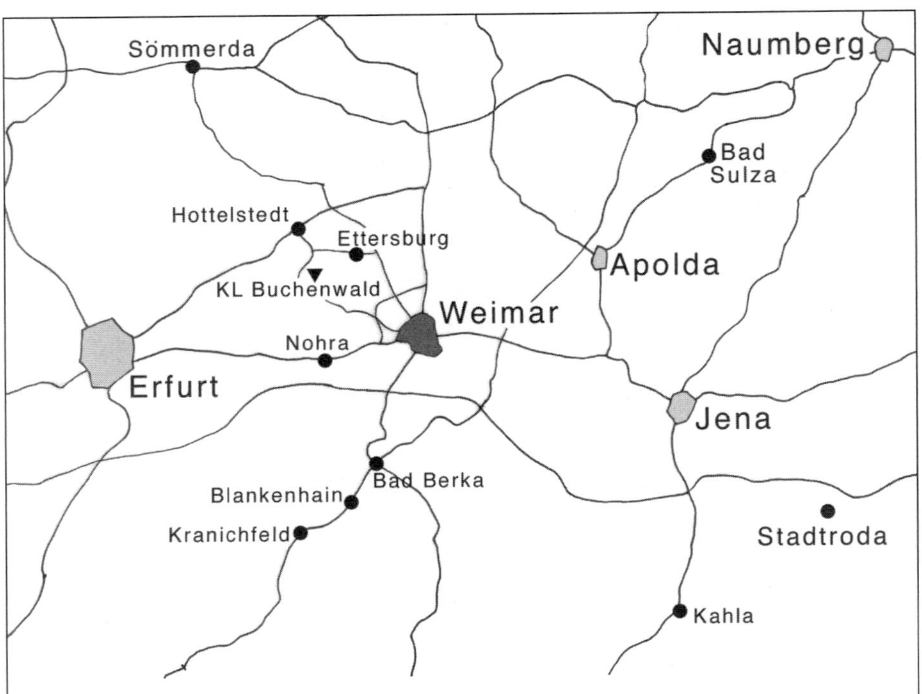

Map of the Weimar area

leadership school for young SS officers. The camp, however, was wholly inadequate for, with only one building, it could hold only 250 inmates.*4

Because Nohra was quickly outgrown, Himmler ordered a larger detention facility built at an abandoned gunpowder factory in the Munich suburb of Dachau; it opened in August 1933 and became the model for the system around which most of the later camps were based. The daily routine—roll call, harassment, assignment of work details, the duties of the SS guards; the establishment of the *Kapo*** system; the striped uniforms and "color-coded" classification of prisoners; the sub-standard housing, sanitation, and dietary conditions; and the public punishment and humiliation designed to keep inmates in a constant state of mental stress and anxiety—were all perfected under Theodor Eicke at Dachau. But who was this Eicke?

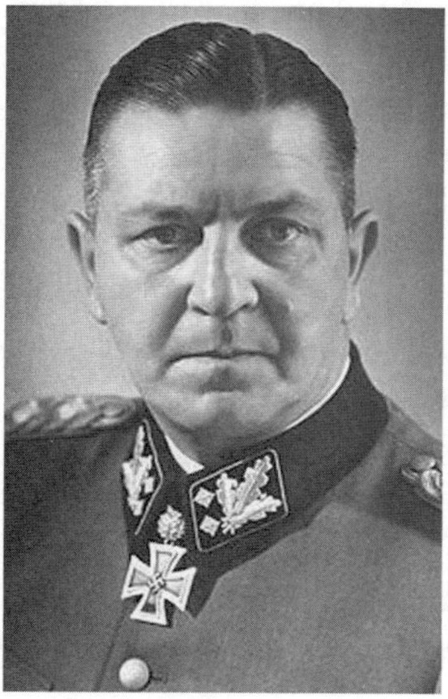

Theodor Eicke, supervisor of concentration camps (U.S. National Archives)

Theodor Eicke was one of Hitler's "hard men" and *alte Kameraden* (old comrades)—a brawler who had been with Hitler since nearly the beginning, and the man perhaps most directly responsible for how the guards at Buchenwald and the other camps treated (and mistreated) their prisoners.

The son of a railroad stationmaster, the no-nonsense Eicke was born October 17, 1892. He served in the German army in the Great War and, after being discharged, discovered

* Run by the Ministry of the Interior for nearly three years, KL Nohra was turned over to the SS on April 1, 1936. (Stein, p. 25) With city jails and detention centers rapidly filling up, and Nohra too small to satisfy the demand, two pre-Nazi-era detention camps—Borgermoor and Esterwegen, both near the northwest German city of Papenburg—were re-opened and pressed into service. Borgermoor took in its first prisoners in July 1933, while Esterwegen went into operation the following month. Like Nohra, both Borgermoor and Esterwegen proved to be too small, and the camps were closed—Borgermoor in April 1934 and Esterwegen in December 1936. Bigger camps were coming on line. (www. jewishgen.org/forgottencamps/Camps/EsterEngl; www. edwardvictor.com/Holocaust/2005/Borgermoor)

** A *Kapo* was a concentration camp prisoner chosen by the SS to be a sort of foreman or trustee and given the responsibility of overseeing other inmates. Many had been common criminals before being incarcerated and dealt with those beneath them with exceptional harshness. *Kapos* were also appointed to be overseers of the various work details, known as *Arbeitskommando*. As "privileged" prisoners, the *Kapos* were allowed to strut around the enclosure, their uniforms a little better and their hair a little longer than the underlings who were their victims, acting in especially cruel ways in the hopes that, through their brutality, they would impress their SS masters and be allowed to keep their relatively cushy jobs. (www. jewishvirtuallibrary. org/jsource/Holocaust/kapos)

that he was temperamentally suited for a law-enforcement career. Eicke worked in police administration, political police, and criminal police fields in Thuringia and Ludwigshafen in the early 1920s before joining I.G. Farben in their anti-industrial-espionage service. With the emergence of Hitler, Eicke became an ardent Nazi, joining the Party and the SA in 1928; he was accepted for membership in the SS in August 1930.

Eicke's zeal for discipline and unquestioning obedience to orders soon caught Himmler's eye and he was promoted to *SS-Standartenführer* (Colonel) and, in November 1931, given command of an SS regiment in the Rhine-Palatinate area. Not everyone thought he should hold high office. Josef Burkel, the area's Nazi *Gauleiter*, or governor, labeled Eicke a "dangerous lunatic" and would later order him committed to a psychiatric clinic in Würzburg.

On June 26, 1933, Himmler appointed the forty-year-old Eicke to command KL Dachau, where he established a set of rules and regulations that became the standard for all future concentration camps.[5] In the Introduction to his rules for camp personnel, Eicke wrote, "Tolerance means weakness. In light of this concept, punishment will be mercilessly handed out whenever the interests of the Fatherland warrant it." And punishment *was* mercilessly handed out, with whippings, floggings, beatings, solitary confinement, and outright torture applied for even minor offenses committed by camp inmates. Death by hanging was permitted and, if a prisoner attempted to escape, Eicke commanded, "he is to be shot without warning." Rudolf Höss, one of Eicke's trainees and later the commandant of Auschwitz, recalled that his mentor stressed, "There was no place in the ranks of the SS for men with soft hearts and any such would do well to retire quickly to a monastery. [Eicke] could only use hard, determined men who ruthlessly obeyed every order."[6]

Described by one historian as being "ever-suspicious, quarrelsome, cruel, humorless, and afflicted with a cancerous ambition," Eicke soon became the epitome of the "perfect" SS man—a man who set about molding a pitiless paramilitary formation in his own pitiless image.[7] In fact, so impressed was Himmler with Eicke's hard nature and dedication to Nazi and SS ideals that, in May 1934, he put him in charge of the entire concentration camp system; two months later, he was given the title *Inspekteur der Konzentrationslager und SS-Wachverbande* (Inspector of Concentration Camps and SS Guards) and promoted to *SS-Gruppenführer*—the second-highest commissioned rank in the SS—in addition to being made Himmler's immediate subordinate in matters pertaining to the camps.[8]

IN NOVEMBER 1933, a small detention camp at Bad Sulza, northeast of Weimar, was opened but quickly became overcrowded; the SS planned to close it and relocate the prisoners elsewhere until, on May 20, 1936, the Gauleiter of Thuringia, Ernst Friedrich Christoph "Fritz" Sauckel (who became a Nazi in 1921), had other ideas. He met with Eicke to discuss expanding the camp in order not to lose its economic benefit to the community. Eicke agreed, and decided to transfer the inmates from the concentration camp at Lichtenburg Castle at Prettin to Bad Sulza. After obtaining Himmler's approval, the transfer was made, but not before approval was also granted for Eicke to build an entirely new and larger camp closer to Weimar, using Dachau as the model. Eicke specified that this new, as-yet-unnamed camp should cover at least sixty hectares* and be able to house from 3,000 to 6,000 inmates.[9]

Hellmuth Gommlich, police chief of the Thuringian Ministry of the Interior, was tasked with finding a suitable site. After several had been considered, Gommlich called a meeting of representatives of the Reich Agricultural Bureau on April 26, 1937, to recommend the heavily wooded hill five miles northwest of Weimar known as the Ettersberg. At the beginning of May, this recommendation was passed on to Eicke, who gave it his stamp of approval; construction of the camp would soon commence. It is not clear if Eicke knew the history of that particular spot, or of Weimar in general, but no matter; it was the future, not the past, that was his primary focus.

And quite a past the Ettersberg had. In the 1770s, a magnificent baroque building known as the Tiefurt Palace, surrounded by an English-style garden in the nearby village of Ettersburg, was built near the summit of the Ettersberg for the Prussian Dowager Duchess Anna Amalia of Saxe-Weimar-Eisenach. She used the facilities as her summer residence, as well as turning it into a retreat for artists, writers, and musicians—her so-called "Court of the Muses."

A niece of Frederick the Great, Duchess Anna Amalia was a wealthy patroness of the arts. In 1775 she invited Johann Wolfgang Goethe, the most prodigious German "Renaissance man" of his day, to spend time at the Tiefurt Palace, and he quickly became the central figure around whom the Court of

* A hectare is 10,000 square meters; an acre is 4,840 square yards. Thus, one hectare is the equivalent of 2.471 acres. Sixty hectares is the equivalent of 148.263 acres. By the time it was fully built out, the Buchenwald camp complex would cover 480 acres.

the Muses revolved; Goethe even staged several of his plays at the duchess's summer palace. Because of Goethe's fondness for Weimar, the city soon attracted the *glitterati*—cultural icons such as Friedrich Schiller, Felix Mendelssohn, Johann Sebastian Bach, Robert and Clara Schumann, Franz Liszt, Richard Wagner, Richard Strauss, Friedrich Nietsche, and many, many more—whose presence made Weimar the cultural capital of Germany up until the early twentieth century.

According to local legend, a tall oak tree at the summit of the Ettersberg was said to be Goethe's favorite retreat—a leafy spot where, it is said, he worked on his masterpiece, *Faust*, a work which took him sixty years to complete. So well known was the tree to locals that it even had its own name: the *Goethe Eiche*, or Goethe Oak.

In 1900, a landmark stone tower known as the Bismarckturm, honoring the memory of Otto von Bismarck, the first chancellor of a unified Germany in 1871 (the "Second Reich"), was constructed above the southern slope of the Ettersberg. With its panoramic views and a restaurant at its base, the Bismarckturm was a popular holiday spot for locals.

But Weimar also had its darker side. Early on, the city developed an association with Adolf Hitler and the National Socialist German Workers Party. In fact, on July 4, 1926, the first Nazi Party Rally Day, following Hitler's 1925 release from Landsberg prison, was held in Weimar. A frequent visitor to Weimar (he was there thirty-five times), the future dictator reviewed ranks of marching Nazis from his balcony at the elegant Hotel Elephant overlooking the Marktplatz (Market Square).

Hitler also bestowed honors on his loyal supporters from Weimar. One of the *Altekämpfer* ("old fighters"—members who joined the Nazi Party before 1933) was the afore-mentioned Fritz Sauckel, who was appointed *Gauleiter* of Thuringia in 1925 and, in 1933, became its governor; he also held senior honorary rank in the SS and SA.[10] Another leading Nazi, Baldur von Schirach, head of the *Hitlerjugend* (Hitler Youth) organization, was born in Weimar.[11]

Despite Weimar's long association as a cultural mecca, the Ettersberg seemd to be the perfect spot for a concentration camp. It was close enough to a major city that it would be easy to transport SS personnel and inmates in and out, yet remote enough to keep prying eyes from seeing exactly what was going on behind its electrified barbed-wire fences.

The first few buildings erected atop the Ettersberg—temporary barracks—were built by members of *SS-Totenkopfstandarten 3 "Thuringen"* (3rd SS

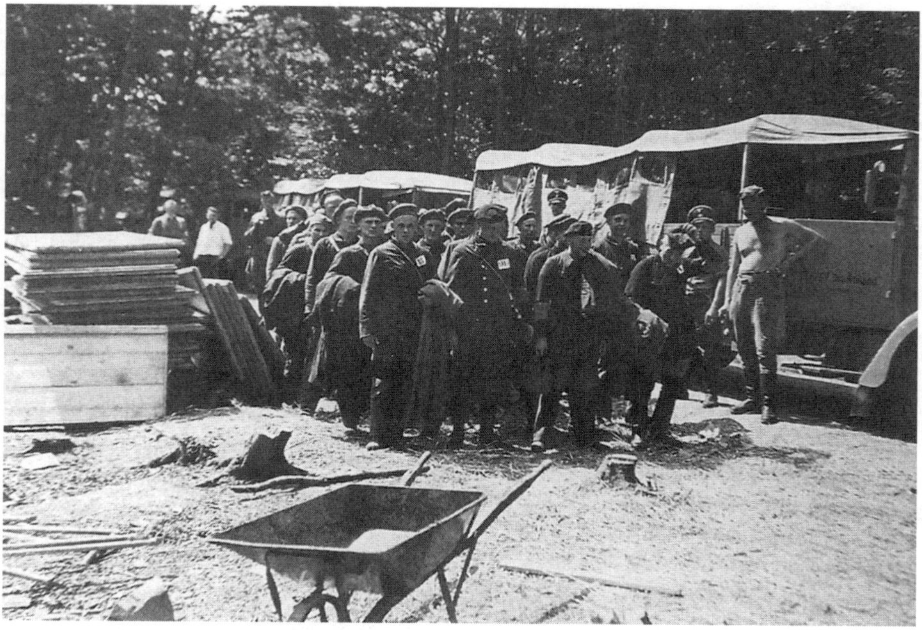

The first inmates arrive by truck at their hilltop prison, July 15, 1937. (Courtesy Buchenwald Memorial)

Death's Head Regiment, Thuringia)* under the command of *SS-Standartenführer* Paul Nostitz.

Other, less enthusiastic, workers soon arrived. On July 15, 1937, a convoy of trucks carrying 149 carpenters and other craftsmen—all of them political prisoners—came up the hill from Weimar and the men, previously inmates at KL Sachsenburg, a small camp southeast of Weimar near the Czech border, were immediately put to work. They were followed the next day by another seventy prisoners; three days later, an additional sixty-six men from KL Lichtenburg, between Bremen and Berlin, joined the work party. By August 6, 1,400 men—most of them prisoners—were working atop the Ettersberg.

And much work needed to be done. With the exception of the so-called "Goethe Oak," much of the land on the northern summit of the Ettersberg was cleared of trees, revealing a rocky ground. The camp streets needed to be surveyed and graded; water and sewage lines laid; fences, guard towers, barracks,

* The unit was formed in 1937 with an authorized strength of some 1,200 men (a year later more than 2,200 men were in the unit) from various *Totenkopf Wachtruppen* (guard troops), mostly the *SS-Wachtruppe* "Sachsen" and *SS-Wachtruppe* "Elbe." By year's end, it would have seven *Sturmbannen* (battalions). (Sydnor, *Soldiers of Destruction*, pp. 37-63; Stein, pp. 37-38)

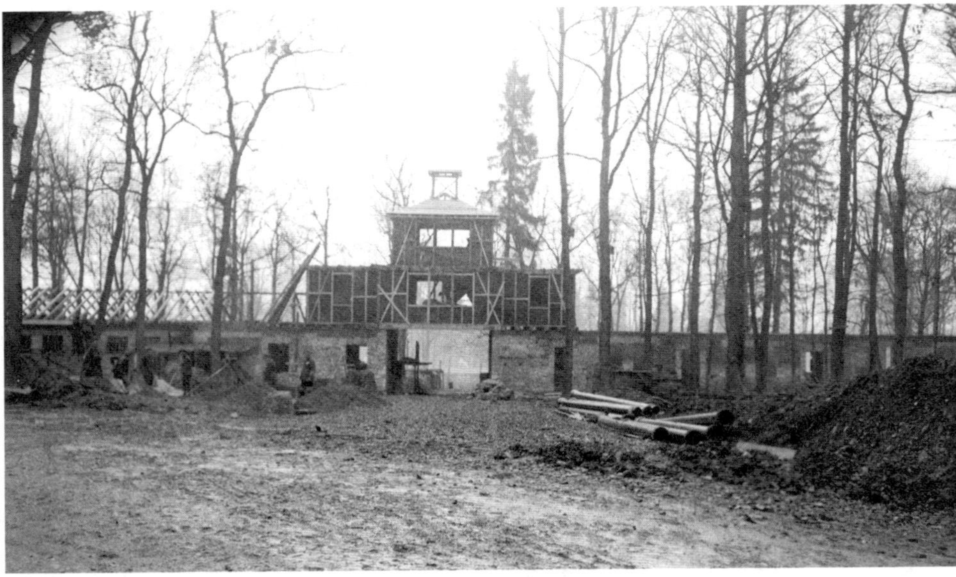

The gatehouse under construction (Buchenwald Memorial)

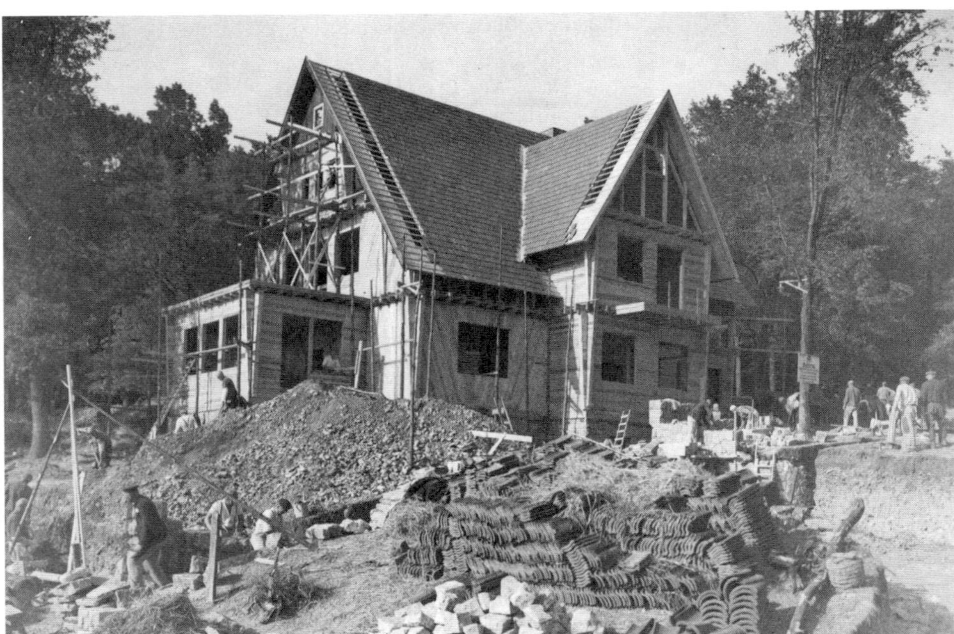

The commandant's residence, known as Haus Buchenwald, under construction (Buchenwald Memorial)

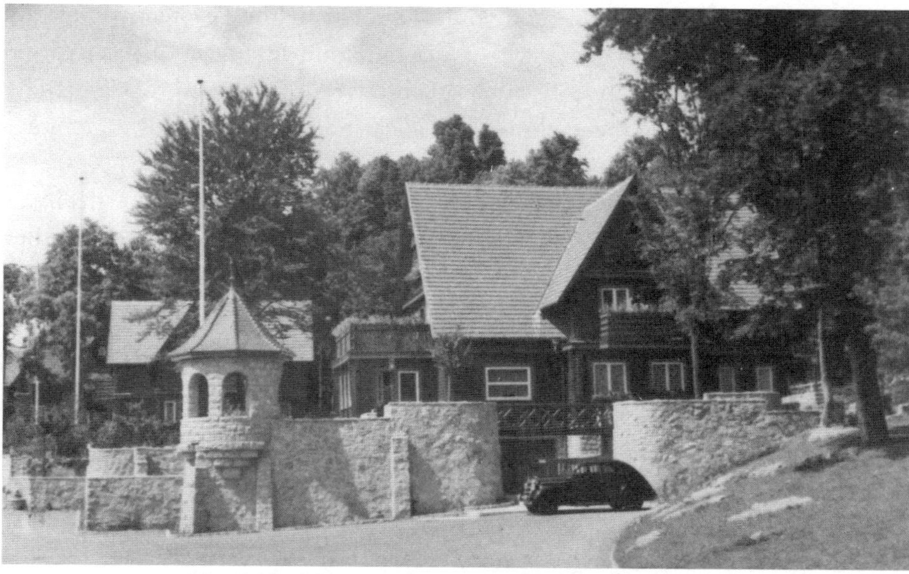

The finished Haus Buchenwald (Buchenwald Memorial)

latrines, administrative offices, storehouses, barracks for the guards, and attractive homes for the officers and administrators constructed along with a gatehouse complete with a clock tower and a sinister wing known as the *Zellerbau* or "Bunker"—an inmates' prison-within-a-prison that contained a number of tiny cells where prisoners often would be tortured in the hours before their scheduled executions. Later would come garages, a gas station for SS vehicles, a stable for horses and an indoor riding arena, a movie theater (the only one in a concentration camp), troop casino, guard-dog kennels, falconry, inmate library, inmate infirmary, troop hospital, shooting ranges, depot for building materials, and, most chillingly, a pathology laboratory and other places where medical experiments would be carried out on living prisoners without their consent. In mid-1940 a six-oven crematorium was built when the Weimar municipal crematorium proved incapable of keeping up with the increasing number of deaths.

Buchenwald, like most of the other camps, was designed and built on the "Dachau model," the Nazis' first major camp, but with several notable exceptions. Instead of having the barracks constructed in straight rows as at Dachau, the natural hump of the top of the Ettersberg lent itself better to curved streets. The gatehouse stood at the top of the hill where it could be seen by the prisoners from almost everywhere within the compound, known as the "protective custody camp," and from which a guard with a machine gun in Tower One could see much of the camp below. Twenty other guard towers surrounded the camp. The barbed wire surrounding the enclosure was electrified and the guards were under orders to shoot to kill any prisoners who approached the wire fence.

In time there would be "amenities" at Buchenwald, too, such as a small zoo for the enjoyment of the SS and their families, a feature not found at other camps. Another change was the sign on the main gate to the prisoner compound. Whereas Dachau, Auschwitz, Sachsenhausen, Flossenbürg, Ravensbrück, and others had the cynical motto *Arbeit Macht Frei* ("Work Makes You Free")* set in welded steel letters on their main gate, the sign at the entrance to Buchenwald read *Jedem Das Sein*, which translates as "To Each His Own."[12]

The choice of the person to run such an establishment was also symbolic. The Nazis wanted someone who would be unafraid of trampling the center of German emotion and intellect, and who could turn a beautiful, bucolic spot into a hideous patch of evil weeds, a place full of fear-inducing brutality. They found just such a man working for them outside Berlin—Karl Otto Koch.**

---

* The phrase *Arbeit Macht Frei* can be interpreted in a variety of ways. It could give the prisoner hope that, if he worked hard and obeyed the rules, he might be released one day. It could also mean that, no matter how terrible your existence here may be, by working hard and concentrating on your job, you can temporarily free your mind from the misery of your life in the camp.

** Pronounced like "coke" or the Scottish "loch," not "kotch."

2
THE BEASTS OF BUCHENWALD

"As I hung there I prayed for death to put an end to my misery."

Jacob Werber
Buchenwald inmate

IN THE SUMMER of 1937, the man selected to be commandant of the new camp was forty-year-old *SS-Standartenführer* Karl Otto Koch. He had already gained considerable notoriety within the SS as a breaker of men and, since September 1933, a no-nonsense administrator at several camps.[1]

A veteran of the Great War, Koch was, as a civilian, a failure in all the professions he had tried, but it was in bending men to his will that he finally found his true calling. In 1931 Koch joined both the Nazi Party and the SS, discovering in himself a penchant for cruelty that was unique even by SS standards. A star graduate of Eicke's school for sadists at Dachau, he went on to ply his trade at KL Sachsenburg, Lichtenburg, Hohnstein, Esterwegen, and the Gestapo's Columbia-Haus prison in Berlin. In 1936 he was assigned to his most important post to date: the sprawling Sachsenhausen Concentration Camp located twenty-two miles north of Berlin in the suburb of Oranienburg. In the summer of 1937, after apparently impressing SS chief Heinrich Himmler with his ability to hand out harsh discipline while at KL Sachsenhausen, the new camp at Weimar became his; he was ordered to report to his new assignment in August. [1] Before leaving Sachsenhausen, the divorced, paunchy, balding Koch married a thirty-year-old red-haired stenographer by the name of Margerete Ilse Köhler in an impressive SS wedding ceremony on May 29, 1937, complete with flaming torches and pagan pageantry.[2]

In many ways, Karl and Ilse Koch were so plain, so ordinary, so undistinguished, that they would be virtually invisible walking down the aisle of any supermarket or discount store today. Yet their power over life and death made them two of the most dangerous people in Nazi Germany, where psychopaths and social misfits populated the halls of power. Before long, Ilse Koch's name would become as synonymous with cruelty and terror as that of her husband.*[3]

---

* The lives of Karl and Ilse are detailed in the author's *The Beasts of Buchenwald* (Cable Publishing, 2011).

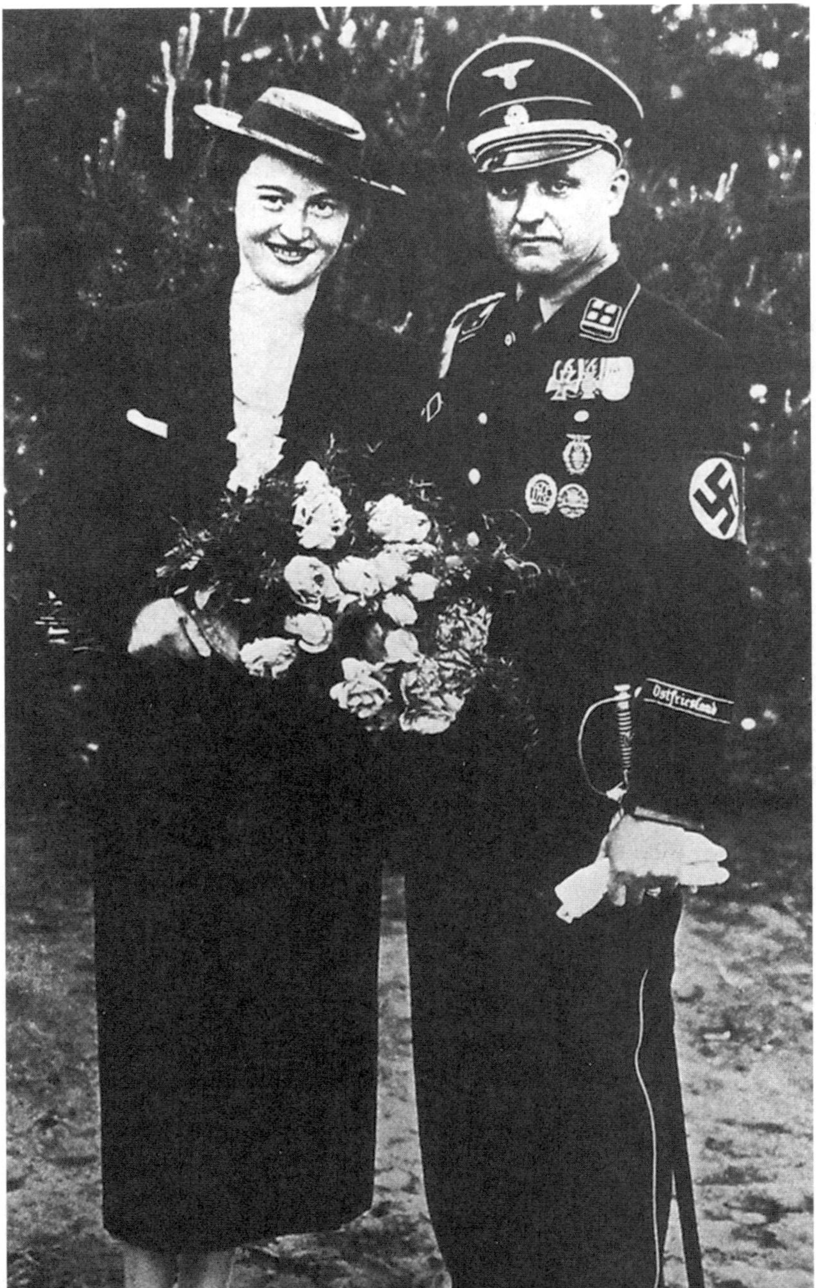

Ilse and Karl shown after their wedding at Sachsenhausen. The cuff title on his left sleeve reads "*Ostfriesland*," the name of the SS regiment assigned to the Sachsenhausen camp. (Koch photo album, U.S. National Archives)

The camp was already taking shape by the time Koch and his bride arrived. Made aware that locals had protested naming the new camp "KL Ettersberg" because the Ettersberg had certain cultural connotations, Koch saw the profusion of beech trees on the hill and so proclaimed it KL Buchenwald, the name by which it would forever be known. It was probably also the last time that he ever took into account anyone else's feelings.

Life at Buchenwald was cheap under the Kochs—as disposable as tissue paper. The camp's *Totesbuch*, or death registry, records that the first inmate to die was Hermann Kempeck, a twenty-three-year-old laborer, who committed suicide on August 14, 1937, by hanging himself. Two days later, Richard Groschke, a forty-year-old bricklayer, was shot "while attempting to escape"—a common SS euphemism for outright murder. Over the next three weeks, six more inmates would die; they were but the tip of the iceberg. Of all the concentration camps before the war, Buchenwald had the highest mortality rate.[4]

One of the main reasons was the complete disregard for safety practices in the Buchenwald workplaces. Throughout the remainder of 1937, and for the next several years, construction was the main activity of the inmates at Buchenwald. One after another, the barracks, or "blocks," went up with as much haste as possible. And, as soon as each one was completed, a new shipment of inmates arrived, filled that barrack, and was put to work building even more barracks.

ON THEIR FIRST day of incarceration, prisoners were quickly brought down to the level of livestock with treatment designed to break the spirit, inspire instant obedience to commands, erode any will to resist or escape, and reduce them to little more than automatons.

The first order of business was registration. Each inmate had his name, nationality, address, date of birth, reason for arrest, and other personal information typed onto a file card. If he died while at Buchenwald, that fact would be noted on his card and his name listed in the camp's *Totesbuch*. No matter how one died, the cause was inevitably listed as "Shot while escaping."

After registration, the inmate had all his body hair shorn by other inmates wielding dull clippers (the hair was collected and used for stuffing mattresses). One Buchenwald inmate recounted the ritual: "My barber started by placing clippers on my forehead and running them to the base of my neck. Five strokes and the job was done.... With dull clippers, underarm, genital, and anal hair was also removed, leaving us nicked and bleeding."[5]

One of the major health problems throughout the entire Nazi camp system was endemic typhus, a louse-borne disease that not only affected the prisoners but could easily spread to the guards, administrators, and the nearby civilian population. So, shortly after the camp was opened, large tanks of delousing solution were installed where new prisoners were dunked shortly after arrival. When a young German Jew named Paul Heinz Victor arrived at Buchenwald, he, like thousands of others, went through the disinfection process: "Once we were inside the campground," he said, "we were led to what turned out to be a bathhouse. We had to strip naked. Our clothes had to be dropped to the floor, and SS guards would walk through the aisles with carts and collect them all. There were bathtubs so large that they could hold about ten people at a time. They were filled with some sort of chemical, apparently disinfectants, judging by the odor. We had to swim or paddle through the pool in front of us, then step under a cold shower and pick up a towel to dry off."[6]

After being sheared and deloused, each inmate was then issued the standard prison uniform—a thickly woven cotton shirt and pants of dull gray and white stripes and a similarly striped bill-less cap.* The prisoner was given an identification number that was stenciled onto a white tag and sewn onto the shirt and pants. (The practice of tattooing numbers on the forearms of Jewish prisoners was carried out only at Auschwitz.) The prisoner was then photographed and the picture attached to his card, which was filed in the camp administration office. Shaven and reduced to merely a number, the process of dehumanization had begun.[7]

The inmates were assigned to a particular block, or barrack, run by a *Kapo* and a *Blockältester* (an "elder" assigned to be the chief of each barrack. Occasionally less brutal than the *Kapos*, the *Blockälteste* kept order in the barrack and even became sort of "father figures" to some of the inmates). The *Kapo*s were to be feared. One of the inmates said, "We soon learned that *Kapo*s were just glorified prisoners who, for extra rations and privileges, ran our barracks. Many of them

* For the first months, prisoners at Buchenwald were issued worn-out police uniforms; the familiar striped uniforms were not introduced until 1938. Footwear was whatever the prisoners had brought with them, and frostbite became a common winter ailment at Buchenwald and throughout the entire concentration camp system as the leather shoes wore out. Inmate-carved wooden shoes, which were painful and proved to be of only minimal value against the elements, soon became the normal footwear in Buchenwald and elsewhere. It was not until September 1941 that prisoners would be allowed to receive packages from home, packages that often contained shoes, socks, and long underwear. Even then, the camp administrators regularly confiscated most of the packages. (Stein, pp. 91-92)

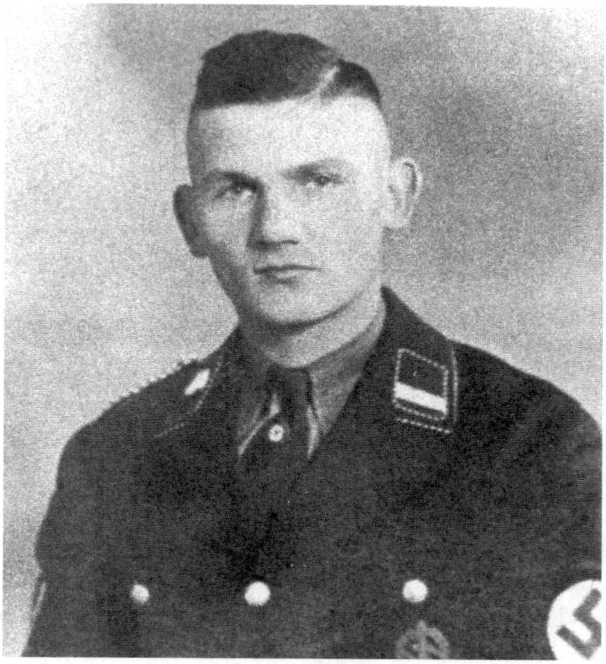

Buchenwald's chief jailer, *SS-Hauptscharführer* Martin Sommer (Buchenwald Memorial)

had been criminals before they'd been sent to Buchenwald. The Nazis allowed them free rein to punish us any way they wished."[8]

Prisoners were also segregated by their status and/or nationality, which was denoted by the triangular cloth patches of various colors (known as *Winkeln*) that the inmates sewed onto their striped shirts. A red triangle, for instance, indicated a prisoner being held for political reasons (more likely than not, a communist or socialist). Someone with a green triangle was a common criminal (thief, murderer, etc.), while a black triangle signified someone accused of being "asocial" (such as a Gypsy, a vagrant, habitually unemployed, or a "non-conformist"). Homosexuals wore pink triangles while the color for Jehovah's Witnesses was purple. Jews were required to wear a yellow triangle, point up, which was sometimes combined with another yellow triangle, point down, to form a six-pointed Star of David—unless the Jewish prisoner was included in one of the other categories of prisoner, such as criminal or asocial, in which case he wore a yellow triangle combined with the other color. Eicke's system of issuing different-colored cloth triangles to be sewn onto the uniform jackets was established at Dachau and standardized throughout the entire camp system in 1936 and 1937.[9]

The barracks were overcrowded from the very start as construction could not keep pace with the growing influx of prisoners. As a consequence, the living conditions were abominable; most barracks in the later years were overcrowded to the extreme—two thousand men in a building designed to hold perhaps eight hundred. The wooden bunks were four "shelves" high, with four or five prisoners, whose personal hygiene was kept at the level of livestock, sleeping pressed together on each shelf. There were few blankets and no pillows or mattresses—just straw that was infested with lice. Dysentery was a common problem in the camps, and so the prisoners' fitful sleep was continually interrupted by inmates scrambling down from the shelves and dashing for the latrine. The smell of each barrack was, as might be imagined, revolting.

ALL OF THIS would have been bad enough, but Koch added to the misery by bringing with him several of his most brutal assistants from Sachsenhausen; they and he, along with Ilse, instituted a personal reign of terror over the inmates. Koch gave his subordinates free rein to treat the prisoners in any manner they wanted. As a result, the names of such men as Martin Sommer, Heinrich Hackmann, Josef Kestel, and a whole host of doctors who would become associated with medical experiments on the helpless prisoners began to build reputations within the SS as men unrestrained by any thoughts of human decency or compassion. The inmates were their private stock of slaves, to use and abuse as they saw fit.

Martin Sommer, the camp's chief jailer, was notorious for the whippings he performed on barebacked prisoners stretched over a special table known as a *Prügelbock* ("flogging goat") in front of the entire camp during roll call. Sommer also gained the nickname "Hangman of Buchenwald" because he was fond of tying prisoners' wrists together behind their backs and then hanging them by their hands a few inches off the ground—a torture that produced excruciating pain and disabling injuries.

Inmate Jacob "Jack" Werber, a Polish bricklayer from Radom, recalled being subjected to this punishment. He noted that, after committing a minor offense against camp rules, he and two other inmates had their hands tied behind their backs and were suspended from a tree branch by their hands. "With my feet hanging free," he said, "the weight of my whole body was on my shoulder joints and the pain was excruciating beyond description. As I hung there I prayed for

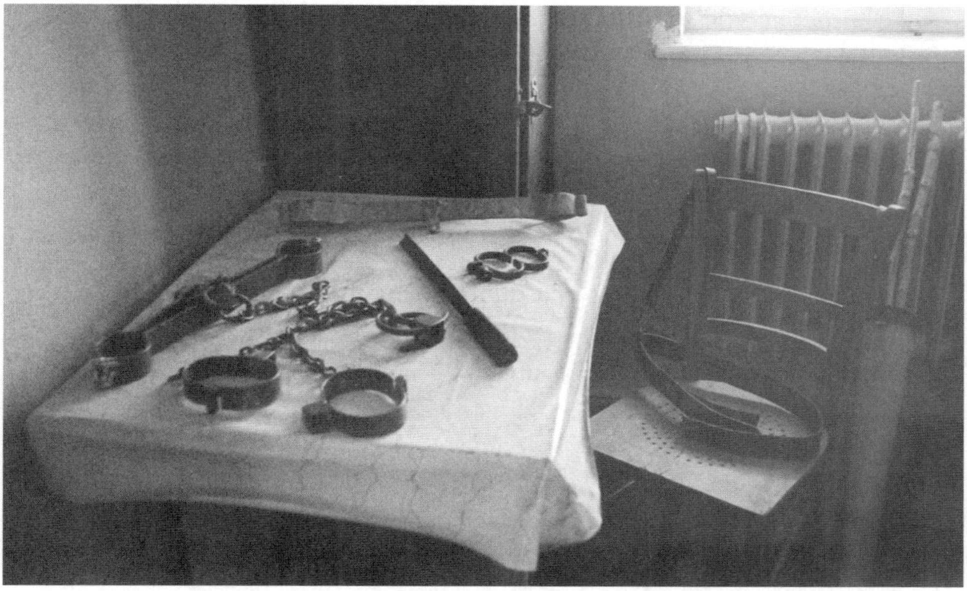

Martin Sommer's tools of torture on display in the "Bunker" (Author photo)

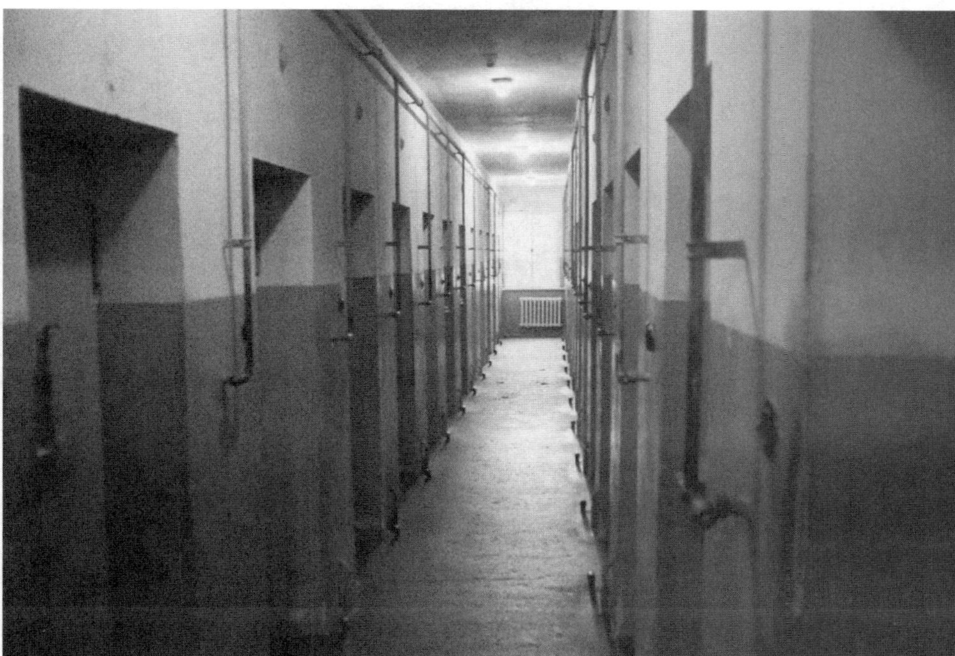

Interior view of the "Bunker" located at the main gate (Author photo)

death to put an end to my misery. Finally, after several hours, I was cut loose from the tree."[10]

Sommer had a variety of torture tools in his office within the Bunker inside the gatehouse—tools he often used to inflict great suffering on any prisoner he felt deserved it. When he was tired of torturing, he would often end the session by murdering the inmate using instruments such as a special vise that could crush a man's skull, lethal injections of phenol or carbolic acid, or his bare hands. There were few methods of murder that the sadistic Sommer did not employ on those unfortunate enough to fall into his hands.

First Lieutenant Heinrich Hackmann was as feared as Sommer. He enjoyed attacking inmates standing at roll call with his fists, boots, whip, or cudgel without warning. He reportedly had two inmates place a fellow prisoner in a beech tree at the lip of the quarry, bend the tree like a catapult, and then launch the inmate to his death. Like Sommer, he enjoyed hanging prisoners—but by the neck instead of by the wrists—from a portable gallows in front of the assembled prisoners.

SS-Hauptsharführer Josef Kestel was the SS man in charge of the Buchenwald quarry operations and, as such, had the power of life or death over the inmates

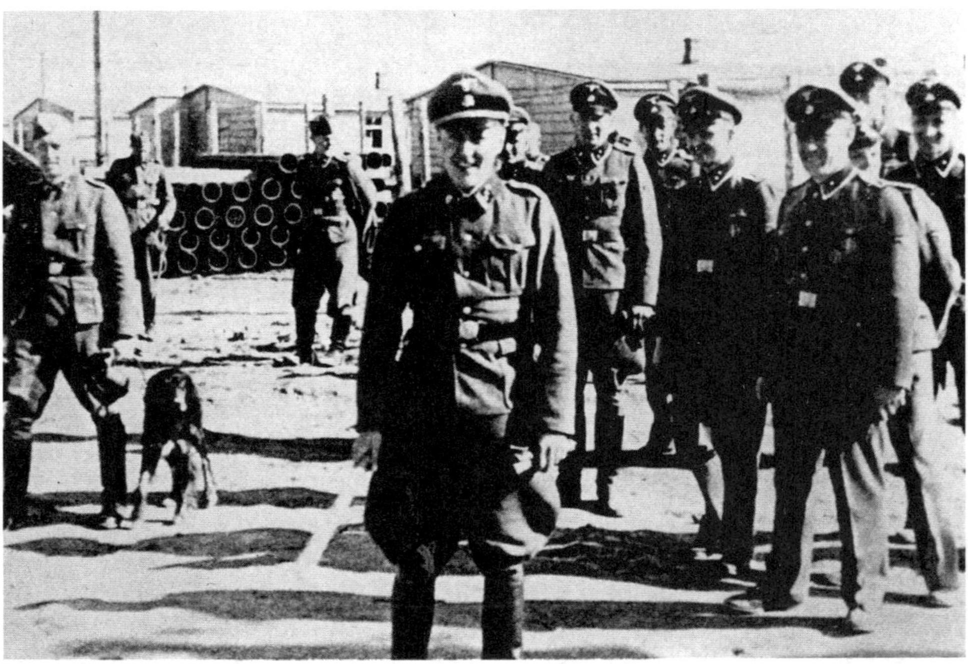

Heinrich Hackmann (center) with a group of smiling SS guards (Buchenwald Memorial)

working there. Greatly feared, Kestel was notorious for beating prisoners to death, throwing stones at them, even holding the head of one prisoner between his legs while a *Kapo* beat the man senseless.[11]

The whole gang of sadists at Buchenwald amused themselves through the suffering of their fellow humans.

THE KOCHS LIVED in grand style atop the Ettersberg. Villa Koch, their residence, had the finest furniture, carpets, draperies, china, and silverware. The larder in the cellar was stocked with an extensive variety of all sorts of products: wines and champagnes from Germany and France; fine beef, veal, hams, and sausages; fruits and vegetables; and other exotic items that were only dim memories to the inmates. Karl built Ilse an indoor equestrian arena the size of a football field to satisfy her passion for horseback riding. Stories are told, too, of drunken orgies that took place at Villa Koch that resembled carnal scenes out of ancient Rome. Karl had affairs (including one with a dancer in Weimar) while Ilse carried on simultaneous affairs with camp adjutant Hermann Florstedt and one of the physicians, Dr. Waldemar Hoven.[12]

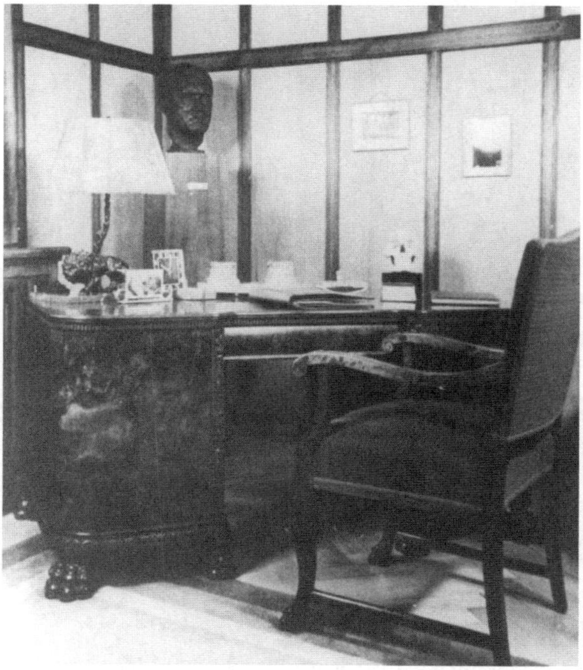

A large bust of Adolf Hitler overlooks Karl Otto Koch's desk in his Buchenwald office. (Buchenwald Memorial)

Some of the prisoners reported in sworn testimony after the war that Ilse liked to ride on horseback to the camp fence or wherever a work party was slaving away on some project and, flaunting her sexuality, whip prisoners in the face with her riding crop when they dared to look at her. One of the inmates who worked as a servant in the Koch household told of a time when Ilse shamelessly exposed herself to him while lying on her bed.[13]

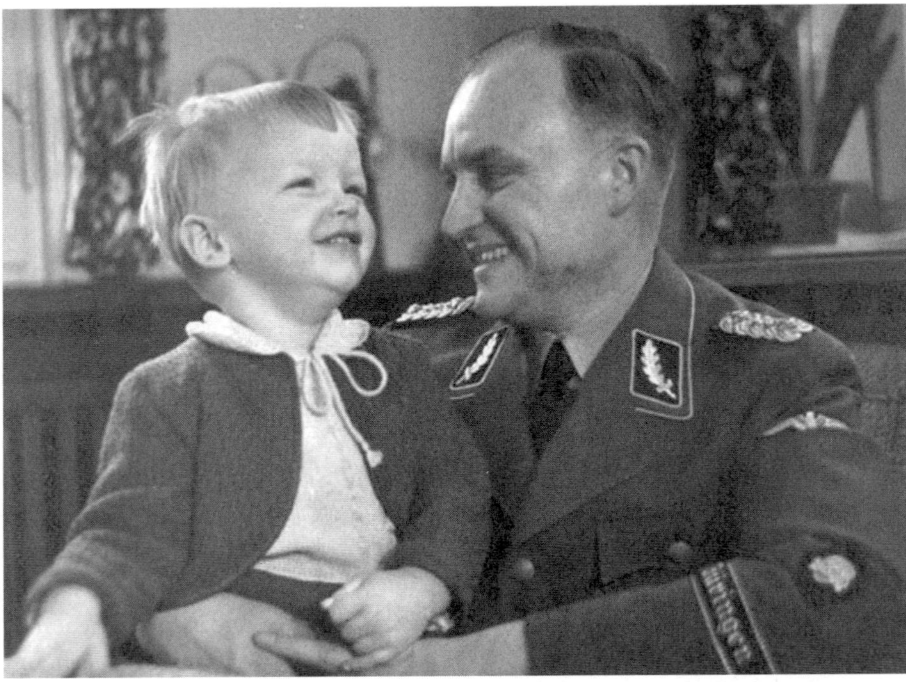

Karl Otto Koch looks lovingly at his son Artwin, early 1940. (Buchenwald Memorial)

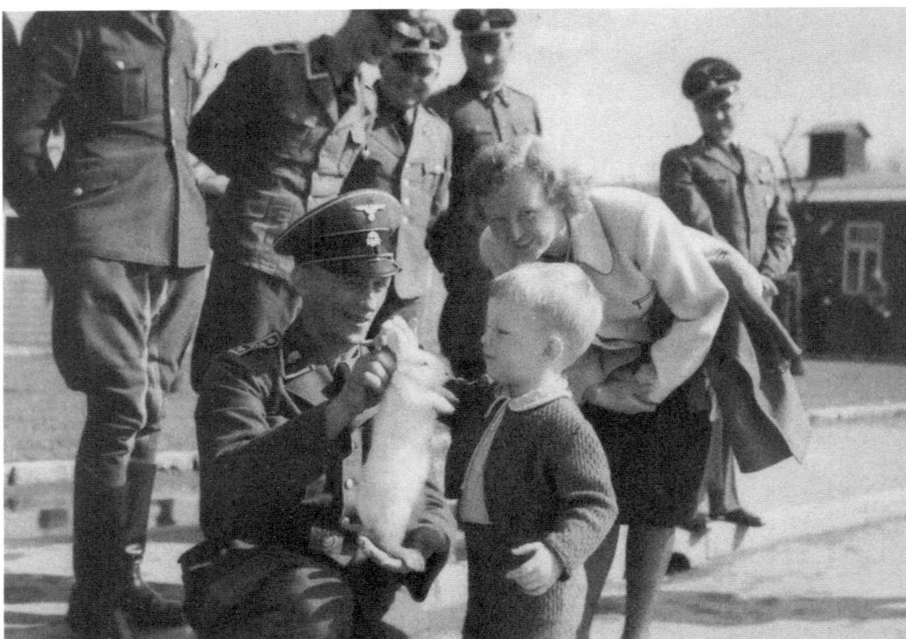

Artwin and an SS man play with the "Easter bunny," 1940, while Ilse and Karl (right) look on. (Koch photo album, U.S. National Archives)

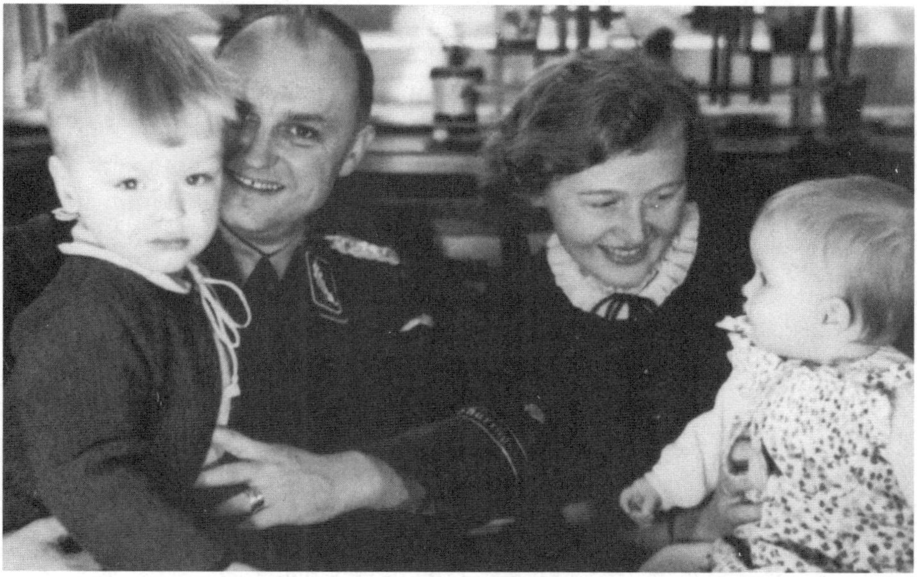

Karl and Ilse Koch and their two children, Artwin and Gisele, photographed at their Buchenwald home, 1940. (Koch photo album, U.S. National Archives)

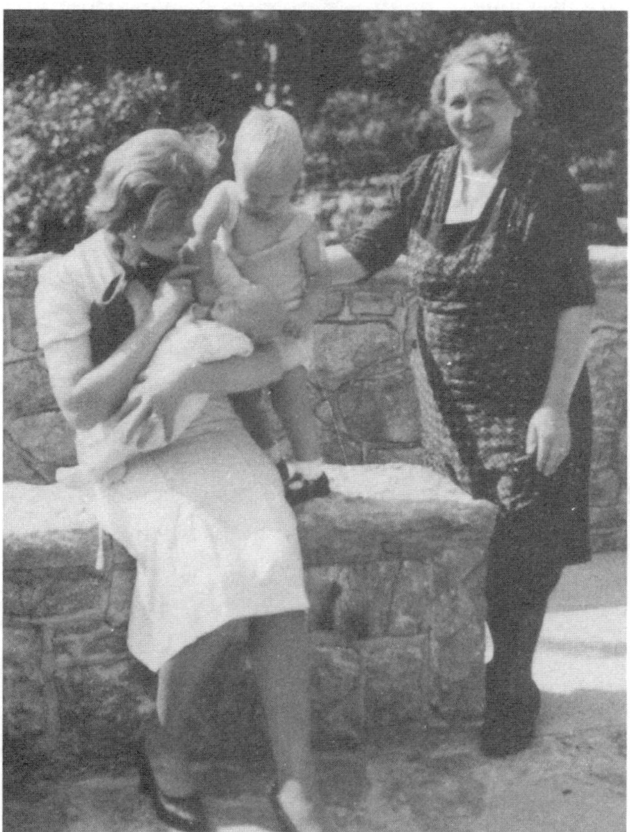

Karl's stepsister Erna Raible (right) watches Ilse and Artwin play with baby Gisele at Haus Buchenwald, summer 1939. (Buchenwald Memorial)

It wasn't long before Karl and Ilse began to enrich their bank accounts at the expense of the prisoners—and the Nazi state. Karl was involved in black-market operations, skimming profits from the staff mess and the prisoners' canteen, and demanding a ransom from the relatives of prisoners in order to secure their early release. He also charged families a fee for the return of the ashes of their cremated relatives. Gold and silver watches and other jewelry confiscated from arriving inmates went into his personal account, and even dental gold extracted from the mouths of dead prisoners was melted down and handed over to the Kochs. Eventually the SS learned of the Kochs' schemes and, before long, the SS investigators were building a case against the *Kommandant* and *Kommandeuse*.[14]

In the meantime, the Kochs were raising a family at Buchenwald. On January 1, 1938, Ilse gave birth to a son, Artwin; on April 26, 1939, she had another child, a daughter named Gisele. (A second daughter, Gudrun, was born the following year but died in infancy.) From the photographs that survive in the family album, Karl and Ilse look like typical loving parents—which make the crimes carried out at during their tenure at Buchenwald all the more chilling.[15]

After the war, several ex-prisoners testified during the Buchenwald war-crimes tribunal held at Dachau about some of the excesses in which Ilse was involved. Some witnesses said that she delighted in ordering the SS guards to require prisoners on work details to strip naked or roll in the mud or perform ridiculous calisthenics while she, other SS wives, and sometimes even her children looked on with great amusement.[16]

But perhaps the most disturbing aspect of all was the contention that Ilse was involved in the gruesome business of ordering the manufacture of lampshades, knife sheaths, the sails of model ships, and other household artifacts made from the skin of tattooed Buchenwald prisoners, a practice allegedly begun by SS Captain Dr. Erich Wagner. In the winter of 1939-40, Wagner had been treating a contagious eye disease intentionally spread to Sinti-Roma (Gypsy) patients whom he treated with injections and after which the patients were killed. Following this experiment, in 1940 Wagner became fascinated in determining if there were a connection between criminality and prisoners with tattoos.[17]

A former prisoner named Paul Grünewald said that he had helped Wagner write a doctoral thesis on the subject of "Do Tattooed Human Beings Show Any Criminal Inclinations Because of The Tattoos?" for presentation at the University of Jena.* Grünewald was also told that "the wife of Colonel Koch

---

* Wagner was captured by American authorities at the end of the war but managed to escape in 1948. He then lived under a false name for six years, eventually working as a doctor in his wife's private practice. He was once again arrested in 1958 and committed suicide on March 22, 1959, while in custody. (Herbert Stolpmann in dachaukz.blogspot.com /2011/11/buchenwald-kz-1937-1945-part-1)

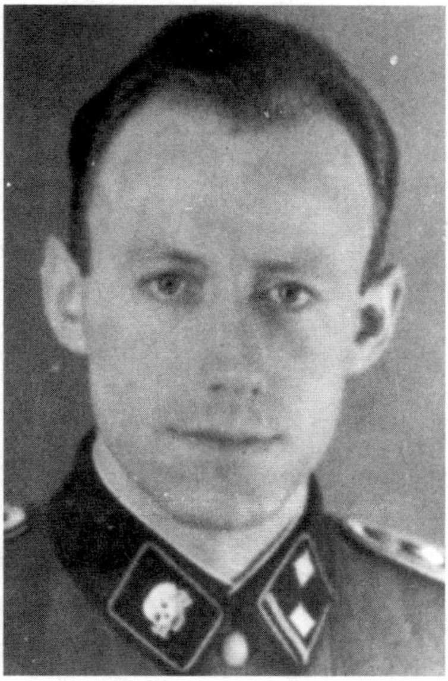

The interest in artifacts made from tattooed human skin was begun by Dr. Erich Wagner, a Buchenwald physician. (U.S. National Archives)

had the idea of utilizing the skin of tattooed prisoners for objects of 'industrial art, which she also did.'"[18] Ilse's connection to this practice allegedly came from her noticing the tattoos on prisoners' bodies during her horseback riding excursions to observe and torment work parties, the recording of those prisoners' numbers, and a request to the SS to have them killed so that their decorated skin could be turned into décor.[19]

These tattooed objects reportedly became all the rage within the SS, with orders pouring in to Buchenwald from SS officers and other Third Reich officials in all corners of the Nazi world; items made from sexually explicit tattoos were in particular demand. A special section was set up in Buchenwald's pathology lab where tattooed inmates were killed, the skin from their bodies stripped, tanned, and then turned into an *objet d'art*. Dr. Kurt Sitte, a German physician incarcerated at Buchenwald from September 1939 to April 1945, was one of several former inmates who testified to a U.S. Senate subcommittee after the war that he worked in the pathology lab and thus was personally familiar with the situation: "As to the lampshade story, I had direct evidence from a man who was not only an eyewitness of its existence but had done much finishing work on it.... His story confirmed and completed what was told by the prisoners of the pathology department and by those who had seen the shade in the Koch house. When I came to the pathology department in 1942 to work, I still met some of the prisoners who had been compelled to tan tattooed skins used for this lampshade. A second lampshade had been ordered, a little after the first had been such a success with the Kochs, by another SS officer. It was never finished but its frame was still in the storeroom of the pathology department when I came there....

"There can be no doubt that in many cases when men with picturesque tattooing died in the Bunker a few days after she [Ilse] had been passing their work detail, their deaths were not another 'accident,' but a deliberate action of Ilse Koch to increase her precious collection of tattooed objects."[20]

It was for reasons like these that Ilse Koch became known to thousands as "the Bitch of Buchenwald."

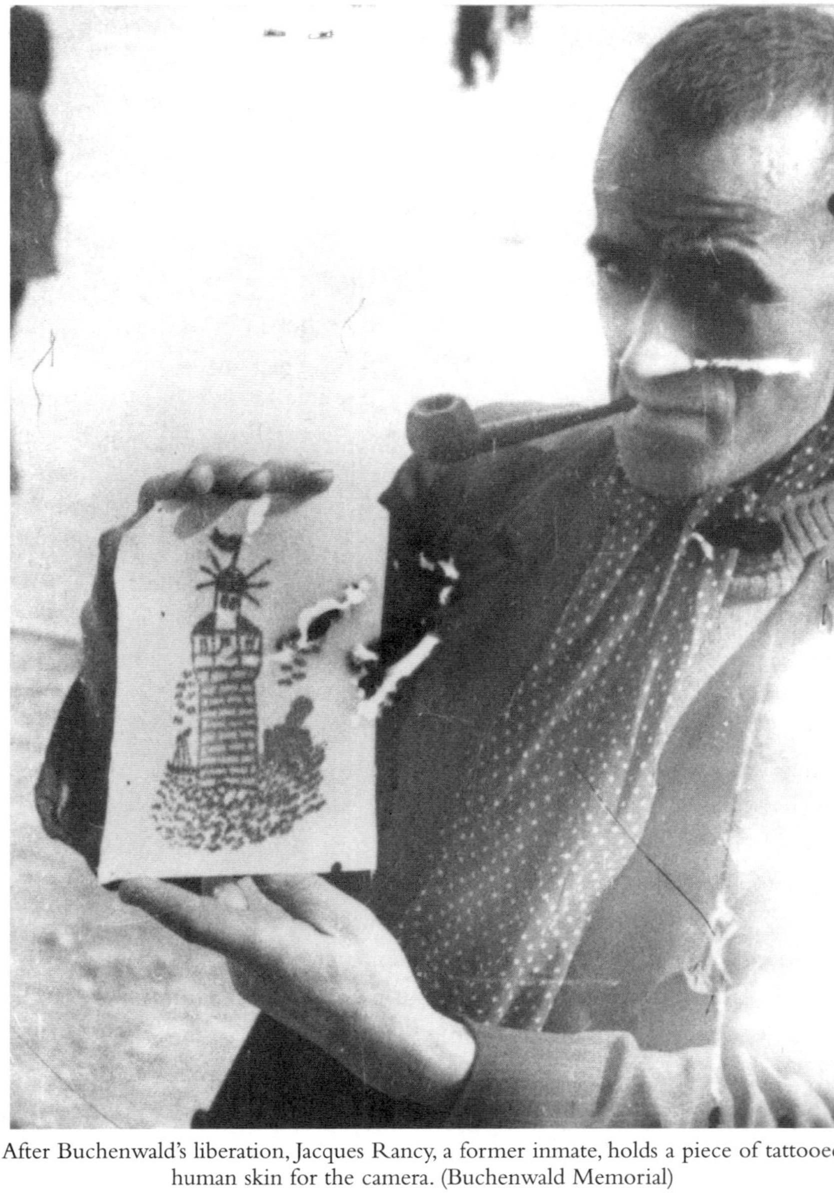

After Buchenwald's liberation, Jacques Rancy, a former inmate, holds a piece of tattooed human skin for the camera. (Buchenwald Memorial)

THE JEWS OF Germany, who became more and more threatened as Nazi laws tightened the screws against them, saw their existence become even more tenuous on the night of November 9/10, 1938, a night of terror known as *Kristallnacht*, when Nazi goons encouraged the civilian populace to go on a rampage throughout the country—burning synagogues, destroying Jewish-owned businesses, and beating and murdering Jews—ostensibly in reprisal for a German diplomat gunned down in Paris by a Jewish student. A few days later, after a widespread roundup of Jews, Buchenwald found itself bulging with nearly 10,000 new inmates; the brutal treatment continued unabated.[21]

Martin Blumenson noted in his book *Kristallnacht* that a former Buchenwald prisoner "wrote of how an older prisoner had been so knocked about by the SS guards that at night, in the shed in which the men slept, 'he kept up a continuous moaning. The brute in charge of this shed hit this man in the face repeatedly, telling him to stop the noise. By morning the old man was dead.' An estimated 350 of the Jews arrested on Kristallnacht died in Buchenwald that winter."[22]

ON APRIL 29, 1939, the *Deutsche Erd- und Steinwerke, GmbH* (German Earth and Stone Works, Inc.) was founded. The mission of this organization was to mine stone from quarries at the concentration camps of Buchenwald, Flossenbürg, Mauthausen, Groß-Rosen, and Natzweiler-Struthof for use in the creation of Hitler's, and chief architect Albert Speer's, grand visions of a fresh, sparkling Germany.

No place at Buchenwald was more dangerous than the *Steinbruch* (quarry)—a place to which almost every inmate was assigned upon first arriving in camp—located just inside the camp's southwestern perimeter. Here men were treated worse than animals, and it was here that most of the early fatalities at Buchenwald occurred. From dawn until dusk, with only a brief break for the thin gruel soup that passed for lunch, the limestone quarry teemed like a human anthill, with 400 to 500 men toiling in unbelievably harsh conditions, chipping great blocks of stone from the earth, carrying them by hand to ore carts positioned on an impossibly steep track, and then pushing the heavily laden carts with all their strength up the incline—all accompanied by the shouts of the foremen who were not shy about applying their whips and truncheons to their charges.

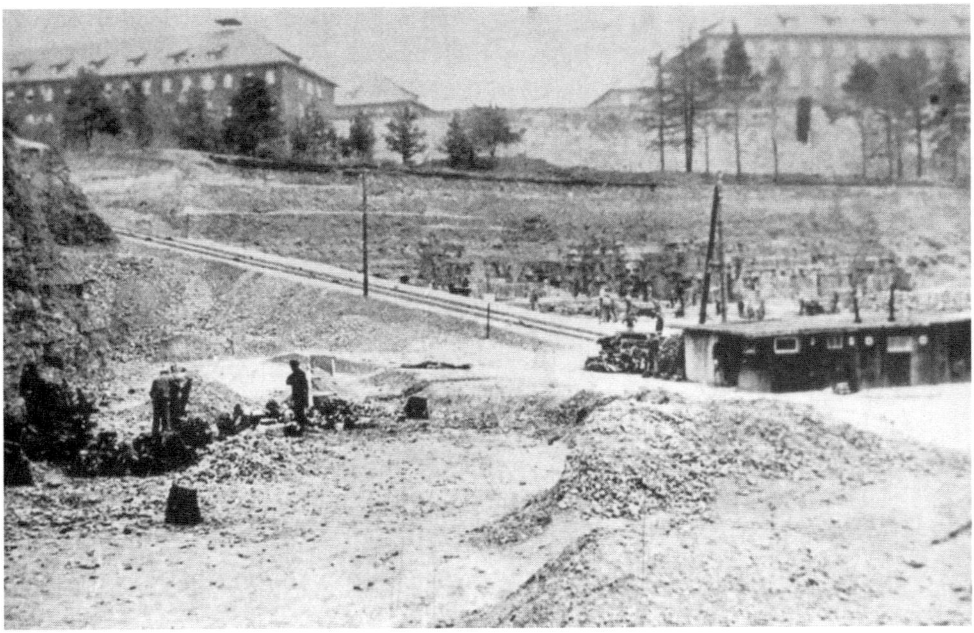

The quarry at Buchenwald, circa 1943. SS barracks are in the background. (Buchenwald Memorial)

Accidents—often fatal—occurred here on a daily basis. Some were caused when inmates lost control of a cart, which then careened back down the track at high speed, crashing into inmates below. Other deaths were the result of stone blocks falling on workers. Some prisoners died after trying to carry stones that were too heavy for them, while others were beaten and even killed for shirking and carrying stones that were too light. Still others were caused by the SS guards beating inmates to death, shooting them if they tried to escape, or pushing them from the cliff at the top of the quarry just "for fun."[23] Eugen Kogon related one incident when a group of SS men standing at the edge of the quarry placed bets on which of them could hit prisoners, slaving below, with stones. When their arms proved inaccurate, they decided to pick off the inmates with pistols and rifles; the toll for the day was seventeen dead and wounded.[24]

Working in the quarry was always a job fraught with peril, as one of the former inmates described: "Under the escort of some *Lagerschutz* [camp police], we were taken to the quarry, where we discovered a veritable calvary of suffering men who were either dying or would soon die of exhaustion. Our job down in this quarry that clattered loudly from the impact of steel tools on hard granite was to choose a stone, shoulder it, and carry it up the long incline to a particular place in the camp for some reason that was not explained to us; how the stone was to be used was irrelevant. There were no breaks allowed, and work began immediately.

"The key point was to make a quick selection of a 'good' stone—one that was neither too small nor too large. Select a too-small stone and you ran the risk of being beaten for being a shirker…while carrying a stone that was too large would be a severe ordeal over the long distance between quarry and camp and, secondly, would attract the censure of colleagues who were ready to label anyone being overly zealous an 'arse-licker.' In fact, however, whatever the size of the stone, it always proved to be too heavy on tender shoulders for the long walk to the camp.

"To complete the punishment, once we delivered our stone, we were required to run back down to the quarry to retrieve another one, running through a gantlet of *Kapos* and SS men all too willing to beat us with truncheons, sticks, whips, and rubber hoses if we were not moving fast enough to please them."[25] Inmates who were able to bribe or otherwise curry favor with the SS escaped the quarry ordeal and were placed in positions of power. Many were given "soft" jobs, such as clerical work in the clothing depot, or as barbers, medical orderlies, kitchen duties, laundry, and general administrative duties. Others were appointed by the SS to act as camp and block seniors, *Kapo*s, and foremen.[26]

But whether their jobs were "soft" or "hard," Buchenwald was no picnic spot. Just surviving the daily routine was more than countless prisoners could do.

3
CHAMBER OF HORRORS

"When a prisoner received twenty-five lashes with a cane, he had to bend over and stick his head in the SS toilet that was filled with excrement."

Richard Gritz
Buchenwald inmate

IN THE MID-1930s, Theodor Eicke devoted himself to a major reorganization of the *SS-Totenkopfverbände*—the concentration camp guards. SSTV was, at Eicke's insistence, expanded in March 1936 from 1,800 to 3,500 men as the camp system itself expanded. It was Eicke's intention to create an "elite within an elite" and have his SSTV, identifiable by the macabre skull-and-crossbones insignia on their uniforms, be considered the pinnacle of the Nazi Aryan ideal.

Until the outbreak of war in 1939, the guards, who had enlisted for a term of from four to twelve years, were required to be young German citizens between seventeen and twenty-two years of age, physically imposing (no less than five feet, ten inches in height), in perfect health, physically and mentally tough, fanatically devoted to the Nazi cause, and be able to supply genealogical proof of at least one hundred years of "racial purity" (i.e., no evidence of Jewish relatives in their families)—each recruit the supreme example of the perfect Aryan warrior.*[1] Any lack of discipline shown by any officer or enlisted member of the SSTV was dealt with almost as ruthlessly as if it had been committed by an inmate; rules-breakers within the ranks were sometimes even sentenced to Buchenwald as inmates![2]

According to author Charles W. Sydnor Jr., "By late 1937, Eicke's energy and drive clearly had transformed the SSTV into a crack paramilitary [Nazi] Party formation. The concentration camp guards developed into Eicke's mold: ruthless, fanatical, pitiless creatures who obeyed every order with reflex instinctiveness, and who, like Eicke, became inured to the cruelties they practiced and indifferent to the sufferings they inflicted."[3]

---

* As the war went on, however, and combat losses began to mount—especially among the *Waffen-SS* formations that were often employed as shock troops—the strict requirements for joining the SS were relaxed. In time there would be SS men drawn from supposed "Aryan" or "Germanic" populations from Scandinavia, Hungary, and Romania, and whole SS units were formed of Ukranians and Latvians. Several times during the war, able-bodied guards and headquarters staffs were reassigned to front-line units of the *Waffen*-SS; gradually, the young guards were replaced by older, often war-wounded, men. (Stein, pp. 38-39)

AS MENTIONED EARLIER, the first guards at Buchenwald were members of 3rd *SS-Totenkopfstandarten* (3rd SS Death's Head Regiment) "*Thuringen*," but shortly before the war broke out in September 1939, the regiment was reassigned to the Wehrmacht for the invasion of Poland.* Twelve days later, the unit was transferred to Poland between Upper Silesia and the Vistula river for "police duties"** behind the lines of the advancing German Army, where it was responsible for numerous atrocities including massacres at Nisko, Rawa Mazowiecka, and Ciepielów, and where it remained through October. After its departure, the 3rd SS-Totenkopf Regiment was replaced at Buchenwald by the 14th SS-Totenkopf Regiment, which was formed by an amalgamation of the 2nd Battalion, 9th SS-Totenkopf Regiment; 3rd Battalion, 6th SS-Totenkopf Regiment; and 4th Battalion, SS-Totenkopf Recruitment Regiment.[4]

IN THE HEADY, early years of the Nazi regime, it seemed that nothing and no one could stop the juggernaut that would eventually consume almost all of Europe. Hitler, through bluff and bluster, and backed up by his formidable, goose-stepping minions, began expanding his Third Reich. First, on March 7, 1936, he tested the resolve of the Great War victors when he sent troops to occupy the demilitarized Rhineland area along the border with Belgium and France, thus violating some of the restrictions imposed by the Treaty of Versailles and Treaty of Locarno. Except for some feeble protests, no one lifted a finger to stop him. Next, two years later, he swallowed up his homeland Austria with a bloodless Anschluß (annexation) and incorporated it into Germany. Third, in October 1938, he threatened Czechoslovakia with invasion

* In October 1939, a month after Germany invaded Poland and sparked the European phase of World War II, the 1st, 2nd, and 3rd Totenkopf Regiments were turned into combat units and consolidated into the 14,000-man SS Totenkopf Division, with Eicke as its commander. The division saw action in Poland (where it was used primarily to terrorize the civilian populace), France, and the Soviet Union. In the fall of 1942, it was reorganized as the 3rd SS Panzer Division. On February 26, 1943, while flying to inspect his troops on the front lines at Orelka, Russia, Eicke's plane was shot down and he was killed. (Heiber and Glantz, p. 993; Sydnor, pp. 37-62; www. holocaustresearchproject. othercamps/eicke)

** "Police duties" meant hunting down Polish soldiers separated from their units, terrorizing civilians, and murdering political leaders, priests, intellectuals, and Jews. The 3rd SS-Totenkopf Regiment was later incorporated into the SS-Totenkopf Division and served in the invasions and occupation of Denmark and Holland in the spring of 1940. (Stein, pp. 37-39)

if the government of Edvard Beneš did not allow the citizens of the German-speaking portion of that country—known as the Sudetenland—to vote on whether or not they desired to be annexed by Germany. Hitler's lust for *Lebensraum*—living space for the German people—was temporarily sated when French Prime Minister Édouard Daladier and British Prime Minister Neville Chamberlain stabbed the Czechs in the back by persuading Beneš to avoid war and appease Hitler's demands.[5]

It was all so easy, Hitler thought; Europe was rolling over and giving in to his demands whenever he rattled his saber at them. Like an alcoholic who craves just one more drink, power-drunk Hitler began hungrily eying some future takeover candidates—France, Belgium, Norway, Denmark, Poland, Great Britain, and the Soviet Union. To lull Josef Stalin into thinking that Germany represented no threat, Hitler had his foreign minister, Joachim von Ribbentrop, negotiate a cynical non-aggression treaty with the Soviets in August 1939—a treaty that also allowed Germany and the U.S.S.R. to carve up Poland between them in the event of a German invasion.[6]

On September 1, 1939, the event came true when Hitler sent his army and air force into neighboring Poland in a swift and violent assault known as *Blitzkrieg*, or lightning war. Britain and France responded by declaring war on Germany.[7] Concentration camps soon filled up with persons captured during the onslaught, and Buchenwald grew like a cancerous tumor on its hilltop, swiftly becoming the very symbol of the evil Nazi state.

Behind its grim, barbed-wire fencing, the camp was a chamber of horrors—in its own way even worse than the six major killing centers that would spring up in Poland after 1941; at least at these killing centers death came relatively swiftly for the victims. After arriving by rail at Auschwitz and the other extermination camps, they were herded directly from the train platforms into the changing rooms, where they were stripped of their clothing, valuables, dignity, and hope, and marched into the gas chambers where their lives were snuffed out within minutes. The whole process of extermination, from arrival to gassing, often took less than an hour.

Not so at Buchenwald. Those unfortunate enough to have been sent there were sentenced to a purgatory with an indeterminate period of hunger, disease, degradation, hard labor, and, often, torture and a slow, agonizing physical and spiritual death. At Buchenwald in the coming years, many prisoners would be used as involuntary human guinea pigs and subjected to painful medical and pseudo-scientific experiments. Thousands more were used as slave laborers to build weapons of war for the Nazi state. The depths of depravity to which the administrators of Buchenwald sank knew no limits.

AT BUCHENWALD, JUST as at Dachau, Sachsenhausen, and the other concentration camps, daily life followed an unvarying pattern. Prisoners, on their first day of incarceration, quickly discovered that they had lost their liberty and identity, and that failure to follow the often arbitrary rules to the letter brought them punishment beyond imagining.

The barracks themselves were of the most Spartan and depressing design, no more luxurious than a cattle barn. Dim light bulbs provided a dull, lifeless glow to the scene. A small stove gave off a modicum of heat only to those nearest it. Some barracks had the most rudimentary toilet and washing facilities; others had none at all.

Then there was the dreaded daily routine. Each day before dawn, the inmates were rousted out of their bunks with shouts from their *Blockälteste*. The inmates scrambled to the latrine and washroom, where they were only allotted very few minutes to take care of their personal business. There a pitifully weak stream of cold water was all the men could use to wet their faces and perhaps splash onto their stinking bodies.

Once the morning ablution was finished, it was off at a run to the mess hall, where thousands of famished men, their stomachs growling audibly, fought over the meager scraps of food provided to them by their masters. It was a stretch to even call the slop "food," for rarely was it fit to feed even barnyard animals. One small loaf of sawdust-laced bread might be divided among five or more men, each one thinking the man next to him received a slightly larger slice than did he; fights over a scrap of bread broke out often. On rare occasions, if the SS men were feeling generous, there might be a small piece of sausage, which was often rotten and made from "condemned" meat. A lukewarm cup of *ersatz* coffee or tea and a bowl of thin, nearly inedible "soup" (usually made from grass and rotten turnips) was ladled out.

The inmates then rushed back to their barrack to sweep it clean and insure that every bed was made and every bunk was perfectly aligned. If anyone had defecated in his bed during the night (a not-uncommon occurrence, given the high incidence of dysentery), the bed had to be scrubbed clean. And if so much as one piece of straw was found on the floor, or one bunk was out of alignment, beatings by the *Kapos* would be meted out to the innocent and guilty alike.

Then it was time for *Appell*, or roll call, a twice-daily exercise in terror. The entire inmate population was marched eight abreast from their barracks to the *Appellplatz*, or roll-call square, adjacent to the main gate, passing a gantlet of SS guards with rubber hoses who lashed out at them as they dashed past; anyone who tripped and fell on the rocky, uneven ground was subjected to a real beating. Prisoners too weak or too ill to run were carried by their block-mates. At the *Appellplatz*, it was common for the SS men to beat any inmates claiming they were sick. Inmates too ill to work (and an inmate needed to be on the verge of death to be excused from work details) reported to the *Häftlingskrankenrevier*, or infirmary—a place from which very few inmates ever returned alive. Guards with loaded automatic weapons watched over the square from the watchtower above the gatehouse, ready to dispatch anyone who fought back or attempted to escape.

There was always much pushing and shoving at roll call by the *Kapos* and their assistants to align the rows perfectly, just the way the SS liked them. Every man stood stiffly at attention, his fingers straight, his thumbs lined up with the seams of his trousers, no matter if the day were warm and sunny, windy or rainy, or if it was freezing and snowing fiercely. Anyone who moved, talked, coughed, sneezed, urinated, or collapsed from the ordeal was sure to receive a savage beating.

From the watchtower over the main gate ("Tower One"), an SS man with a microphone broadcast over loudspeakers the command "*Mutze...ab!*" ("Caps off!"), the prisoners had to whip off their small cotton caps with military precision and hold them against their right pant leg; anyone slow in obeying the order could count on a beating with rubber hoses by the *Kapos*. The next order—"*Mutze...auf!*" ("Caps on!") was similarly scrutinized. Again, slowness in executing the command would bring verbal and physical harassment. As getting thousands of persons to perform this cap-off, cap-on maneuver with military precision was virtually impossible, it was repeated over and over again until everyone—thousands of sick, starved, and brutalized men—performed the action in unison, like a well-rehearsed drill team.

SS men with the rank of *Scharführer* (sergeant) then counted the inmates assembled from each barrack. Once the counting was finished (and rarely was it finished within an hour), the scraps of paper on which the numbers had been written were gathered up and taken to the gatehouse, where SS men added up the numbers. Only during this time were the prisoners allowed to relax from their rigid postures. If the numbers were not correct—and seldom were they correct on the first count—the roll was retaken. This process—in every type of weather—normally took hours. The SS personnel had a fetish for accuracy; if anyone died during the night, their corpses had to be present as well, for no one was allowed to be officially declared dead until after the evening roll call.[8]

Next came the dreaded order for some inmates who had received a note from the orderly room the night before to report to specific numbered places outside the gatehouse. There they waited in fear, sometimes for hours, to learn why they had been summoned; the summons could be something as innocuous as correcting some paperwork or as sinister as being jailed and tortured or murdered in the gatehouse's cellblock, the dungeon known as the Bunker.

After the morning counting, announcements, and beatings were concluded, the assembled prisoners were quickly broken down into their work groups, or *Arbeitskommando* and, with the camp band playing lively tunes, marched off to begin their twelve-hour workday. Work could be anything from the backbreaking, often fatal, labor in the rock quarry just inside the camp's southwestern perimeter to "easier" tasks at the camp zoo, hospital, lumberyard, pig farm, or as *Kalfaktorn* (servants) in the SS officers' quarters. Other inmates with specialized skills might be put to work in relative comfort in the camp's library, kitchen, photography department, printing and bookbindery shop, art and woodcarving studios, laundry, clothing and equipment depot, machine shop, leatherworking shop, or to some other make-work project the SS had dreamed up to keep the prisoners occupied and degraded. No matter what their chores, however, brutality usually accompanied them; prisoners could be whipped or clubbed for the slightest of offenses—or none at all—based on the mood of their guards.[9]

One of the worst details was the "Gardening" or "Landscaping" *Kommando*. While the name sounds idyllic, inmates assigned to it were always in mortal danger. An especially feared SS lieutenant by the name of Dumböck (more about him in Chapter 7) was in charge of the gardening detail, and he wanted to make sure that no one thought that his *Kommando* was a cushy job. In fact, so brutal was Dumböck that he allegedly killed at least forty prisoners with his own hands and drove others to suicide.[10]

Jacob Werber recalled that the Landscape *Kommando*'s main job "consisted of pulling out roots and tree stumps. All of us tried to avoid [being assigned to the *Kommando*] like the plague but once you were chosen for it, there was no alternative." He said that everyone feared Dumböck—"an animal who enjoyed beating and killing people. If you fell, he would step on your throat until you died."[11]

Throughout the camp's existence, the sanitation system was less than primitive. There were open latrine pits twenty-five feet long, twelve feet deep, and twelve feet wide. Prisoners, up to fifteen at a time, sat over the pits on logs; no toilet paper was provided. The SS had great sport in knocking seated prisoners off the logs into the filth. Eugen Kogon reported that in October 1937 ten prisoners were drowned by the SS after being thrown into the excrement.[12]

Inmates assigned to the latrine detail were also at particular risk. Ironically dubbed the "4711 *Kommando*," after a particular brand of German cologne, these men were often abused by their masters to the point of death by being thrown into the cesspools and having their heads held under the "water" until they drowned. Inmate Richard Gritz recalled one disgusting incident: "There were two toilets in the [punishment Bunker]: one for the prisoners and one for the SS. When a prisoner received twenty-five lashes with a cane, he had to bend over and stick his head in the SS toilet that was filled with excrement. After the punishment was completed, he was not allowed to wash off the excrement. In the half-minute 'morning wash,' it was hardly possible to wash adequately, so the prisoner…had to run around covered with excrement for weeks."[13]

Commandant Koch devised one particularly agonizing punishment for a Gypsy who had attempted escape in 1938. Koch ordered built a small, wooden box covered on one side by chicken wire. The other wooden sides and top had long nails driven through them so that the effect was like the inside of a pincushion. Unable to stand or lie down, the prisoner was forced to remain in a crouching position inside the box. Kogon's description: "He was kept in the roll-call area for two days and three nights, without food. His dreadful screams had long since lost any semblance of humanity. On the morning of the third day he was finally relieved of his sufferings by an injection of poison."[14]

One of the most grueling tasks was the construction—entirely by hand—of the *Blutstraße* ("Blood Road"), a concrete road more than three miles long that ran downhill from the Caracho Weg at top of the Ettersberg to the bottom. Using crude wagons, two hundred Jewish inmates began in June 1938 to haul heavy limestone slabs that would form the sub-base. Because their foremen often made them sing as they worked, the teams of men pulling the wagons from the limestone quarry to the work site were called the "singing horses."[15]

AFTER A THIRTY-minute break for lunch (which invariably consisted of ersatz coffee or tea and a watery bowl of soup flavored with grass, turnip greens, or decaying vegetables) it was back to work until evening.

Once the workday had ended, rather than being allowed to rest, the exhausted prisoners were subjected again to another long, mind-numbing evening roll call that, like the morning *Appell*, could last for hours, and in all sorts of weather, while the SS made sure that their numbers were correct and no one had escaped. (Inmates who had died during the day were required to be present before being carted off to the crematorium.) If the count were not accurate, then, according to Eugen Kogon, the SS lost their tempers and let their fists and boots fly. Most *Appells* lasted ninety minutes or longer. He noted one particularly memorable *Appell*, on December 14, 1938, when the temperature stood at five degrees above zero Fahrenheit and the thinly clad prisoners were required to stand at rigid attention in the cold for nineteen straight hours; twenty-five men froze to death that evening; a further forty-five were found dead the next morning.[16]

On occasion the inmates were ordered to stand at roll call and empty their pockets; much money and tobacco ended up in the possession of the guards. Another time, in February 1938, the prisoners were ordered to strip and stand unclothed for three hours, despite the freezing weather. Ilse Koch, wife of the commandant, reportedly showed up outside the fence with the wives of four other officers to amuse themselves at the sight of the naked, shivering men.[17]

Even after evening roll call had concluded, there was still no rest for the weary, for public punishments—usually twenty-five lashes with a leather whip on a bare-backed inmate stretched over the whipping table or even an occasional hanging on the portable gallows—were then meted out.[18] A former inmate recalled that the entire camp was forced one day to witness the lynching of a Pole who had tried to escape from a *Kommando* but was recaptured: "Coming back from work one day at six o'clock, we found the gallows set up on the roll-call platz.... Standing before the gallows was a Polish prisoner wearing a very short rope around his neck with a slipknot. In his hands he held a sign that said...'On my return from my trip, this evening I shall be hanged....'

"This particular figure, in our world without justice or judgment, faced certain death. The scene had been set and he had the principal role. He now stood there: Still, calm, almost absent, going through his last hours, pinned there between the gallows and the ironic sign he carried. It was an unbearable expression of the hell we were in.... We were ordered to keep our eyes on the hanging and to observe silence. Such were the rules for this kind of entertainment.... With superhuman effort, the condemned Pole moved towards the little stool, alone, his hands tied behind his back. He stepped onto the stool, more and more isolated from the rest of the world. How did he have the courage?

Had he taken something? He seemed to be living his last moments completely removed from the rest of the world. The SS duty officer seized the end of the rope and passed it over and around the hook of the gallows, with an assumed air of casualness. Then, slowly and deliberately, as if to chase a fly, he pulled the stool away. The rope stretched and the condemned man's death began."[19]

Once the evening roll-call activities were concluded, the prisoners were allowed to return to their barracks and consume their evening meal—normally cold—of the usual thin broth, perhaps flavored with scraps of rotten meat and perhaps some sort of salad made from moldy greens of unidentifiable provenance. (At Buchenwald, prisoners received an average of 800 calories or less per day.) Mealtimes were rarely peaceful, either, as some SS guards delighted in disrupting the supper to order the inmates to perform calisthenics, or crawl under the tables, or perform other humiliating activities.

Once the evening meal was finished, the prisoners might get a chance to visit the latrine and relax. But the fear was always there that something would happen during the night—which it sometimes did—when a drunken guard or block leader would roust everyone out of bed and into the camp street in their shirts (the only garment the prisoners were allowed to wear to bed, no matter what the temperature) for an impromptu roll call or a little calisthenics session.

A variety of intimidations, both large and small, kept inmates continually on edge, distrustful of each other and fearful of their own shadows. The small forms of intimidation were the constant verbal and physical humiliations—screaming orders into the face of an inmate as a form of belittlement; making prisoners stand at attention for hours on end at *Appell*; SS guards, *Kapos*, or *Blockältestern* flying into tirades at the slightest breach of camp rules; the withholding of food or privileges, etc. Kogon noted that even in the barracks, the inmates always feared the next tirade at any moment.[20]

And so it went—the daily, deadening routine rarely varying, a dehumanizing process that not only turned the inmates into automatons but also made it possible for the SS to regard the prisoners as less than animals.

For decades, a rational explanation has been sought to understand by what process or flaw in the human psyche men can be turned into monsters capable of mistreating other human beings without feelings of guilt or compassion. Has the answer been found? The next chapter may provide some clues.

4
TURNING MEN INTO MONSTERS

"We have the moral right—we have the duty *to our people to do it—to kill this people who wanted to kill us."*

Heinrich Himmler
Reichsführer-SS

SO MANY BOOKS have been written about the horrible concentration camp conditions and the excessive ruthlessness of the guards that it seems almost redundant to repeat those accounts here. What has been less studied and understood is who the guards were and how they could treat other humans the way they did. First-hand accounts by guards are almost non-existent; what little they have said about their activities and mindset has come mainly from war-crimes-tribunal transcripts and a few letters and diaries.

The question often asked is: "How could ordinary, law-abiding Germans become the murderous monsters who ran the camps and killed millions of human beings with impunity?" There are several answers. First, an organization's character is almost always a reflection of its leadership. The SS was the product of Hitler's and Himmler's insistence on unquestioning obedience to orders, and a vision of a Nazi Germany cleansed of all negative elements. The SS leadership also included Theodor Eicke. As author Charles Sydnor noted, "Like many of the concentration camp commanders he trained, Eicke basically was pitiless and cruelly insensitive to human suffering, and regarded qualities such as mercy and charity as useless, outmoded absurdities that could not be tolerated by the SS."[1]

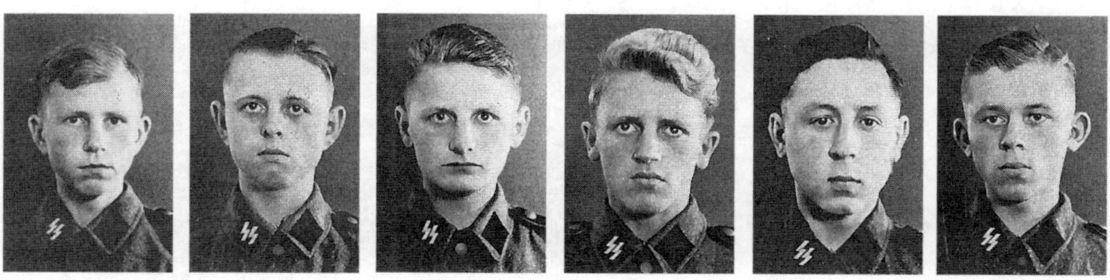

Their official SS identification photos reveal that some of the SS guards at Buchenwald appear to be no more than teenage boys. (Courtesy Louis Gros)

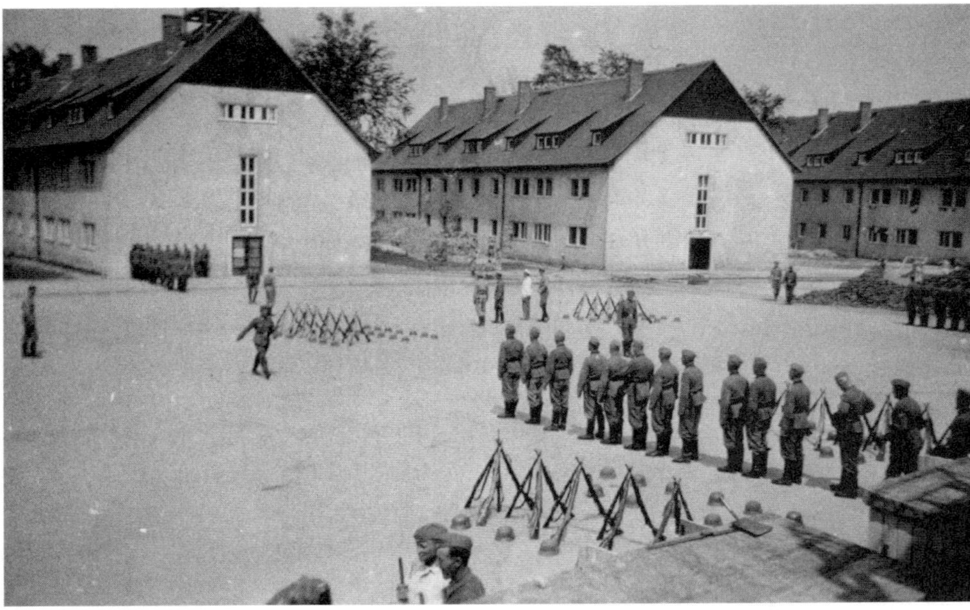

Guards line up on their parade ground for an inspection (Buchenwald Memorial)

A number of psychologists studying the phenomenon confirm this theory. According to John P. Sabini and Maury Silver, "Perhaps the most potent technique of degradation is to make the individual filthy, to make him stink.... In modern Western culture the requirement that one remain clean (both of contamination by mud, dirt, and other environmental sources of pollution and, perhaps more importantly, of one's own excrement) is a first and central demand.... To withdraw [baths, showers, and toilets] or forbid their use makes it inevitable that the individual will be unable to sustain the immediate, compelling appearance of a worthy self, and makes it easier for another to ignore the moral fact that such a spoiled appearance has no bearing on the question of value or worth."

Sabini and Silver also noted, "Starvation, along with reducing the economic burden of the slaves to the slave masters, destroys the body's capacity to produce the range of expressions we take as a sign of affective life. Constant hunger, like constant pain, removes the individual from the social world, fixates attention of the internal state, and hence dehumanizes."[2]

It was *streng verboten*—strongly forbidden—for a guard to show any friendliness or compassion toward an inmate. Having any "non-official communication" with an inmate, or even using the familiar German form of "you" (*Du*) toward a prisoner, was regarded as a breach of the "anti-fraternization" rules that would

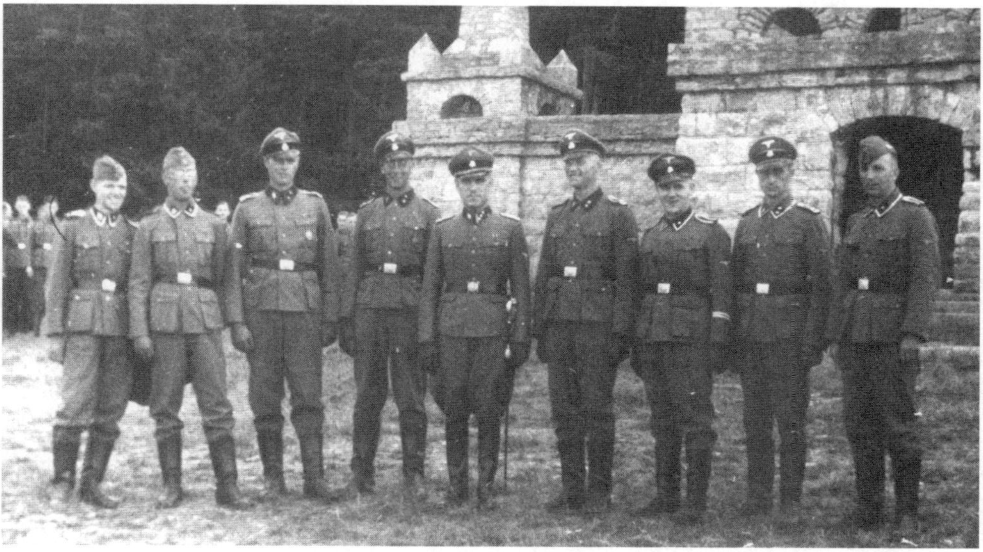

A group of SS guards from Buchenwald pose in front of the Bismarckturm in an undated photo. (Buchenwald Memorial)

result in the punishment of the guard (which could include being transferred to a combat front).

As Buchenwald historian Harry Stein wrote of the Death's Head guards, "Their heroic self-image as 'political soldiers' stood in sharp contrast to the banal military routines, the demagoguery, the comradeship and the cruelties that constituted their daily lives."[3]

IN MANY WAYS, of course, the guards were just ordinary men who were simply making a living by doing the jobs assigned to them—not unlike guards at any American jail or prison. They got up in the morning, put on their uniforms, ate breakfast, and went to work. They had mothers and fathers. Some were married and had children. They followed the news of the war and the fortunes of their favorite soccer teams.* They chatted with each other over lunch in the mess hall about current events and, like soldiers everywhere, grumbled about their pay and long hours and unreasonable sergeants. They had their own daily

* During the war, professional soccer continued to be played in Germany, as it did in the other warring countries, primarily to keep up the home-front morale and give the war-weary population a diversion from their increasingly difficult lives. But in April 1945, with defeat looming for Germany, the professional leagues suspended play. (www. abseits-soccer.com/essays/nazi)

inspections and roll calls. Some who were wounded combat veterans told war stories of their time on the Eastern Front, North Africa, or wherever.

Most of the guards probably enjoyed a cold beer and a plate of wurst and sauerkraut at the end of the day. They suffered through the mindless bureaucracy of the military organization, caught colds, saw the dentist, had their boots and uniforms repaired, and took out the trash. They had financial difficulties and marital problems. They worried about family members who lived in cities that were being bombed by the Allies. Most were simple country folk, not terribly well educated, intellectual, self-aware, or introspective. Many guards were coarse brutes, others not so much. As an anti-religious organization, the SSTV discouraged its soldiers from attending church. Eicke "aimed to create among his men a hatred for the churches as enemies of National Socialism," wrote Sydnor. "By late 1936, Eicke's efforts resulted in official renunciation of Christianity by a substantial majority of the men in the SSTV."[4]

Germans have traditionally loved to sing, and so the guards at KL Buchenwald most likely entertained themselves in a service club or Weimar pub with songs—bawdy, patriotic, and sentimental. Many played games—cards, chess, skittles. Some engaged in athletic pursuits during off-duty hours. And they laughed and played with their children, if they had them, and made love to their women.

The guards were treated to movies—musicals, light comedies, newsreels, and serious propaganda films with a heavy anti-Semitic message (such as the vile, anti-Semitic film *Jud Süß,* which compared Jews to an over-breeding horde of sewer rats and expressed the need for Germany to stamp them out for the good of humanity)—on a regular basis; with anti-Semitic attitudes rife in Europe for centuries, it did not take much to turn mistrust into disgust, and dislike of Jews into outright hatred.

Also, the hard military training the SS received had two fundamental purposes: first, to strengthen the awareness of belonging to an "elite, racially superior" group and, secondly, to teach guards how to deal with prisoners in a cold, brutal, and unfeeling way. After all, as their officers and non-coms continually drilled into their heads, these prisoners wouldn't be in the camps if they weren't inferior. "Just look at those filthy pigs," their officers and non-coms would tell them while surveying the emaciated, foul-smelling, feces-stained wretches lined up for the twice-daily roll calls. "They are not human. No self-respecting human would eat slop out of bowls, submit meekly like a sheep or a cow to our punishments without resisting, or wear shit-stained clothes that look like rags," was the dehumanizing message that made it easier for the guards to hold the inmates in contempt and to feel few or no qualms about abusing or even killing them.

And with their heads, moustaches, and beards shaved, the inmates could be viewed by their guards as being anonymous creatures with no identifying characteristics or personalities, as indistinguishable as one ant from another. The filthy prisoners, the guards came to believe, *were* the sub-humans, the *Untermensch*, that they—the tall, strong, spotlessly uniformed SS guards, representatives of the Master Race—had been hearing about for so long.

The lives of the guards at Buchenwald were, without a doubt, similar or identical to the lives of the guards at Auschwitz, Sachsenhausen, Dachau, Mauthausen, Ravensbrück, and the hundreds of other camps. As such, the members of the *Totenkopf* formations, whether engaged in simple "prison-guard" duties or the more horrendous "death-camp" duties, are inextricably linked. As Sybille Steinbacher wrote in *Auschwitz: A History*: "Domestic peace did not contradict the professional everyday life of the SS members. In fact the insistently nurtured family idyll may actually have encouraged the killing in the camp, because it gave the SS men the psychological stability they needed. We should not be surprised that SS men could be both mass murderers and loving fathers. The façade of family happiness revealed nothing whatsoever about the men's humanitarian convictions.

"Rather, the extermination of 'inferior' people was given moral legitimacy by the idea that it was securing the existence of the 'Aryan race,' and against a background of a biological and genetic value system it was seen as entirely necessary. Mass murder and respectability were not opposites, but were closely interwoven. So to see mass crime as the result of pathological states of mind seems just as implausible as assuming that the perpetrators had fallen victim to a collective split personality. SS family life—like mass extermination—served the construction of the 'racially pure' ethnic community."[5]

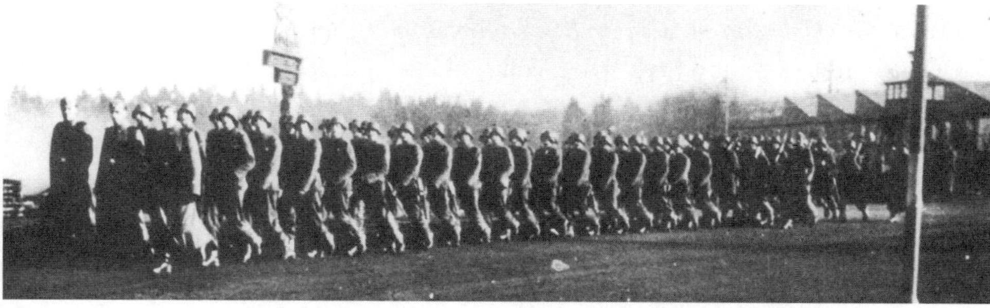

Guards marching to work, winter 1943-44. (Buchenwald Memorial)

OF COURSE, HUMAN beings are not cold, unfeeling automatons, and the Nazis' attempts to exorcize them of feelings of compassion and empathy were not always successful. Reflecting on the fact that German soldiers and citizens went on a furious rampage during *Kristallnacht*, John P. Sabini and Maury Silver wrote: "The German state annihilated approximately six million Jews. At the rate of 100 per day this would have required nearly 200 years. Mob violence rests on the wrong psychological basis, on violent emotion. People can be manipulated into fury, but fury cannot be maintained for 200 years. Emotions, and their biological basis, have a natural time course; lust, even blood lust, is eventually sated. Further, emotions are notoriously fickle, can be turned. A lynch mob is unreliable, it can sometimes be moved to sympathy—say by a child's suffering. To eradicate a 'race,' it is essential to kill the children."

The Nazis' brilliantly calculated answer, according to Sabini and Silver, was to replace the mob with a bureaucracy, rage contained within the structure of obedience to authority. If the leader of a country (such as Adolf Hitler) made it a national requirement for the preservation of nation and race to persecute and eventually establish a government-sanctioned program of extermination, then certain persons would be more likely to follow that path rather than resist or disobey; "I was only following orders," was the common refrain uttered by defendants at the many war-crimes trials in the wake of World War II.[6]

BECAUSE THERE IS little written by SS camp guards on their experiences, we must look elsewhere to get into the minds of the perpetrators. One such revealing source in which one finds participants' accounts is *"The Good Old Days:" The Holocaust as Seen by Its Perpetrators and Bystanders*, first published in German and edited by Ernst Klee, Volker Riess, and Willi Dressen.

To massacre in cold blood thousands of Jews, communists, Gypsies, and partisans in Poland (and later in the Soviet Union) after the front line of combat troops swept through, the German SS and Gestapo organized groups of *Einsatzkommando*—mobile killing squads made up of special police battalions supposedly psychologically hardened in order to perform such ghastly duties.

Kurt Möbius, a German policeman who had been involved in *Sonderaktion* (special action) mass murders in Poland noted, "...the orders to exterminate the Jews had been issued by Hitler and Himmler. We had been drilled in such a way that we viewed all orders issued by the head of state as lawful and correct. We police went by the phrase, 'Whatever serves the state is right, whatever harms the state is wrong.' I would also like to say that it never even entered my head that these orders could be wrong. Although I am aware that it is the duty of the police to protect the innocent, I was, however, at that time convinced that the Jewish people were not innocent but guilty."[7]

Karl Kretschmer, an *SS-Obersturmführer* (first lieutenant), wrote many letters to his wife and children in which he detailed some of the atrocities he was "forced" to witness or commit in Russia and how it affected him: "I am in a very gloomy mood [September 27, 1942]. I must pull myself out of it. The sight of the dead (including women and children) is not very cheering. But we are fighting this war for the survival or non-survival of our people." A few days later he wrote, "We have got to appear to be tough here or else we would lose the war. There is no room for pity of any kind." On October 15, he wrote, "I have already told you about the shooting—that I could not say 'no' here either.... But you can trust your Daddy. He thinks about you all the time and is not shooting immoderately." And, four days later, he noted, "We have to eat and drink well because of the nature of our work, as I have described to you in detail. Otherwise we would crack up.... It's not very pleasant stuff."[8]

An Austrian policeman, one of a group ordered to clean out a Byelorussian ghetto, was even more blunt in a letter to his wife: "So I joined the great slaughter the day before yesterday. With the first vehicles (which brought the victims), my hand shook at the moment of firing, but you get used to it. By the tenth, I was aiming calmly and shooting with a steady hand—women, children, and infants. I had in mind the fact that I also have two infants at home, and that this pack of wild animals would have acted in exactly the same way with them, maybe even ten times worse.... The infants flew through the sky in big arcs and we shot them in midair before they fell into the pit or in the water. We have to finish off these beasts that have dragged Europe into war." One can only wonder what his wife's reaction was to receiving such a letter.[9]

Not everyone succumbed to blood lust or followed orders blindly. It was commonly believed by members of the SS that they would be severely punished—perhaps even put to death if they did not torture or kill their victims—but such apparently was not always the case. A member of Third

Police Battalion 307 was ordered to kill civilians in Brest-Litovsk but refused. "Nothing happened to me as a result of my refusal," he said. "No disciplinary measures were taken."

Another *Einsatzkommando* policeman reported, "We could refuse to obey an order to participate in the *Sonderaktionen* without adverse consequences." Another policeman said he refused an order to kill Jews in Hrubieszow, Poland; he went to his superior, a man named Kozar, and said he would not comply: "I had no desire to shoot defenseless people. I had no wish to become a murderer.... I did not experience any disadvantage as a result of refusing to be involved in the shooting. Although I said to Kozar that he could send me to the front or anywhere else but that I would not shoot any defenseless Jews, there were no such consequences."[10]

IT IS AN interesting and revealing exercise to imagine oneself as an SS guard at a place like Buchenwald and wonder how someone could go from being an ordinary human being to someone who seemed to delight in the savage mistreatment of others. Many people will claim that they could never, under any circumstance, harm or torment another person. They are, no doubt, sincere in that belief. Yet, the question—*how close is the average person to being capable of committing the same sorts of crimes the Nazis committed?*—is one that must be answered in order to begin to understand Buchenwald, the Nazis, the concentration camps, and the Holocaust.

A groundbreaking experiment in obedience to authority was conducted in 1961 by Stanley Milgram, a professor of psychology at Yale University. Beginning just a year after the trial of ex-Nazi Adolf Eichmann in Israel had sparked considerable worldwide interest and debate, Milgram wanted to find out if the Nazis' defense in their war-crimes trials—"We were just following orders"—was a legitimate defense, or if something darker and deeper was at work. The results of the study were published in Milgram's 1974 book, *Obedience to Authority: An Experimental View.*

To carry out his experiment, Milgram told volunteer "subjects" that they could administer an electric shock whenever a "victim" gave an incorrect answer to a question. In fact, no victim was actually hooked up to the shock-generating device. Despite convincing screams of pain delivered by actors who were performing the role of victims, the subjects were told by the "person in authority" conducting the experiment to keep increasing the amount of voltage. Sixty-five percent of the volunteers obeyed the experimenter's orders to increase the voltage all the way up the realistic-but-fake shock generator's maximum setting of 450 volts.

On the basis of his experiment, Milgram concluded that many ordinary people were indeed willing to torture a protesting victim simply because someone in authority commanded them to do so—in spite of the fact that the victim had not done anything to warrant such punishment. (To absolve them of guilt and worry, the volunteers were told at the end of the experiment that no actual harm had come to the victims.)

As Milgram later concluded, "Stark authority was pitted against the subjects' strongest moral imperatives against hurting others, and, with the subjects' ears ringing with the screams of the victims, authority won more often than not. The extreme willingness of adults to go to almost any lengths on the command of an authority constitutes the chief finding of the study and the fact most urgently demanding explanation."[11]

THE STANFORD PSYCHOLOGY professor Dr. Philip G. Zimbardo would likely argue that everyone has a capacity for evil. Ten years after Milgram's study, Zimbardo conducted an experiment showing that research participants were often more than willing to obey authority figures, even when doing so violated their personal ethics.

Wanting to replicate the premise of Milgram's experiment in a different way, Zimbardo built a fake prison in the basement of the Stanford psychology building and recruited student volunteers, who were then randomly assigned to play the roles of either prison guards or inmates. The guards wore uniforms and carried nightsticks; Zimbardo himself played the role of the prison superintendent. The experiment was to last twenty-four hours a day for two weeks.

On the first day, nothing much happened but, on the second day, the prisoners staged a revolt and barricaded themselves in their cells. Perceiving the inmates as "dangerous," the guards cracked down hard on the rebels in order to establish who held the power. Said Zimbardo, "At first, guard abuses were retaliation for taunts and disobedience. Over time, the guards became ever more abusive, and some even delighted in sadistically tormenting their prisoners.

Though physical punishment was restricted, the guards on each shift were free to make up their own rules to demonstrate their dominance over their powerless charges."

The experiment was planned to continue for a full two weeks but lasted less than one when Zimbardo, caught up in the role-playing himself, unexpectedly terminated it. When he took his girlfriend to view the experiment, she became upset because of the abuses she saw taking place. Despite trying to calm her and reassure her that the experiment's setting was only artificial and of important scientific value, Zimbardo was persuaded that "human beings were suffering, not prisoners, not experimental subjects, not paid volunteers. And further, *I* was the one who was personally responsible for the horrors she had witnessed.... She also made it clear that if this person I had become—the heartless superintendent of the Stanford prison—was the real me, not the caring, generous person she had come to like, she wanted nothing more to do with me."

Jolted by the departure of his girlfriend, Zimbardo realized that he—and his experiment—had, indeed, gone over the edge, and that he was receiving some unexpected, visceral pleasure at being in power, at seeing others suffer. He terminated the experiment after only six days, then went into a long period of soul-searching, trying to find answers to the questions his brief test had created in his mind. In retrospect Zimbardo realized, "The situation won; humanity lost. Out the window went the moral upbringings of these young men, as well as their middle-class civility. Power ruled, and unrestrained power became an aphrodisiac. Power without surveillance by higher authorities was a poisoned chalice that transformed character in unpredictable directions. I believe that most of us tend to be fascinated with evil not because of its consequences but because evil is a demonstration of power and domination over others."[12]

Zimbardo, in effect—and Milgram, too—had created a concentration-camp atmosphere in microcosm, a place where those "in charge" were permitted, even encouraged, to go beyond the bounds of human decency and morality, to inflict pain and suffering on those without the ability to resist, to unquestioningly obey authority in the exercise of their duties.

Obviously, the environment in which both the Milgram and Zimbardo experiments were conducted was artificial. Unlike the concentration and death camp guards, none of those who performed the roles of persons in authority actually had unlimited power of life or death over their victims. Everyone involved in the psychological experiments knew their roles were of a short, temporary duration.

Not so the *SS-Totenkopfverband* camp guards who professed total obedience to the state and the Führer. They had had years of conditioning to regard Jews, communists, homosexuals, Gypsies, and others as undesirables and sub-humans, and a blot on the concept of Aryan supremacy in Germany. They had been "brain-washed" by books and lectures and films for a considerable period of time to believe that what they were doing—i.e., persecuting others—was for the national good, indeed, *essential* for Germany's survival and triumph.

The actual concentration-camp guards lived in a rarified atmosphere where human kindness was punished and hardness rewarded. Reacting without pity to suffering imposed upon others was the SS guard's expression of superiority. If an SS guard were seen to be "soft" toward prisoners, he feared that he would be demoted, transferred, dismissed from the service, or otherwise censured for his kind act. Heinrich Himmler recognized this "flaw" in the human character—the tendency in most people toward compassion—and the need for the SS to expunge it.

Speaking to an audience of Nazi officials and high-ranking SS officers in Posen, Poland, on October 4, 1943, after the mass extermination of the Jews was well underway, he said: "One basic principle must be the absolute rule for the SS men: We must be honest, decent, loyal and comradely to *members of our own blood* and to nobody else. What happens to a Russian, to a Czech, does not interest me in the slightest. What other nations can offer in the way of good blood of our type, we will *take*, if necessary, by *kidnapping their children and raising them here with us*. Whether nations live in prosperity or starve to death interests me only so far as we need them as slaves for our culture; otherwise, it is of no interest to me. Whether 10,000 Russian females fall down from exhaustion while digging an anti-tank ditch interests me only insofar as the anti-tank ditch for Germany is finished.

"I am now referring to the evacuation of the Jews, the extermination of the Jewish people. It's one of those things that is easily said: 'The Jewish people are being exterminated.' Says every Party member, 'this is very obvious, it's in our program, elimination of the Jews, extermination, we're doing it, hah, a small matter.' [....] But of all those who talk this way, none had observed it, none had endured it. Most of you here know what it means when 100 corpses lie next to each other, when 500 lie there or when 1,000 are lined up. To have endured this and at the same time to have remained a decent person—with exceptions due to human weaknesses—have made us tough. This is a page of glory never mentioned and never to be mentioned. [....] We have the moral right—we have the *duty* to our people to do it—to kill this people who wanted to kill us."[13]

There was also the matter of peer pressure and mob mentality; if everyone around you is doing something, even if violent or morally repugnant, it is difficult to resist the pressure to go along with the crowd. One of Himmler's biographers wrote, "Such was the empire of the camps: all who were sucked in, whether guards, doctors, or inmates, were caught up inevitably in the living nightmare and adapted and lived the parts ascribed and expected of them or went insane or died or were killed, or themselves killed. It was outside imagination, a nether world where primal, forbidden urges for blood, sacrifice and subjection were licensed and given free rein on non-persons; it was the inversion of love, the ultimate fantasy of the superman and the master race where 'sub-humans' were reduced to '*Musselmen*'* and '*Musselmen*' were dispatched 'to the chimney' and reduced to ashes."[14]

Former Buchenwald inmate Dr. Victor Dupont, however, gave the guards and doctors the slightest benefit of the doubt when he told the court during the Nürnberg International War-Crimes Tribunal, "The degree of uniformity in the way in which the camps were run is clear evidence of orders from higher headquarters. In the case of Buchenwald in particular, the personnel, no matter how rough it might be, would not have done such things on their own initiative. Moreover, the camp chief and the SS doctor himself always pleaded superior orders [from Himmler]."[15]

No matter whether Dr. Dupont's assessment was right or wrong, the fact is that the abuses continued and were becoming worse. But what did the world know about the camps? More importantly, what, if anything, was anyone going to do about them?

* In the jargon of the camps, a *Musselmann* was a person reduced to skin and bones, profoundly apathetic, totally indifferent to his surroundings, and exhibiting a complete lack of interpersonal response. It was usually the last stage before the inmate expired of "natural causes." (Dimsdale, p. 169)

5
WHAT THE WORLD KNEW

"We are in the presence of a crime without a name."

Winston S. Churchill
British Prime Minister

BEGINNING IN THE autumn of 1939, the Nazis operated a secret euthanasia program known as "T-4," the name deriving from the address of the program's Berlin headquarters, Tiergartenstrasse 4. Obsessed as he was about eliminating people who did not fit the strong, robust Aryan stereotype from his soon-to-be racially pure nation, Hitler authorized T-4 to rid Nazi Germany of mentally and physically disabled persons. It is estimated that between December 1939 and August 1941, some 50,000 to 60,000 German men, women, and children were put to death by lethal injection or carbon monoxide gassing.[1]

In October 1941, the Nazis threw the machinery of human destruction into high gear as preparations began that would convert an old mansion in the Polish city of Chelmno, some eighty miles west of Warsaw, into a place of mass murder. Chelmno's first commandant, Herbert Lange, was an old hand at the game, having gassed thousands of persons while he was head of the T-4 program. (Gassing operations at Chelmno, using carbon monoxide gas piped into trucks packed with Jews, began on December 8, 1941, and operated until March 1943. Chelmno then reopened in 1944 to liquidate Jews from the Łódź ghetto.)[2]

After invading Poland, Hitler set his sights on the West, invading and conquering Norway, Denmark, France, and the Low Countries with relative ease in the spring of 1940. Next, it was the Soviet Union's turn to be on the receiving end of *Blitzkrieg*. On June 22, 1941, after lulling Stalin to sleep with a non-aggression pact, Germany launched Operation Barbarossa—a three-million-man attack into the U.S.S.R. along a 1,800-mile front. Within a matter of weeks, the Germans had the Soviets reeling and a Nazi victory seemed imminent. The shock troops were followed by special killing squads known as *Einsatzgruppen* whose mission was to slaughter any Jews and partisans who might have survived the initial attack.[3]

With the Nazis stepping up their mass killings, it seems impossible that such an enterprise could have remained secret for long. And it wasn't. Yiddish dailies in New York in July 1941 first began reporting well-substantiated rumors that the Nazis had murdered hundreds of Jews in Minsk, Lvov, and other cities inside the Soviet Union. (In October, the *New York Times* would also report the massacre of up to 15,000 Jews in Galicia.)[4]

Lest anyone think that reports of atrocities were known only by Jewish communities, British Prime Minister Winston Churchill was outspoken about the fate of the Jews. On August 24, 1941, Churchill noted in a radio broadcast: "Whole districts [of the Soviet Union] are being exterminated. Scores of thousands—literally scores of thousands—of executions in cold blood are being perpetrated by the German police-troops upon the Russian patriots who defend their native soil. Since the Mongol invasions of Europe in the sixteenth century, there has never been methodical, merciless butchery on such a scale, or approaching such a scale. We are in the presence of a crime without a name." Furthermore, in a message to the *Jewish Chronicle* on November 14, 1941, he wrote: "None has suffered more cruelly than the Jew, the unspeakable evils wrought on the bodies and spirits of men by Hitler and his vile regime."[5]

Much of the information about the mass murders of the Jews came from the British being able to crack the Germans' secret "Enigma" code, but having this information suddenly put Churchill and the British in a difficult position; if they disclosed too many details, the Germans would know that their codes were being broken and their messages read. The Germans must have had some suspicions because, on September 28, 1941, Kurt Daluege, head of the *Ordnungspolizei*, issued instructions that field commanders were to make their reports by courier and not by radio.[6]

Nine days earlier, German troops had entered the ancient Ukranian city of Kiev on the Dnieper River—the Soviet Union's third-largest city. At first seen as liberators freeing them from Stalin's heavy-handed rule, the citizens of Kiev soon saw that their liberators were in fact worse than their previous oppressors, and began to fight back. Partisans made a series of bomb attacks against German offices in Kreshchatik Street, killing several Nazi officials. Believing that the bombings were the work of Jews, the Nazis launched a campaign of retaliation. On September 28, the Germans ordered the entire Jewish population of Kiev to report the next day with all their money and valuables to an appointed location at an appointed time; anyone failing to comply would be shot. Most of the Jews complied, believing—or at least hoping—that they were going to be resettled.

The following day, tens of thousands of Jews were marched to the northwest outskirts of Kiev and herded into a deep ravine—a ravine known as Babi

Yar. There, along the rim of the ravine, they were lined up and shot *en masse*, their bodies toppling into the chasm below. According to an *Einsatzgruppe* Operational Situation Report, 33,771 Jews were killed at Babi Yar in two days.

Not content with merely slaughtering Jews, the Nazis next rounded up Gypsies and also killed them at Babi Yar. In keeping with their policy of euthanizing those with mental infirmities, 700 patients of a local psychiatric hospital were gassed, their bodies dumped into the gash in the earth. Soviet prisoners-of-war, too, were brought to Babi Yar and shot; thousands of other Kiev civilians also lost their lives there. For months the mass grave at Babi Yar continued to fill up with corpses. It is estimated that 100,000 people were murdered or dumped there, turning the ravine of Babi Yar into a human landfill.[7]

AS 1941 CHANGED from fall into winter, Karl Otto Koch, who thought he was no longer under suspicion by the SS for corruption, received some good news. He was informed in November that he would be transferred in January 1942 to the sprawling Maidanek Concentration Camp near Lublin, Poland, where he would be responsible for enlarging the camp to accommodate up to 150,000 prisoners, mostly captured Soviet soldiers, but also Polish Jews. It was an assignment he relished; Ilse would stay behind with the children at Buchenwald until he received orders allowing her to join him. He could lead a bachelor's life until then.

Before leaving Buchenwald, though, Koch made the mistake of taking care of some unfinished business; he arranged to have two medical inmate-orderlies murdered. They had been involved in treating him for the syphilis that he had contracted while in Norway the previous year, and he wanted them silenced permanently. But the unauthorized killings waved a red flag in front of his immediate superior, Prince Josias Erbprinz Georg Wilhelm Adolf von Waldeck und Pyrmont, a general in the SS headquartered at Kassel. He and Koch had long had a contentious relationship, and Waldeck saw this matter as the perfect way of getting rid of him.

In late 1941, at the prince's urging, the SS opened a secret, formal investigation into the Kochs' financial dealings, with SS lawyer and judge Georg Konrad Morgen as the chief bloodhound. After some preliminary investigations that showed Koch had been skimming money from the prisoners' canteen, helping himself to funds that should have gone into camp improvements, and operating several black-market schemes in Weimar, Morgen was convinced of Koch's guilt and had him arrested on December 17. Koch was released after spending only one day in the Gestapo's Weimar prison, but he now knew that the SS was hot on his trail.[8]

TEN DAYS BEFORE Koch was arrested, however, the law of unintended consequences drastically altered the trajectory of world history. On December 7, 1941, forces of the Japanese Empire struck at U.S. naval and air force bases in Hawaii and the Philippines, thus guaranteeing America's entry into the war.

In a burst of misplaced optimism at Japan's attack, the Third Reich celebrated by brutalizing its political prisoners. At Buchenwald, for example, the inmates stood at attention on the freezing *Appellplatz* from 6:00 A.M. until 9:00 P.M. If any prisoner complained or fainted, he was strung up off the ground for hours by the hands.[9]

The surprise attack also postponed a secret meeting that had been scheduled for December 9, 1941, at a secluded, elegant villa located at No. 56-58 Am Großen Wannsee in the Berlin district of Wannsee. The meeting, whose purpose was to determine the most effective way of annihilating the eleven million Jews of Europe, was pushed back to January 20, 1942.[10]

On December 11, Germany and Italy, in solidarity with their Axis partner Japan, declared war on the United States, thereby effectively committing suicide. With the industrial might of the United States now fully on the side of Britain and the Soviet Union, the Axis stood little chance of victory.[11] But Hitler, not fully comprehending the situation, jubilantly declared, "Now it is impossible for us to lose the war.... We now have an ally [Japan] who has never been vanquished in three thousand years."[12]

The attack also emboldened Hitler to carry out his long-held dream—the "Final Solution" of what he termed "the Jewish problem." A few months earlier, he had made up his mind to proceed with the mass extermination of European Jewry, and authorized *Reichminister* Hermann Göring to move forward and turn the idea into reality. To be sure, tens of thousands of Jews and other "enemies of the state" had already been killed since 1933, but the efforts were haphazard, sporadic, disorganized, and inefficient. A better way must be found so that the murders could be carried out on a massive, unprecedented scale; it was up to his minions to devise a way to do it.

Göring in turn handed the job off to Reinhard Heydrich★, the sinister, ambitious head of the RSHA (*Reichsicherheitshauptamt*, or Reich Central Security Service, which was formed in 1939 when he combined the SD—*Sicherheitsdienst*, or Security Service, with the Security Police Administration, a plain-clothes police force). On January 20, 1942, a high-level meeting of Nazi bureaucrats and cabinet ministers took place. The conference, chaired by Heydrich, put together the mechanics of mass murder and authorized the establishment of the six major killing centers in Poland. Before long, trial runs that expanded upon Herbert Lange's mass killings at Chelmno were underway.[13]

AT SOME POINT in early 1942, a new administrator arrived to take command of Buchenwald: fifty-six-year-old *SS-Oberführer*★★ Hermann Franz Josef Pister. Determined at an early age to pursue a military career, Pister, born on February 21, 1885, in the north German port city of Lübeck, joined the Imperial German Navy in 1901 and served until the end of World War I.[14] After being mustered out in 1918, he started a new life, becoming an apprentice automobile mechanic at the age of thirty-three. This line of work soon led him into automobile sales, but the Great Depression and economic upheaval of the late 1920s and early 1930s was not conducive to the selling of cars.

Missing the military life and seeking financial stability, in 1931 Pister joined the Nazi Party, the SS (SS member number 29892), and was assigned, likely because of his automotive-sales background, to a unit known as the "SS Motor Echelon." Two years later he was assigned to SS Motor Regiment 19 and then, in 1936, to SS Motor Regiment 1. The next year he became a part of Himmler's SS motor pool.[15] On October 9, 1939, Pister embarked upon a new career within the SS—that of concentration camp commandant. He became the first head of *SS Sonderlager Hinzert* (Special Camp Hinzert), a relatively small

---

★ Heydrich himself would meet a violent end. On May 27, 1942, while holding the office of "Protector of Bohemia and Moravia" in Czechoslovakia, he was being chauffeured to his office in Prague's Hradcany Castle when his car was ambushed by Czech partisans; he died of his wounds on June 4. In a burst of typical Nazi retribution, the partisans were hunted down and killed, and two Czech villages—Lidice and Ležáky—were destroyed and all their inhabitants either killed outright or shipped off to concentration camps. (Dederichs, pp. 141-145; Gilbert, *The Second World War*, pp. 331-332)

★★ There is no equivalent U.S. Army or German Wehrmacht rank. *SS-Oberführer* was a field grade between colonel and brigadier general. The exact date that Pister arrived at Buchenwald is unclear. Although Stein (p. 41) says Pister became commandant on January 19, 1942, Pister himself, during an interrogation by a U.S. civilian investigator on March 4, 1947, said he was "appointed only on the 1st February [1942] and took over the camp only in the middle of April 1942."

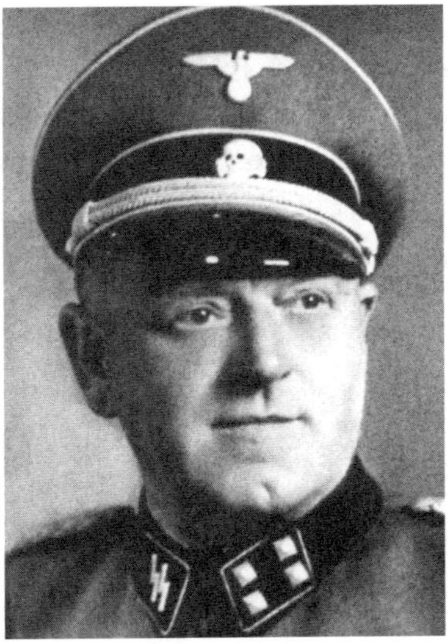

SS-Oberführer Hermann Pister, Koch's successor as commandant of KL Buchenwald (Buchenwald Memorial)

camp near Trier that originally was established as a police detention camp, then as a "re-training camp" for construction workers from *Organisation Todt* who had worked on the "West Wall" fortifications but had been caught drinking on the job or otherwise shirking work. After World War II broke out, the camp was turned into a concentration camp for deportees from German-occupied countries, especially Poland, Luxembourg, and the Netherlands; seventy Soviet POWs were also held (and murdered) there. The status of Hinzert was "upgraded" on July 1, 1940, when it was placed under the jurisdiction of the Inspector of Concentration Camps. During its six years of existence, a total of more than 13,000 persons were interned there; hundreds died from brutality

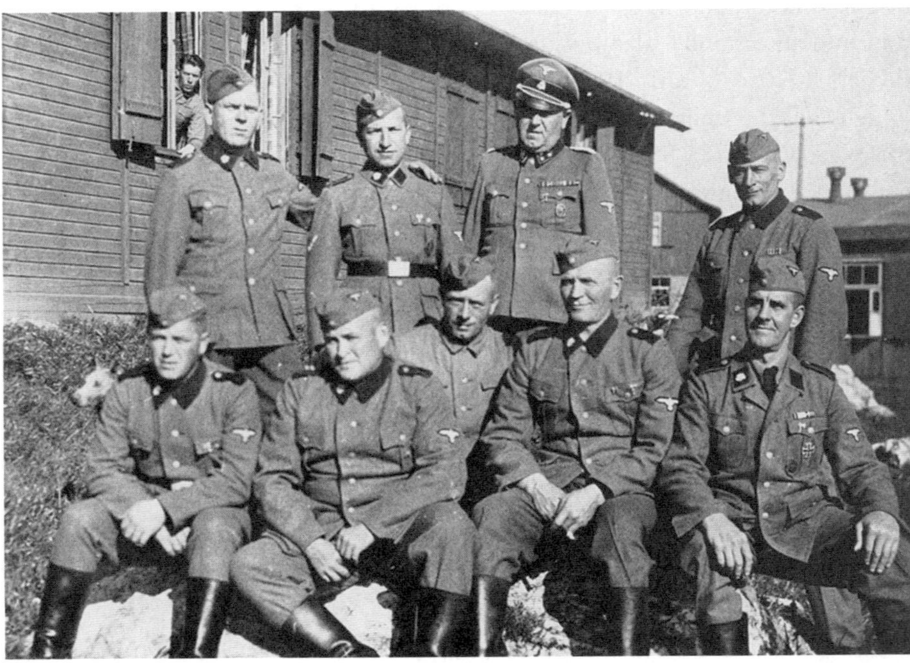

Hermann Pister (standing, second from right) and some of his staff photographed at Special Camp Hinzert (U.S. National Archives)

and lethal injections. In December 1941, Pister was notified that he would be transferred from Hinzert to Buchenwald to replace Koch and assume the duties of commandant.[16]

Although considered by some to be slightly less brutal than his predecessor, Pister was by no means a gentle soul. As a way of stamping his personal mark on the inmates after he arrived, Pister ordered that all inmates would fall out a half hour earlier than before to perform calisthenics—an order that was harmful to all inmates because of their general undernourishment, lack of strength, and the bitterly cold weather. The calisthenics program proved so detrimental that Pister was forced to cancel it after two months.

Other prisoners recalled that Pister, while making conditions in the camp slightly less onerous, still had a penchant for cruelty, beating inmates with a rubber hose, forcing inmates to work through the night, or siccing his dog on them.[17]

ON MARCH 1, 1942, New Yorkers started practicing blackout drills in order to hide the city from German submarines, which had been sinking U.S. ships along the coast from Maine to Florida. On that same day, an estimated 75,000 Christians and Jews showed up at New York's Madison Square Garden for what was billed as a "Stop Hitler Now" rally sponsored by Rabbi Stephen S. Wise's American Jewish Congress; given the Garden's 20,000-seat capacity, 55,000 persons were left to demonstrate outside. Inside, the speakers and crowd demanded that Germany halt the persecution and slaughter of the Jews. They were preaching to the choir; their demands fell on deaf ears.[18]

American and British newspapers, of course, had been running reports of Nazi atrocities and persecutions in Germany since 1933, but now the news took a more somber turn. In the March 1, 1942, *New York Times*, under the headline "Extinction Feared by Jews in Poland," Dr. Henry Shoskes, a prominent Jewish leader who had emigrated to the U.S. from Poland, told reporters that the Jews in the Polish ghettos were dying at a rate of 10,000 a month. Despite this alarming report, the Roosevelt Administration and the general American public did nothing.[19]

One of the major problems was that, other than issuing threats and ultimatums, almost nothing of substance could be done. The ghettoes and concentration camps were beyond the range of the Royal Air Force, and the U.S. Eighth Air Force was only in the early stages of setting up shop in England; it would take many months of construction, training, and assembling the aircraft, bombs, and other supplies before the American B-17s and B-24s could strike targets in Europe. And the possibility of a major invasion of the Continent was still two years off. The sad fact is, the Jews and others trapped in the ghettoes and concentration camps had absolutely no hope of redemption.

Why not open American shores to Jewish refugees? many asked, but this, too, was a non-starter. The U.S. State Department—especially Breckinridge Long—remained dead-set against the idea.

THE JEWISH POPULATION of Poland continued to be decimated. According to an article in the June 25, 1942, edition of London's *Daily Telegraph*, the Germans were planning to murder all the Jews in Poland. There were reports about the deteriorating conditions in the Warsaw ghetto, too; reports about murders committed in the eastern territories of Poland; reports about 50,000 Lithuanian Jews murdered in Vilna; and reports about the use of mobile gas chambers to kill Jews. Still, the Western powers, ever skeptical of such reports, sat on their hands.[20]

DESPITE THE SUMMER heat and humidity, Gerhardt Riegner, a German Jew and the secretary of the World Jewish Congress in Bern, Switzerland, broke out in a cold sweat. In his trembling hands the former lawyer, who had escaped from Germany in 1933, held a telegram dated July 30, 1942, from Eduard Schulte, a sympathetic German industrialist with ties to the Nazi hierarchy, that the plan to exterminate all the Jews of Europe was underway. The telegram read, in part: "In Fuehrer's headquarters plan discussed and under consideration that all Jews in countries occupied or controlled [by] Germany...should after deportation and concentration in east at one blow be exterminated."

Believing his source to be unimpeachable, Riegner, on August 8, 1942, met in Geneva with Howard Elting, Jr., the Vice-Counsel at the American Legation, to pass the information on to him. Perhaps, said Riegner, the Americans, who had not yet planted a single combat boot on German-controlled territory, could do something about the impending disaster. Elting was sympathetic but non-committal; the United States, which was still struggling to take the offensive in the

Pacific and had only recently commenced aerial bombing of Germany, could offer no material help. Riegner pressed on, asking Elting to at least alert Washington and London about the information he had received; Elting said he would. He sent a cable to the Secretary of State that outlined the concerns of a "previously generally reliable" source and noted the information referenced a Nazi plan "to exterminate at one blow this fall three-and-a-half to four million Jews following deportation from countries occupied."

A Legation official named Leland Harrison attached a note of skepticism: "Legation has no information which would tend to confirm this report which is however forwarded in accordance with Reigner's wishes.... The report has earmarks of war rumor inspired by fear and what is commonly understood to be the actual miserable condition of these refugees who face decimation as result [of] physical maltreatment persecution and scarcely endurable malnutrition and disease."

The U.S. State Department was not as convinced as Elting that Riegner's information was reliable, and dismissed it as just a "fantastic" war rumor. Nor did the State Department think the information important enough to pass along to Jewish leaders in America. However, in addition to contacting Elting, Riegner had also informed the British consulate, who cabled the information to the Foreign Office in London, where it was passed on to a member of Parliament, Samuel Sydney Silverman. On August 28, 1942, Silverman forwarded it to Rabbi Wise, president of both the American Jewish Congress and the World Jewish Congress.

Wise was in a dilemma. He desperately wanted to help the Jews of Europe but feared that by appearing to be too militant, he would only end up fueling anti-Semitism in America. Other, more outspoken Jewish leaders and activist groups in the U.S., such as the Bergson Group, had already done that with their forceful demands that the United States come to the rescue of European Jewry, and Wise worried that a backlash would hurt the cause. Slow and steady diplomacy that did not rock the boat was Wise's preferred method (he was opposed, for example, to the Bergson Group's "We Will Never Die" pageant, feeling it was too emotional and inflammatory). A personal friend of President Roosevelt, the rabbi often clashed with Breckinridge Long, Assistant Secretary of State and the main obstacle to immigration at the State Department.

Weary of locking horns with Long, Rabbi Wise, without realizing the State Department already had a copy of Riegner's cable, passed it on to Secretary of State Cordell Hull and Undersecretary of State Sumner Welles, asking that its contents be made public. Welles declined, saying that the Department would need to verify its accuracy—a process that took more than two months.[21]

It must be noted that the State Department's Division of Near Eastern Affairs was considered decidedly hostile toward anything that smacked of Zionism. One reason for this attitude was the very real worry that if the U.S. pressured Britain (which held the mandate over Palestine) to allow large numbers of European Jews to immigrate to Palestine, the Arab nations in the region might side with the fascists. Memories of the violent Arab uprising of 1936-1938, followed by the Grand Mufti of Jerusalem's collaboration with the Nazis, further inflamed these fears.*[22]

Another domestic concern was the fear of the impact that a sudden influx of thousands of refugees would have on America's high unemployment situation, still recovering from the Great Depression. Of course, in the first few months after Pearl Harbor, American industry, much of which had been idle since the crash of 1929, was gearing up to supply ships, aircraft, tanks, guns, ammunition, and other goods for the war effort; millions of workers would soon be needed and a state of nearly full employment would come to pass. The old canard that immigrants would take jobs away from "real Americans" would soon be proven hollow; the U.S. soon would have more jobs than people to fill them. Still, the State Department refused to hang out the "Welcome" sign.[23]

PERSONS LOCKED UP behind bars or barbed wire, whether they be common criminals, prisoners of war, or concentration-camp inmates, spend many of their waking hours plotting, scheming, and thinking about escape. The inmates of Buchenwald were no exception.

During the summer of 1942, in anticipation of the day when they might be able to revolt against their wardens, members of the Buchenwald camp underground began smuggling stolen weapons into the camp from the on-site DAW armaments factory and stashing them in secret hiding places. In some cases, they had complete weapons while, in others, they were able to manufacture weapons out of parts stolen from the factory. Weapons and ammunition was also purchased through bribing guards thought to be sympathetic to the prisoners. The inmates knew, of course, that if the weapons were ever discovered, it would mean instant death for them all.[24]

* The self-proclaimed Grand Mufti, Haj-Amin Al-Husseini, was the most powerful and influential leader of the Palestinians in the 1940s. Ardently anti-Zionist, he was also a great admirer of Hitler. (Lebel, passim)

KARL OTTO KOCH, now commandant of Maidanek, again found himself in hot water. In July 1942, under investigation by the SS for corruption while at Buchenwald, Koch was suspended as commandant of Maidanek. Koch was demoted to administrative posts in postal-service security units on the Eastern Front until he was arrested again the following month on charges of embezzlement, forgery, making threats to officials, and "other charges." After Koch's removal from Maidanek, crematoria were constructed at the camp, and there was an enormous increase in the number of prisoners killed. Like Auschwitz, Majdanek operated as a concentration, slave-labor, and extermination camp; gassing operations began there in October 1942.*[25]

Hermann Pister's Buchenwald, too, was becoming more important in the Nazi scheme of things, and was about to gain increased notoriety as a place where an almost unlimited supply of human guinea pigs existed for use in some of the Third Reich's most disturbing top-secret medical experiments.

IN SEPTEMBER 1942, Hitler decreed that Jews capable of working would have every ounce of productivity squeezed out of them by turning them into slave laborers who would be put to work in war-materials factories, building the network of highways, on defensive fortifications, and on other projects before they were killed.

It didn't take long for the armaments firm of Krupp AG, headquartered in Essen, to submit a request to Fritz Sauckel for over a thousand Jewish workers to be used for assembling artillery fuses at the firm's Auschwitz plant. (By war's end, Krupp would employ some 100,000 slave laborers at nearly a hundred factories in Germany and the occupied countries.)[26]

As an American attorney involved in the post-war Nuremberg War-Crimes Trials noted, Alfried Krupp's "exploitation of slave labor was worse than that of any other industrialist, including I.G. Farben. Nowhere was there such sadism,

---

* In November 1942, the first shipment of hundreds of thousands of Polish Jews arrived at Maidanek; it is estimated that during the camp's existence over 360,000 of the 500,000 persons who passed through the camp lost their lives, mostly from disease, starvation, and brutal treatment. (Gilbert, *The Holocaust*, pp. 498-499) A year later, the deliberate murders were stepped up and most of the Jewish prisoners—some 42,000 of them—were massacred by the Nazis, 18,000 of them in a single day. The camp and the nearby city of Lublin would be liberated by the Soviets on July 24, 1944—the first killing center captured by an Allied army. (*Historical Atlas of the Holocaust*, pp. 100-102)

such senseless barbarity, such shocking treatment of people as dehumanized material."[27]

The SS was more than happy to oblige German industry's requests, for its coffers were growing full from the fees that it charged companies for the use of inmates.*

During the whole of the war, it is estimated that between a half-million to one million concentration-camp prisoners were rented out to German industry. For most of the slave laborers, though, the conditions in the factories were barely better than the conditions in the camps. And, as Allied bombers targeted the German war plants, the slave workers were put in harm's way.[28]

With the need to extract every bit of productivity from the slaves working for German industry, the brutal conditions in the camps in 1942 were somewhat ameliorated. William Manchester noted that, although the Nazis' view of sub-humans remained unaltered, "Germany's requirements for mass labor were so urgent that even the most fanatical members of the hierarchy recognized the need for some restraint. A contented slave, they realized, was a competent slave. Excesses were thus condemned, not because they were unconscionable but because they were inefficient."

Goebbels, it was said, believed that only if a slave received sufficient food could he or she do a proper day's work. Albert Speer, Germany's Minister of Armaments, also argued that all slave laborers be adequately housed and fed "on the grounds that the alternative was hopeless inefficiency." Even Fritz Sauckel, in charge of the slave-worker program, begged his superiors to give the slaves at least enough food, medical care, and decent living conditions to allow them to be more productive. "Slaves who are underfed, diseased, resentful, despairing, and filled with hate," he insisted, "will never yield that maximum of output which they might achieve under normal conditions."[29] If any conditions changed for the better, however, they went unnoticed.

As the war continued, the civilian populace of Germany also suffered; besides the daily and nightly Allied air raids, the average German urban dweller was also required to go on a restricted diet, receiving an average of slightly more than a thousand calories per day—which was still two or three times more than what the average Buchenwald prisoner received.[30]

---

* At the war-crimes trial of Oswald Pohl, the prosecutor noted, "Each SS industry put aside an amount ranging from 30 pfennigs to 5 Reichsmarks per day, ostensibly to be used as prisoner's wages. However, it was never even considered that the inmate should receive any part of the sum. 'Legally' such 'wages' belonged to the Reich treasury. Various schemes, however, were utilized by [Pohl's staff] to enable the WVHA illegally to retain a substantial part of the funds." (Pohl trial transcript, found at avalon.yale.edu)

THE FATE OF Polish Jews was growing more ominous by the day. In the August 10, 1942, issue of *Newsweek*, for example, it was reported that trainloads of Warsaw Jews were vanishing into a "black limbo."[31]

But Polish Jews weren't the only ones vanishing. The Jews of occupied France were also disappearing. On August 20, 1942, the *New York Times* quoted the previous day's edition of the French paper, *Paris Soir*, which stated that French Jews were being deported to "Polish Silesia."[32] As one example of the round-up of French Jews, at nine-thirty in the evening of Wednesday, September 23, 1942, the Gestapo and members of the French police burst into an apartment building at 10 Rue des Deux Ponts, on the Ile St. Louis in Paris. On each floor, up and down the halls, the intruders banged on doors and ordered the Jewish residents to gather their belongings and get on the buses that were waiting for them downstairs. Eventually they would round up 112 inhabitants from that apartment building, forty of them children.

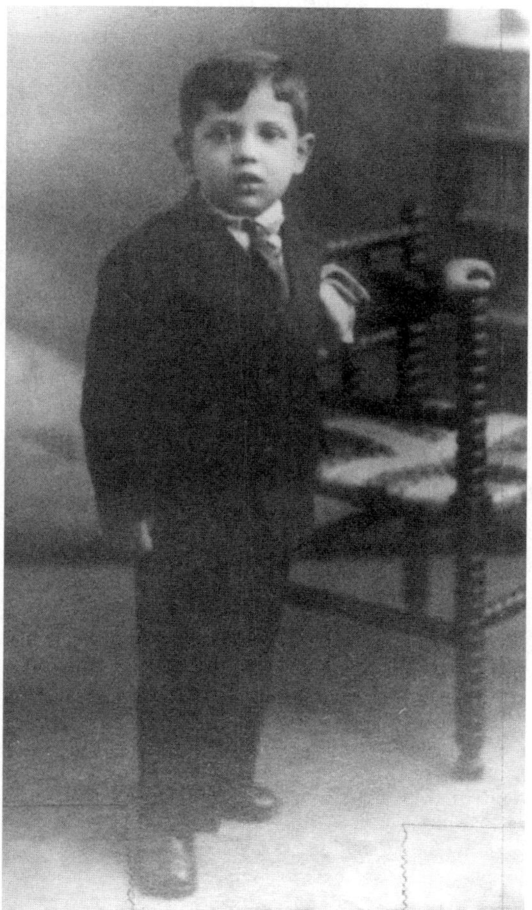

Robert Max Widerman (later to be known as Robert Clary), photographed at age four and a half in Paris, 1930 (Courtesy Robert Clary)

One of the families was that of Moishe Widerman, his wife Baila, their five daughters—Ida, Aimée, Hélene, Cécile, Madeleine—and the youngest child, a son named Robert Max Widerman. A large extended family lived nearby. The Widermans were neither rich nor poor—"middle class" is probably the most apt description. They had a spacious apartment in one of Paris's loveliest neighborhoods, and plenty of food to eat. Moise was an Orthodox Jew and a tailor. The family was law-abiding. There was no reason for them to be arrested, but the Gestapo needed no reasons.

Robert, a natural "ham," precocious singer, dancer, artist, and entertainer, had known nothing but love and support from friends and family; a new reality now intruded upon that innocent childhood. Robert was a teenager—seventeen—and the raid was the most terrifying thing he had yet experienced.

Frightened, the Widermans and other Jewish families in the building promptly complied with Gestapo and police demands. Fresh in their memories was the night of July 16-17, 1942, just two months earlier, when nearly 14,000 Paris Jews were evicted from their homes and apartments, herded onto buses, and taken first to the Velodrome d'Hiver, a bicycle-racing stadium where they were held in horrendous conditions. As rumor had it, the children and parents had been separated, and the parents then transported to Poland—a place called Auschwitz—where they were gassed and their bodies cremated. Five days later, the terrified children were transferred to either Drancy, Beaune-la-Rolande, or Pithiviers, where they remained for weeks behind barbed wire, brutalized and starved, before following in their parents' footsteps into the gas chambers of Auschwitz.*

But who could believe such fantastic tales? Why would the Germans starve men, women, and children? Gas chambers? Mass killings? Impossible! It was only a rumor, a preposterous fable dreamed up by someone with a perverse nature, said the Jews to each other, hoping against hope.

But the rumors, as the world now knows, turned out to be true.

In all the chaos on that September day, Robert Widerman's sister Madeleine managed to find a hiding place in the apartment building, but Robert, his mother, uncle Yankef, sister Ida, her husband Jacques, and two young cousins, Bernard and Edmond, were caught in the Gestapo dragnet, put on the buses, and taken to Drancy. Robert later said, "I didn't know that people were transferred out of Drancy to slave labor and concentration or extermination camps. Nobody was told, nor could they have imagined, that they were going to be put into gas chambers. So we went like cattle to the slaughterhouse."

After a short but frightening night of screaming, crying, and terror, Robert and his relatives and nearly a thousand others at Drancy were bused to a Paris rail siding and packed into filthy cattle cars. Into each car were thrown scraps of food and two buckets to serve as toilets for a hundred people. The train began to move

* Drancy was a "transit camp" established in 1940 by the collaborationist Vichy government of Phillippe Pètain and run by the French police. Its purpose was to serve as a collecting point for Jews who would then be sent on to the concentration camps inside Germany and extermination camps inside Poland. From 1941 to August 1944, more than 140,000 French Jews were sent from Drancy to various Nazi camps, primarily Auschwitz. In July 1943, control of the prison was taken over by the infamous Alois Brunner, Adolf Eichmann's assistant. Thousands of Jews died in Drancy and its satellite camps—Noe, Gurs, and Recebedou. Fifteen hundred inmates were still in Drancy when it was liberated by Allied troops on August 17, 1944. (*Historical Atlas of Holocaust*, pp. 106-110)

eastward. Those crammed into the cars had no idea where they were going, how long the trip would take, or what would happen to them once they arrived.

After three days and nights, the train stopped in Kosel (also spelled Kozle), a small town in Upper Silesia, near where Germany, Poland, and Czechoslovakia come together. The doors to the fetid cattle cars were opened by armed SS soldiers with barking, vicious dogs straining at their leashes, and all the males aged sixteen to fifty were ordered out. Those who didn't move fast enough were met by a rain of blows from rifle butts. The elderly men, women, and young children—including Robert's mother and relatives—were left in the cars, and the doors slammed shut again and locked. Robert's mother's final, unforgettable words to him were, "Do whatever they tell you to do. Don't fight it." The train's whistle mingled with a chorus of wails coming from the cattle cars as it slowly pulled away down the tracks. Those on board were heading toward extermination at Auschwitz.

Robert found himself with 174 others, all trembling with fright, on the station platform. *What will happen to my family?* he wondered. *What will happen to me?* After the train was out of sight, the group was roughly herded by uniformed men with rifles and snarling guard dogs into open trucks and continued their journey into hell. Along the way, while the convoy passed through towns and villages, children stood along the curbs and hurled rocks at the prisoners, yelling "Dirty Jews! Dirty Jew bastards!"

The SS guards just laughed.

The convoy continued on to Ottmuth, a small (four barracks), transient slave-labor camp in Poland. There the prisoners were guarded not by SS but by ordinary Wehrmacht soldiers—older men, or those who had been wounded in battle and were unfit for front-line service; the soldiers did not harass the prisoners too badly, and life was tolerable, even if barely.

Robert Max Widerman remained at Ottmuth working as a shoemaker for nineteen months. Fortunately, his small stature, his sense of humor, and his ability to sing, dance, and entertain made him a favorite of the *Kapos* and *Blockältestern*, and so they watched out for him and made sure that he was not treated roughly or shipped off to some extermination camp. Despite his sense that he was being cared for, Robert Max Widerman was frightened and hungry, never sure that his "privileged" status would not be stripped away from him.

Like millions of other European Jews at that time, he had no idea what had happened to the rest of his family, nor what fate awaited him. What had he done to make the entire nation of Germany so angry at him? He had not yet heard of a camp called Buchenwald, nor realized that he would soon end up there. All he knew was that he was frightened and trembling.[33]

WHILE THE U.S. State Department dithered, stalled, and did its best to avoid doing anything to aid the Jews of Europe, the Nazi plan for their extermination roared ahead at full speed.

During September 1942, while Jews were being rounded up across Europe in ever-increasing numbers and shipped off to their deaths, the confident German army was surrounding Stalingrad, a vital Soviet industrial city on the Volga. General Friedrich von Paulus was certain that his 600,000-man Sixth Army would soon take the city and then head for Moscow. His confidence was misplaced; the Battle of Stalingrad, which would last nearly eight months and cost a million and a half lives, was the bloodiest single battle in history.[34]

Meanwhile in the skies over Germany, American and British bombers, in an unprecedented aerial offensive that would only grow stronger over the next two years, were laying waste to German cities and armament plants.

THE AUTUMN OF 1942 brought more grim news of the slaughter taking place in Poland. In September and October, reports from Nazi-controlled countries continued to pile up on the desk of Secretary of the World Jewish Congress Gerhardt Riegner, convincing him beyond all doubt that the Germans were wiping out the Jews as quickly as possible. For example, on October 5, 1942, the Jewish Telegraphic Agency reported on the systematic deportation of Jews from Lódz, whom, the agency said, were being killed by poison gas. In its November issue, the New York magazine *Jewish Frontier* reported about the murder of Jews in Chelmno in mobile gas vans.

Like a man running to flag down a busload of passengers that was headed full speed for a cliff, Riegner forwarded each of these reports to the U.S. Legation in Bern in hopes that the United States would somehow be shaken out of its bureaucratic inertia and act on them. But pushing against Washington's malaise was an exercise in futility; not until November 1942, after four sworn statements had reached the State Department that fully substantiated Riegner's reports, was the truth finally accepted. Rabbi Wise and a delegation representing the New York Jewish community were asked to come to the State Department and meet with Undersecretary Sumner Welles. Welles began the meeting grimly: "Gentlemen, I hold in my hands documents which have come to me from our legation in Bern. I regret to tell you, Dr. Wise, that these confirm and justify your deepest fears."

Wise noted in his autobiography, "He handed me the original documents from Berne [sic] which confirmed our dreadful apprehensions. The documents' red seals suggested the blood of my people pouring forth in rivers. Mr. Welles added, 'For reasons you will understand, I cannot give these to the press, but there is no reason why you should not. It might even help if you did.'"[35]

IT IS OBVIOUS that President Franklin D. Roosevelt was aware of the wholesale slaughter that was taking place within the Third Reich. On October 7, 1942, he stated, "It is our intention that just and sure punishment shall be meted out to the ringleaders responsible for the organized murder of thousands of innocent persons in the commission of atrocities which have violated every tenet of the Christian faith."[36] The innocent persons wondered when, if ever, that would happen.

ON OCTOBER 17, 1942, an order was issued that directed all Jewish prisoners being held in the Reich, with the exception of 204 workers deemed "essential," be sent to the death camps in Poland for extermination.[37] This order included some 10,000 Jews at Buchenwald. They were transported to Auschwitz and gassed. Joining them in death were 7,000 from Sachsenhausen, and 5,000 more from camps in Holland. In the month of October, another 49,000 Jews were killed at Belzec, 11,000 at Sobibór, and more than 100,000 at Treblinka. Poland had been turned into a charnel house.[38]

FINALLY, THE UNITED States was about to take the first step on the long, hard road that would ultimately lead to the crushing of the Axis powers. On November 8, 1942, 180,000 American soldiers under the command of General

Dwight D. Eisenhower began wading ashore at three widely scattered beachheads along the coast of North Africa. Operation Torch, as the invasion was code-named, was the beginning of the end for Vichy France, Fascist Italy, and Nazi Germany.[39] It would take two-and-a-half more years, but the demise of the Third Reich had finally begun—a demise that would not come soon enough for millions of innocents, however. The gas chambers were working overtime, trying to kill as many Jews, Sinti, Roma, homosexuals, and Jehovah's Witnesses as possible. Crematoria burned night and day, but the mountains of corpses continued to grow at a far faster rate than the ovens could dispose of.

UNABLE TO HOLD back the terrible news any longer, on November 24, 1942, Rabbi Stephen Wise called a press conference in New York City to announce that the Nazis were deporting Jews from German-occupied territory to Poland for mass slaughter. He told reporters that he had learned from his sources overseas that half of the four million Jews in the Nazi-occupied areas of Europe had already been murdered. Although most newspaper editors, perhaps weary of years of persecution stories, buried the news deep inside their editions, it was the first time that the American general public became aware of the scope of the genocide being perpetrated by the Nazi regime.[40]

On December 8, after weeks of trying to get Roosevelt to meet with him, Wise, with a delegation of other Jewish leaders, finally was able to present to the president a twenty-page document ("Blueprint for Extermination") and discuss with him ideas on how to combat the genocide. Donald McKale wrote that Wise and the delegation "urged [FDR] to publicize the German killing of Jews to the world and attempt to stop it. Although the reports from Europe concerned the President and rekindled his prewar interest in finding havens outside Europe for Jewish refugees, his remarks on the subject to Jewish leaders, including Morgenthau, never seemed very realistic or reassuring."

Except for urging Roosevelt to condemn Germany's actions in the strongest terms, Wise's delegation had few concrete suggestions; Roosevelt invited them to return when they did. If nothing else, the President felt that the United Nations, at that time a group of eleven Allied governments at war with the Axis, could come out with a strong statement of condemnation. On December 17, 1942, Anthony Eden, the British Foreign Secretary, delivered a joint Allied statement that called the world's attention to "Hitler's oft-repeated intention to exterminate the Jewish people of Europe" and promised that "those responsible for these crimes shall not escape retribution."[41]

In the meantime, the prisoners at Buchenwald were about to become part of two new Nazi schemes to use their services to the maximum before being discarded on the ash heap growing outside the crematorium—as slave laborers to help keep the German war machine running and as human guinea pigs in terrible "scientific" experiments run by Nazi doctors.

6
THE DEVIL'S DOCTORS

"I must tread with care in matters of life and death. . . .
Above all, I must not play at God."

Hippocratic Oath

FEW CHAPTERS IN the short, violent history of the Third Reich are as repugnant as the one about the Nazi doctors and the crimes against humanity they committed. Life at Buchenwald was terrible enough, what with the back-breaking work in the quarry, the filth and disease, the starvation rations, the callousness, and the never-ending physical and mental torture. To all this was added a new and even more horrendous component: the use of inmates as human guinea pigs for scientific and pseudo-scientific experiments.

To be sure, some of the experiments had a true and worthwhile scientific goal—the discovery of cures or antidotes of diseases such as typhus, for example. But many were conducted in a scientifically slip-shod manner. Others were merely sadistic exercises with no value whatsoever other than to satisfy some ghastly desires of the experimenters. And there was absolutely no justification—medical, legal, moral, ethical, or otherwise—for using live, involuntary human subjects as lab rats.

AT THE END of 1941, the Nazis had instituted a new and more sinister program designed to replace the discontinued T-4 euthanasia program—a program known as "Special Treatment 14f13." Not surprisingly, KL Buchenwald was destined to play a major role in it.

In his opening remarks during the post-war tribunal of perpetrators of the "14f13" euthanasia program, the prosecutor stated, "This case is concerned with the euthanasia program because thousands of prisoners of all nationalities were transported from the concentration camps to euthanasia stations and murdered there. It is also true that camp doctors systematically killed inmates who were no longer able to work under the pretense that they were insane. These killings were usually accomplished by injections of phenol [carbolic acid] or gasoline. The executions were carried out under the code name '14f13,' which apparently was derived from a file number in *Amtsgruppe D* of the WVHA. That office played an essential role in the operation of the program."

Hermann Pister would introduce many new concepts of cruelty, but is perhaps best remembered as the man who was in charge of Buchenwald when it became a major center of the Nazis' conduct of medical experiments on prisoners against their will. Pister had just reported for duty at Buchenwald when he was made aware of "14f13," details of which were contained in a December 10, 1941, letter from the Inspectorate of Concentration Camps, Theodor Eicke. Also receiving the letters were the commandants of Auschwitz, Dachau, Flossenbürg, Groß-Rosen, Mauthausen, Neuengamme, Niederhagen (near the SS castle at Paderborn), and Sachsenhausen. The commandants were informed that, in the near future, a special "doctors' commission" would visit the camps to select prisoners for "Special Treatment 14f13."

On December 15, 1941, the process began at Groß-Rosen, the Sachsenhausen sub-camp located about thirty miles southwest of Wroclaw, Poland. The camp doctors there had selected 293 inmates as eligible for the *Sonderbehandlung* (Special Treatment) *14f13* program and wanted them seen by the doctors' commission. These unfortunate people were classified under such headings as "Poles or Czechs in Protective Custody," "Shirkers," "Jews in Protective Custody," "Jews who were Habitual Criminals," "Jews who were Shirkers," and "Jews who Defiled the Race." (A "Jew who defiled the race" was any Jew who had married or had sexual intercourse with an Aryan.)

This list was sent to Eicke, who informed the Groß-Rosen commandant to expect a visit on January 16, 1942, from Dr. Friedrich Mennecke, one of the so-called experts in the euthanasia program and head of the state mental hospital at Eichberg; Mennecke would then make the final selection. Of the 293 Groß-Rosen inmates listed as eligible, 214—Jews and non-Jews alike—were selected by Mennecke for extermination. One hundred and twenty-seven of those prisoners were then sent to the Bernburg euthanasia station on the Saale River near Dessau and killed. Thirty-six died before the transport left Groß-Rosen and, of the remainder, forty-two were not sent because, as a result of a month-long rest, they were again able to resume work.

Buchenwald was the next to be visited by the doctors' commission. In February 1942, after inspecting a group of inmates at the Ettersberg, a "14f13" euthanasia transport, which consisted of hundreds of mentally ill German inmates, left Buchenwald for Auschwitz, where the victims were gassed.

It was clear that the euthanasia program had not stopped; it merely had acquired a different name.[1]

THE NAZIS PERVERTED everything they touched. Even the sacrosanct medical profession was not immune from their evil deeds. In fact, the annals of Nazi medicine are filled with tales of such terrible experiments as to make B-grade horror films seem tame by comparison. But how did members of the medical profession become such tools of the Nazi regime? One answer may be found in an article in the *Annals of Internal Medicine.*

Drs. Andre N. Sofair and Lauris C. Kaldjian wrote: "Soon after rising to power in 1933, Hitler asked the German medical profession to address the 'race question.' He took control of its professional organizations, restructured the medical schools and the Public Health Department (purging them of non-Aryans), and centralized the insurance and payment systems. Many physicians were attracted to Nazi ideology, and the medical profession had one of the highest rates of party membership of any profession.

"By 1936, 31% of Berlin's non-Jewish physicians had joined the Nazi party, and rates of party membership were similar elsewhere in Germany. Financial incentives encouraged physicians to support the Nazi government. From 1927 to 1932, physicians' average annual income had fallen by 27%, and many were unemployed. The inability of the preceding Weimar government to address this problem was countered by Nazi promises to restore the lost status of physicians.

"By 1935, physicians' average taxable income had increased by 25%. Physicians were also induced to join the Nazi party because a spotless Nazi record was required for a government-sponsored practice. Academic appointments and salary support in German medical schools depended on loyalty to the Nazi party, and Nazis of dubious professional attainment were appointed as rectors and deans. Instruction in eugenics became compulsory for medical students, and by 1935, students were required to wear Nazi uniforms and undergo Nazi indoctrination. Nazi medical propaganda was also directed at practicing physicians."[2]

Caught between the proverbial rock and a hard place, it is perhaps understandable that many doctors joined the Nazi Party—and why so many became the handmaidens of Hitler's twisted philosophy. Taking part in the mandated medical experiments ensured that the doctors—even those who had no fanatical devotion to Nazi ideology—would enjoy a booming practice, a decent income, and respectability within the medical community. The physician's sacred oath contains the phrase, "I must not play at God," yet this foundation of the Hippocratic Oath was violated time and again by the Nazi doctors, whose oath to the Party trumped all other considerations and allegiances.

MANY HISTORIANS BELIEVE that the genesis for the Nazis' medical experiments sprang from their intense interest in the concept of Aryan "racial purity," and that by experimenting on human beings they hoped to unlock the secrets of genetic engineering. "Racial purity" was a subject that had long obsessed Hitler. He often wrote and spoke of it, especially how the mixing of Aryan and Jewish blood would eventually "mongrelize" and thereby destroy the pure German race that he regarded as superior to all others.

To prevent this from happening, laws were passed (i.e., the Nürnberg Laws, or *Nürnberger Gesetze*, of 1935) that restricted Jews from marrying and/or having sexual relations with supposedly "pure Aryan" women and thus producing genetically mixed offspring. A second law, the so-called "Reich Law of Citizenship" (*Reichsbürgergesetz*) made the distinction that only those Germans of pure blood would be considered citizens of the state, while Jews and other non-Aryans would merely be "subjects."[3]

Hitler appointed a crony, the Estonia-born Alfred Ernst Rosenberg, who had joined the Party in 1919 (and whom William R. Shirer described in *The Rise and Fall of the Third Reich* as "dim-witted," "dull," "stupid," "mediocre," and a "muddled pseudo philosopher"), to be the Nazi Party's chief intellectual and racial theorist. Basing his views on the anti-Semitic rantings of the Protestant leader Martin Luther (1483-1546); the French Aryan master-race theorist Joseph Arthur Comte de Gobineau (1816-1882); the German composer Richard Wagner (1813-1883); Houston Stewart Chamberlain (1855-1927)—a British racial theorist and husband of Wagner's step-daughter; and the American eugenicist Madison Grant (1865-1937), among others, Rosenberg lent a kind of intellectual credibility for Nazi Germany's oft-stated belief that only pure-blood Aryans (which included Nordic Scandinavians) were the true "master race" destined to rule the "inferior races," such as Jews, Slavs, Czechs, Poles, blacks, etc.[4]

In an effort to determine the best way to slow down or stop the breeding of these "undesirable" populations, concentration-camp inmates were often used to test various methods of sterilization, usually with painful, deadly results. To determine if millions of people could be sterilized quickly and easily, doctors at

Auschwitz, Ravensbrück, and elsewhere experimented on both male and female inmates. They exposed the genitals of men to high doses of radiation, then castrated them to study the resulting changes in their testes. Women had various types of caustic substances forced into their cervixes or uteri, which caused horrible pain, bleeding, and bursting spasms in the stomach. Thousands who were sterilized and survived underwent untold mental and physical anguish for the rest of their lives.[5]

The gynecological anatomist Professor Dr. Hermann Stieve of the University of Berlin and the Berlin Charity Hospital used female prisoners for his studies on the effect of mental stress—the women's own impending executions—on the menstrual cycle. Before a woman of reproductive age was to be executed by the Gestapo, Dr. Stieve was informed and he thus told her when she was scheduled to die. Stieve would then monitor the effects of the psychic trauma on the doomed woman's menstrual pattern. After the victim was murdered, Stieve had their pelvic organs removed for study.[6]

Just as the Nazis sought ways to stop the "undesirable" races from breeding, so too did they also try to increase the number of Aryan births to populate the "New Germany." After hearing that Auschwitz physician Dr. Carl Clauberg injected hundreds of women with various solutions to see if any of the chemicals would prevent pregnancy and, learning that Clauberg had successfully treated an SS officer's infertile wife, Himmler ordered Clauberg to conduct artificial insemination experiments on inmates. Some 300 women at Auschwitz subsequently underwent artificial insemination at the hands of Clauberg, who reportedly tormented victims strapped down on tables by informing them that he had just inseminated them with animal sperm and that monsters were now growing in their wombs. Many of them went mad before they were killed.[7]

The vast number of other experiments were apparently carried out simply for the sadistic pleasure of the experimenters watching helpless persons suffering and dying in horrible pain. And there seemed to be no shortage of experiments conceived by twisted minds to which unwilling inmates* were subjected: typhus (spotted fever); malaria; yellow fever; smallpox; typhoid; paratyphoid A and B; cholera; diphtheria; mustard gas; tetanus; jaundice; gas gangrene; streptococcus; nerve, bone, and muscle transplants; poison; sea water; high-altitude; freezing; incendiary phosphorous; and more.[8]

* At their war-crimes trials after the war, a number of the defendants declared that many of their subjects in the experiments had volunteered, usually after they were told that they would receive more and better rations, time off from their brutal work details, and possible reduction of their sentences. But, because dead men tell no tales, it is impossible to verify the truth of these statements. (www. mazal.org/archive/nmt)

THE MAJOR CONCENTRATION camps that were selected to be the venues for these horrendous experiments included Auschwitz, Bergen-Belsen, Dachau, Natzweiler, Treblinka, Ravensbrück, Sachsenhausen, and Buchenwald. Chosen—or volunteering—to conduct the experiments were some of Germany's leading scientists and doctors from Germany's major hospitals, clinics, institutes, and universities. These individuals included Dr. Karl Brandt, Hitler's personal physician; Lieutenant General Dr. Siegfried Handloser, Chief of the Wehrmacht (Army) Medical Services; Dr. Oskar Schroeder, Chief of the Luftwaffe (Air Force) Medical Services; Dr. Paul Rostock, Chief Surgeon of the Berlin Surgical Clinic; Dr. Karl Gebhardt, president of the German Red Cross; Dr. Josef Mengele, the so-called "Angel of Death" at Auschwitz; and hundreds more.

There were, of course, even more horrendous experiments that had little or no scientific value being carried out by doctors at other camps. At Auschwitz, for example, Mengele, apparently for his own twisted desires, carried out experiments on twins and dwarfs, and had Gypsy inmates killed and their eyes removed for further study.[9]

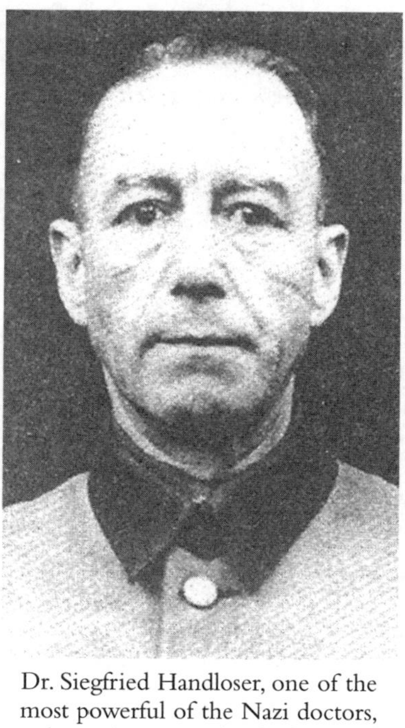

Dr. Siegfried Handloser, one of the most powerful of the Nazi doctors, shown in a mug shot before his 1946 war-crimes trial (U.S. National Archives)

Buchenwald's Block 46 (also known as the "isolation ward" and surrounded by double rows of barbed wire) became the infamous main laboratory for several of the experiments, such as finding a vaccine for typhus, judging the effectiveness of poisons, or determining what medications best treated serious burns. Plying their gruesome trade at Buchenwald were Drs. Handloser (chief doctor for awhile at Buchenwald), Gerhard Schiedlausky, Joachim Mrugowsky, Waldemar Hoven, Erich Wagner, Werner Greunuß, Erwin Ding-Schuler, Gerhard Rose, Hans Eisele, and others whose names were Blies, Ellenbeck, Horn, Rogge, and Neumann—men whose crimes have been lost to history.[10]

IN *THE NAZI Doctors*, author Robert Lifton noted that "The SS doctors assigned to the early concentration camps tended to be medically undistinguished, strong in their Nazi ties, and personally self-aggrandizing."[11]

Other than Karl Brandt, the Reich Commissioner for Health and Medical Services, no doctor in the Third Reich wielded more power than Siegfried Handloser, a fervent Nazi. On July 28, 1942, Handloser was promoted to *Generaloberstabsarzt* (lieutenant general, staff doctor) and appointed by Hitler to hold the twin positions of the German army's medical inspector and the chief medical officer of the field forces. In this exalted position, he did not personally conduct experiments on unwilling subjects but directed others to carry them out.

After the war, Handloser was charged by a war-crimes tribunal with authorizing twelve different experiments involving typhus, poison gas, high-altitude, freezing, malaria, sea water, epidemic jaundice/hepatitis, and bone, muscle, and nerve regeneration and transplantation, as well as participating in biological warfare and gas edema experiments.

As the prosecution at his 1947 war-crimes trial noted, "[Handloser] never used his tremendous power as Chief of the Medical Services of the Armed Forces to stop these criminal acts, which resulted in the murder, torture, and inhumane treatment of thousands of helpless men, women, and children of many different nations."*[12]

TYPHUS IS A virulent, louse-borne disease that is often rampant in unclean environments, such as a battlefield or concentration camp, and thus the Germans urgently sought a vaccine. By the fall and winter of 1941, typhus was running rampant on the Eastern Front, decimating German ranks like Stalin's guns. Handloser, at a conference held at Buchenwald on December 29, 1941, directed the medical chiefs present to conduct experiments with chicken egg-yolk vaccine on inmates who were to be deliberately infected with the typhus virus.[13] The German chemical firm I.G. Farben, manufacturers of the poison gas Zyklon-B that was used in the Nazis' various gas chambers, was contracted to produce the typhus vaccine.[14]

* Handloser was found guilty and sentenced to life in prison. His sentenced was later reduced to twenty years but, as he was ill from cancer, he was released in 1954 and died shortly thereafter.

At that December 29th conference, Buchenwald was selected to become the main facility for testing anti-typhus vaccines (the others being the Typhus and Virus Institute of the Army in Cracow, Poland, and the concentration camps of Schirmeck and Natzweiler-Struthof, both in France). Dr. Joachim Mrugowsky, head of the Hygenic Institute of the *Waffen*-SS in Berlin, directed *SS-Hauptsturmführer* Dr. Erwin Ding, Buchenwald's then-chief doctor, to conduct tests of various anti-typhus vaccines. In response, Ding opened the Typhus and Virus Institute in Block 46 at Buchenwald. During Ding's first experiments, fresh blood was injected into five inmates who had been deliberately infected with the disease; all the subjects died.[15]

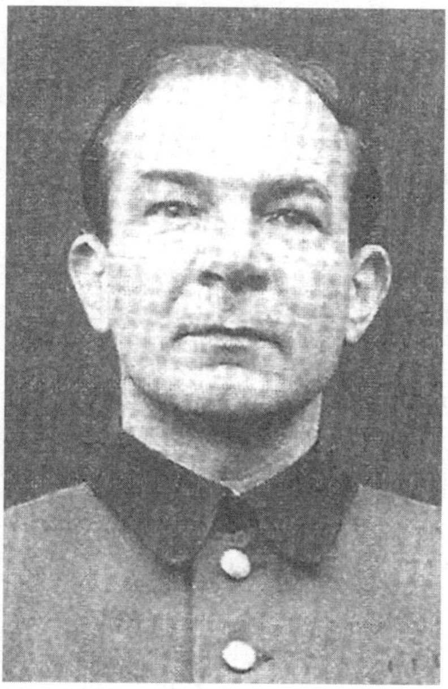

Dr. Joachim Mrugowsky, head of the Waffen-SS Hygenic Institute, and later chief physician at Buchenwald. He was executed by the Allies. (U.S. National Archives)

After supervising typhus experiments at Sachsenhausen, Dr. Mrugowsky joined Ding at Buchenwald where they infected hundreds of inmates with the disease, then tried various vaccines in human-subject trials in Block 46 beginning on January 6, 1942—trials that continued nonstop until March 1945.[16] Dr. Ding (who later changed his name to Schuler) outwardly appeared to be pleasant, intellectual, and gentle—not the kind of evil scientist that one stereotypically associates with Nazi doctors. And yet his gentle smile and relaxed manner made his murderous deeds all that much more chilling.

He was the out-of-wedlock son of a doctor and African explorer by the name of von Schuler. Before the doctor could adopt him and make him his legal heir, he died. His mother eventually married a man named Ding, from Leipzig, and Erwin took his last name. After earning his medical degree (through the assistance of the Nazi Party), he became indebted to the Nazis and was more than willing to do their bidding; he became quite adept at killing inmates quickly with injections of phenol.[17]

Before the war began, Dr. Ding had joined the SS *Totenkopf* Division and served as a surgeon until August 1940, when he transferred to the Hygenic

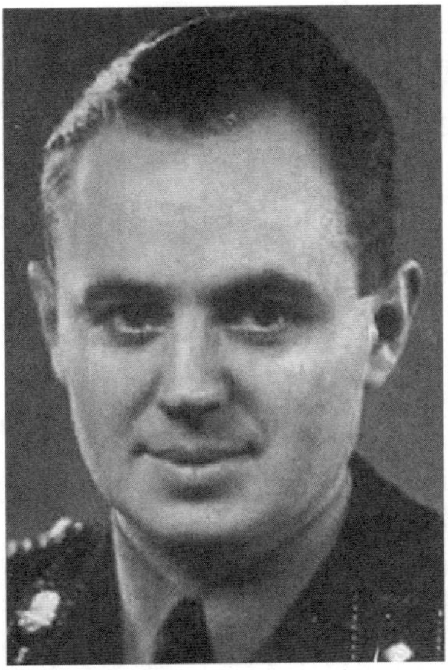

The pleasant-faced Dr. Erwin Ding (who later changed his name to Schuler), one of numerous SS doctors who performed medical experiments on inmates at Buchenwald. (Buchenwald Memorial)

Institute of the *Waffen* SS and was assigned to study the typhus problem.[18] This led Ding to Buchenwald, where he replaced the camp's previous chief doctor, *SS-Hauptsturmführer* Hannes "Hans" Eisele. At Buchenwald, Ding soon acquired a reputation as one of the most sadistic of the camp doctors. One post-war assessment said that he was "a very ambitious man who was apparently willing to engage in any professional activity which he thought might further his medical career. He gladly seized upon the opportunity to conduct experiments on concentration camp inmates in connection with the vaccine study. Every German officer holding a position comparable to that held by Dr. Ding was required to keep a journal or diary showing his official activities. It appears that Dr. Ding kept two diaries. Ding's personal diary containing official and personal entries and work reports had disappeared; his official log or journal concerning his work at Buchenwald is the document in evidence [at his war-crimes trial]."[19]

Vivien Spitz, a court reporter at the Nuremberg War Crimes Tribunal and author of *Doctors From Hell*, noted, "In the beginning, subjects were infected artificially by lacerating the skin and introducing a typhus culture from contagious lice. This changed in 1943 when subjects were injected with fresh blood containing the typhus virus intravenously or intramuscularly. Of twenty-five subjects, nineteen died."[20]

Eugen Kogon,* an inmate working as Ding's clerk in Block 46, recalled a far higher number. Kogon noted that, "All in all, about a thousand prisoners passed through Ward 46. Some of them had the good fortune to be used only in blood-bank tests, or in other experiments that, for one reason or another, stopped short of actual infection. Of the remainder of some 450 persons, 158 died...."[21]

* Kogon had been one of Ding's "favorites" since early 1942, and had assisted him in making his journal entries; in April 1943 Kogon was officially assigned to be Ding's clerk. When the camp was liberated two years later, Kogon obtained possession of the diary and kept it as evidence in the event a future trial of Dr. Ding was ever held. (Kogon, pp. 146-168) Ding cheated the hangman by committing suicide in prison on August 11, 1945. (Sydnor, p. 339)

Dr. Alfred Balachowsky, an inmate working in the Buchenwald typhus laboratory, was required to take part in obtaining cultures of the typhus germs with which the human guinea pigs were infected. He noted, "A constant supply of these cultures was kept in Block 46 by means of the contamination of healthy individuals through sick ones. Now, it is well known that artificial inoculation of typhus by intravenous injection is invariably fatal. Therefore, all these men who were used for bacterial culture during the whole time such cultures were required died, and we counted 600 victims sacrificed for the sole purpose of supplying typhus germs."[22]

In another typhus experiment, a group of inmates, selected from the healthier ones who had developed some resistance to the disease, was injected with an unproven vaccine. Thereafter, all the persons in the group were infected with typhus. At the same time, other inmates who had not been vaccinated were also infected for purposes of comparison—a so-called "control" group. Still others were intentionally infected for the sole purpose of keeping the typhus virus alive and generally available in the bloodstream of the inmates for future research. The experiments continued until November 1944. Ding's underlings—Buchenwald physicians Dr. Arthur Dietsche and Dr. Waldemar Hoven, the latter one of Ilse Koch's lovers—selected the test subjects from the inmate population and assisted Ding.[23]

Another of Ding's clerks was a German political prisoner named Walter Poller. He described Ding as being "a highly intelligent man, who was well-mannered, of an agreeable disposition, friendly, and sometimes actually genial. His features were rather pleasant than stern, his eyes lively and observant. Above all, he was exceptionally self-assured, and I was repeatedly surprised at the ease with which he always found a way out of the most complicated situation.... Nobody who knew Dr. Ding could avoid the impression that he was a man of undoubted talent and even fine character."[24]

EUTHANASIA WAS COMMONPLACE at Buchenwald. As Ding himself testified after the war, prisoners were often selected to be murdered without any explanation to the person assigned to do the killing. "I do not remember a diagnosis as to why euthanasia was to take place, but probably I did not ask about it, either," Ding admitted at trial. "They [the victim] sat down quietly on a chair.... A male nurse blocked the vein in the arm, and Dr. Hoven quickly

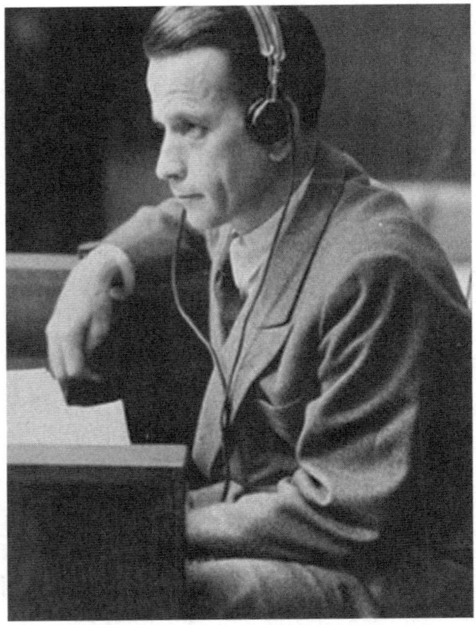

Dr. Waldemar Hoven, Buchenwald physician and one of Ilse Koch's lovers, on the stand during the "Doctors' Trial" at Nuremberg, December 1946–August 1947. He was found guilty of committing atrocities and hanged on June 2, 1948, at Bavaria's Landsberg Prison. (U.S. National Archives)

injected the phenol. They died in an immediate total convulsion during the actual injection without any sign of other pain. The time between the beginning of the injection and death [of the inmate] I estimate at about one-half second."*[25]

Dr. Hoven admitted after the war, "In some instances I supervised the killing of these unworthy inmates by injections of phenol at the request of the inmates. These killings took place in the camp hospital.... On one occasion Dr. Ding came to witness the killings with phenol and said that I was not doing it correctly, therefore, he performed some of the injections himself. At that time three inmates were killed with phenol injections, and they died within a minute.

"The total number of [inmates] killed was about 150, of whom 60 were killed by phenol injections, either by myself or under my supervision in the camp hospital, and the rest were killed by various means, such as beatings, by the inmates." **[26]

Killing their human test subjects quickly and quietly via injection was something at which the camp doctors became quite adept. Inmate Eugen Kogon recalled that SS Dr. Hoven "finished off a whole row of prisoners with injections of sodium evipan," then "strolled from the operating room, a cigarette in his hand, merrily whistling 'The End of a Perfect Day.'"[27]

* Dr. Ding/Schuler was arrested by American military authorities after the war and charged with being responsible for the deaths of nearly 600 inmates. (Sydnor, p. 339)

** Hoven implied that the "request by inmates" came from inmates who, for political or personal reasons, wanted a fellow inmate killed. In 1943, Hoven was arrested by SS authorities and charged with poisoning a material witness in the corruption investigation of Karl and Ilse Koch; he was found guilty by the SS and was sentenced to death but, after spending eighteen months in prison, was given a reprieve due to the shortage of doctors and restored to his post at Buchenwald. After the war, Hoven was arrested and tried by the Allies on a charge of committing war crimes. He was hanged at Landsberg Prison on June 2, 1948, along with Joachim Mrugowsky. (law2.umkc.edu/faculty/projects/ftrials/nuremberg/NurembergDoctorTrial)

TYPHUS WAS NOT the only disease to be deliberately inflicted on humans at Buchenwald; in January 1942, Buchenwald became the testing facility for experimental spotted fever serums. Yellow fever, too, found its way into the bloodstreams of involuntary subjects. Beginning in January 1943, batches of the vaccine were sent to Drs. Ding and Hoven to be tested on inmates who had been intentionally infected with the virus. Experiments involving human subjects and vaccines against diarrhea and cholera were also conducted at Buchenwald.

Ding and Hoven were also involved in research to determine why soldiers were dying after receiving a serum to combat the effects of gas edema—a disease resulting from a bacterial infection of wounds on the battlefield. Four or five Buchenwald inmates died in the process of the experiment, which also consisted of deadly intravenous injections of phenol.[28] Further experiments involving old blood plasma were conducted on inmates in Buchenwald's *Kleinelager* or "Little Camp," for the benefit of the Military Medical Academy. Not surprisingly, the experiments reached no effective solution.[29]

BECAUSE PHOSPHORUS MUNITIONS produce devastating burns when they come in contact with the skin, Drs. Mrugowsky and Ding conducted experiments on Soviet prisoners-of-war from November 1943 to January 1944 to test the effect of various pharmaceutical preparations, salves, and emollients on phosphorus burns. Naturally, this meant subjecting inmates to phosphorus material extracted from unexploded incendiary bombs. In November 1943, five inmates were deliberately burned with phosphorus material removed from an English incendiary bomb, permanently injuring them and causing unbearable agony. The screams of the victims carried far beyond Block 46.

In another study, Russian POWs were used as lab rats to study the effects of phenol and cyanide injections; all died.

Block 46 was also where doctors experimented to study the effect various poisons had on living subjects, and so, also beginning in November 1943, a three-month-long test was run at Buchenwald during which poison was secretly slipped into the food of specially chosen inmates. In another Mrugowsky experiment, the efficacy of various poisons was tested by shooting certain selected prisoners in the thigh with bullets tainted with aconitin nitrate. If the victims did not die during these experiments, they were killed afterwards and their bodies autopsied.

The internal organs of hundreds of victims from these experiments were kept in jars of formaldehyde in the Pathological Department in Buchenwald. It is said that over 30,000 organs were thus preserved.[30]

NOR WERE DING, Hoven, and Mrugowsky the only doctors who played God at Buchenwald. After working at Sachsenhausen, Natzweiler, and Dachau, Dr. Hannes Eisele moved to Buchenwald, where he conducted vivisections on healthy subjects, along with unnecessary operations and amputations before murdering his victims; it is said that he killed at least 300 people at Buchenwald. Eisele also murdered, with injections of the poison evipan natrium, hundreds of inmates suspected of being infected with tuberculosis. According to William Denson, the American prosecutor at the Buchenwald war-crimes tribunal held at Dachau in 1947, Eisele started off as "a good doctor" and was referred to as "the Angel" by prisoners. But he steadily became cruel and sadistic until he was known as "the Butcher" because of the medical experiments he carried out on prisoners, allowing them to die slowly after injections of cyanide.*[31]

A doctor named Heinrich Plaza killed many patients with lethal injections. Another doctor by the name of Neumann is known to have performed vivisections—removing portions of inmates' livers for study. And others at Buchenwald and Neuengamme experimented with "cures" for homosexuality; many of the test subjects died as a result of castration or the injection of synthetic hormones.[32] Florence Tamagny, author of *A History of Homosexuality: Europe Between the Wars*, noted that the Nazis were quite interested in studying homosexuality in order "to gain absolute control over the homosexuals and to prove that they had an 'illness' that was 'curable....'" She also said that Nazis were most anxious to "rehabilitate" them so that they could be reintegrated into society but, more importantly, could fill the ranks of the army being rapidly depleted on the battlefields.[33]

* Eisele was found guilty at the tribunal and sentenced to death. But his sentence was commuted and in 1952 he was freed from Landsberg Prison—with compensation for time served. He established a medical practice in Munich but fled in 1958 when he was warned he was about to be arrested again. He managed to escape to Cairo, Egypt, where, under the assumed name of Carl Debouche, he opened a medical practice and lived quietly and in anonymity until his death in 1967. (Fisk, "Butcher of Buchenwald in an Egyptian Paradise," *The Independent*, August 7, 2010)

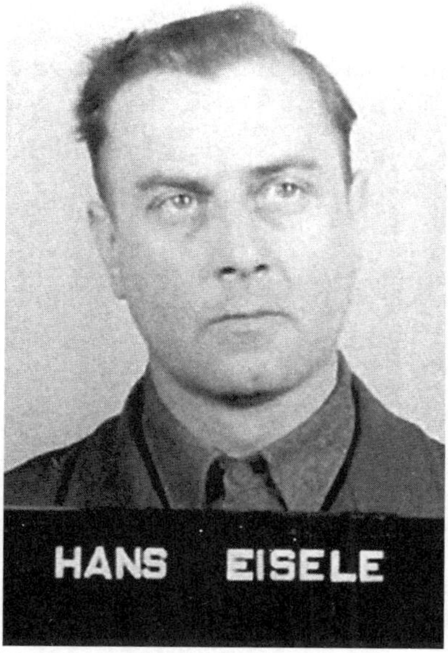

Dr. Hannes "Hans" Eisele was notorious for killing prisoners at Buchenwald with poisonous injections. He was tried by the Allies and sentenced to death. His sentence was reduced to life in prison but he was released in 1952, after which he fled to Egypt and lived there in freedom until his death in 1967. (U.S. National Archives)

To aid in these homosexuality-cure experiments, in 1942, with Himmler's blessing, a Danish endocrynologist and SS major by the name of Dr. Carl Peter Jensen (alias Carl Vaernet) came to German-controlled Prague from Copenhagen in hopes of being able to conduct experiments in search of a cure for homosexuality. SS Captain Dr. Gerhard Schiedlausky, Chief Garrison Physician at Buchenwald, began corresponding with Jensen/Vaernet, going so far as to offering to provide Jensen/Vaernet with human "guinea pigs" from among Buchenwald's population.[34]

In July 1944, believing that a combination of castration and hormonal (testosterone) treatment was the key to a homosexuality cure, Jensen/Vaernet selected six inmates based on their records; Schiedlausky's assistants castrated them. The results were inconclusive; there were tremendous problems with conducting the experiment by long-distance and many of the tests were botched. That fall, with Himmler's permission, Vaernet came to Buchenwald to test and operate on a number of subjects. In December, six more were castrated. Only an outbreak of yellow fever that resulted from a camp experiment gone bad ended the experiments. No final reports apparently survive to document the outcome of the homosexuality-cure experiments, nor detail those who may have died.[35]

Of course, not all medical experiments were carried out at Buchenwald; many of the other camps served as laboratories for the gruesome, deadly, and pseudo-scientific work. At these camps, doctors interested in seeing how people died from poison gas, injected poisons, burns, gangrene, bacterial infections, diseases, starvation, high altitudes, hypothermia, and a variety of wounds and injuries plied their gruesome trade. Other doctors, seeking mass sterilization methods that would stop "undesirables" from reproducing, tested various ways to prevent conception. Conversely, some physicians, such as the notorious Dr.

Josef Mengele at Auschwitz, did research with twins in order to find ways to more effectively multiply the Aryan race. At Ravensbrück, Nazi doctors, wanting to know if severed arms and legs could be transplanted onto soldiers who had lost limbs in battle, amputated the arms and legs of female inmates and attached them to other inmates. Not surprisingly, the experiment failed, and the few victims who lived through it suffered severe pain, mutilation, and permanent disability.[36]

In virtually every experiment, the human subjects died outright, were terribly maimed, or were left in ineluctable pain. Once their value as human guinea pigs was over, most of these subjects were murdered. The Nazi doctors suffered the self-delusion that they were somehow advancing the frontiers of medical science when, in fact, they were doing little more than playing God for their own sadistic amusement, twisted gratification, and the advancement of the Nazi state.

Brigadier General Telford Taylor, a prosecutor who later tried dozens of Nazi doctors in 1946-1947 at Nürnberg for these and other barbaric medical crimes committed under the guise of scientific research, said, "We will christen this macabre science 'thanatology'—the science of producing death."[37]

PRISONERS DID NOT need to be part of a medical experiment to fear visiting the doctors at Buchenwald—just being sick was enough to strike terror in the hearts of inmates. They knew that rarely did anyone ever return alive from a trip to the infirmary.

And no wonder—stories told by inmates about the quality of care given at the infirmary are frightening in the extreme. According to the official report of the tribunal of camp personnel, "Medical care was lacking and it was almost impossible to get into the hospital [as a legitimate patient]. Inmate doctors were not allowed to treat other inmates in the hospital until 1942 or 1943. SS doctors were in charge of the hospital. Prior to the time that the inmate doctors worked in the hospital, untrained inmates performed operations on other inmates. It was a matter of general knowledge among the inmates of the camp that the camp physician frequently called healthy inmates to the camp hospital and performed surgical operations on them. These inmates were usually killed by injections shortly thereafter....

"If an inmate patient did not have cigarettes, food or other gifts for the chief

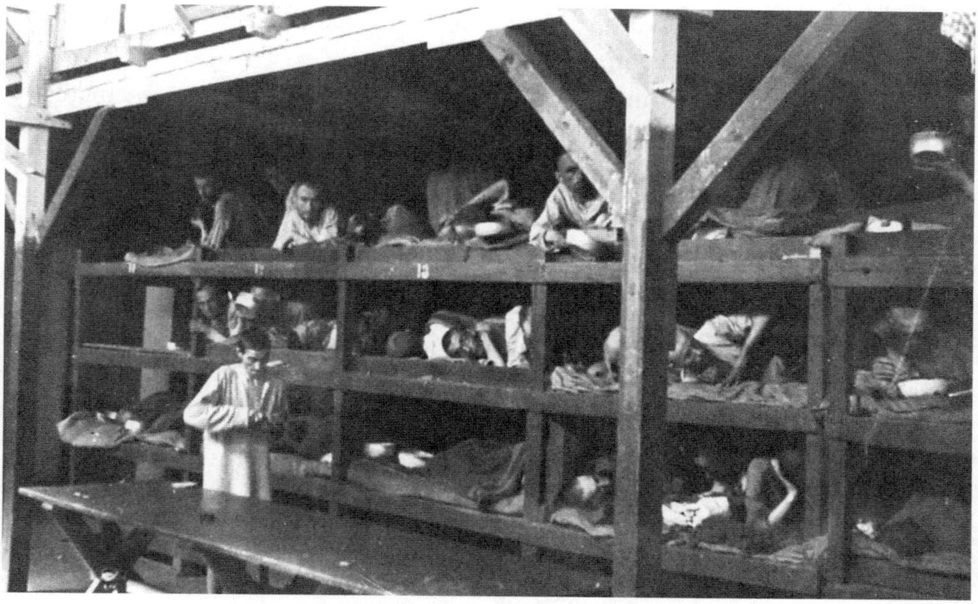

Buchenwald infirmary (U.S. National Archives)

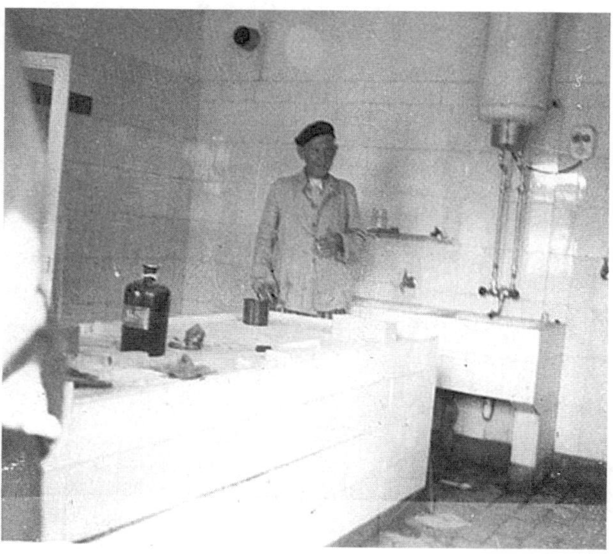

A former inmate stands at the autopsy table in the pathology laboratory, where gold teeth were extracted from corpses and tattooed skin was removed before cremation. (Photo by Edwin Bonde, June 24, 1945, courtesy Alan Bonde)

doctor of the small camp [Edwin Katzen-Ellenbogen], he would not treat him. [Katzen-Ellenbogen] sold medicine supplied for inmates on the black market. When asked by inmates why he refused to treat them, he answered, 'You are here in a concentration camp and not in a sanatorium. You are just like your comrades here to die like a dog and not to be cured.' French inmate doctors in the [Little

Camp] were not permitted to treat the sick. They were threatened with punishment if they treated the inmates."[38]

Dr. Petr Zenkl, the former Lord Mayor of Prague, a minister in Czech president Edvard Bénès' government, and a political prisoner incarcerated in Buchenwald from 1939 to 1945, recalled, "It was very difficult to reach the infirmary even by the most ingenious devices. One had to have permission from the foreman of the block, and the SS overseer on duty had to approve it. At the entrance to the infirmary stood a prisoner-porter. He chased away the majority of petitioners, or he healed them by strokes [i.e., beating them with a stick]. From those who could reach the entrance, the porter made his selection. He often beat the sick with a cudgel so hard that some of them ran away while others just collapsed. The remainder came to be examined. The porter broke the arm of a co-prisoner on one such occasion. When the man fell, a note fell out of his pocket. It was the recommendation of another prisoner to the porter, the reasons being political. The porter grew very excited and abused the mutilated man for not having shown him the slip earlier proving that he was a Communist."[39]

As disturbing as these tales of criminal physician behavior are, few are as strange as one doctor in particular.

7
THE DEMENTED DOCTOR

"I can help you only, Doctor, if you will forget that I am a prisoner and you are the SS doctor."

Edwin Katzen-Ellenbogen, M.D.
Buchenwald prisoner

THEN THERE IS the disturbingly curious case of the afore-mentioned Dr. Edwin Katzen-Ellenbogen, a naturalized American citizen and inmate/doctor at Buchenwald.

Katzen-Ellenbogen was born in 1882 in Stanislawow, a part of Austria-occupied Poland. He earned his medical degree in psychiatry at the University of Leipzig in 1905, then sailed for the United States, where he met and married Marie A. Pierce, the daughter of a prominent Massachusetts judge. After securing money and letters of introduction, he returned to Europe for two years to associate with some of the leading names in the field of psychiatry, including Sigmund Freud. With credentials in hand, he sailed back to the U.S. in 1907, became a naturalized American citizen, and began work at the Danvers State Hospital of Massachusetts (also known as the State Lunatic Hospital), and lectured at Harvard University.

After Woodrow Wilson became governor of New Jersey in 1911, Katzen-Ellenbogen was named to the post of Scientific Director of the State Village for Epileptics at Skillman, New Jersey. He also became co-editor of an international journal, *Epilepsia*. Wilson even asked the doctor to draft the New Jersey law allowing for the involuntary sterilization of epileptics and "mental defectives."

Although it seems unbelievable today, the field of eugenics in the early twentieth century enjoyed widespread acceptance in the United States. As author Edwin Black noted, "Hitler and his henchmen victimized an entire continent and exterminated millions in his quest for a co-called 'Master Race.' But the concept of a white, blond-haired, blue-eyed master Nordic race didn't originate with Hitler. The idea was created in the United States, and cultivated in California, decades before Hitler came to power. California eugenicists played an important, although little known, role in the American eugenics movement's campaign for ethnic cleansing."

Black called eugenics a "racist pseudoscience" that could create a master race by sterilizing and segregating persons who did not fit the Nordic stereotype. To accomplish this goal, in the early 1900s twenty-seven states enacted forced sterilization and segregation laws, and even marriage restrictions that prohibited marriage between Aryans and certain races and other classes of people. Eventually, some 60,000 Americans were coercively sterilized.

"Eugenics would have been so much bizarre parlor talk," Black noted, "had it not been for extensive financing by corporate philanthropies, specifically the Carnegie Institution, the Rockefeller Foundation and the Harriman railroad fortune. They were all in league with some of America's most respected scientists hailing from such prestigious universities as Stanford, Yale, Harvard, and Princeton. These academicians espoused race theory and race science, and then faked and twisted data to serve eugenics' racist aims.

"Stanford president David Starr Jordan originated the notion of 'race and blood' in his 1902 racial epistle, 'Blood of a Nation,' in which the university scholar declared that human qualities and conditions such as talent and poverty were passed through the blood. In 1904, the Carnegie Institution established a laboratory complex at Cold Spring Harbor on Long Island that stockpiled millions of index cards on ordinary Americans, as researchers carefully plotted the removal of families, bloodlines and whole peoples. From Cold Spring Harbor, eugenics advocates agitated in the legislatures of America, as well as the nation's social service agencies and associations."[1]

Katzen-Ellenbogen enthusiastically embraced the study of eugenics, becoming a charter member of the Eugenics Research Association at the Carnegie Institution's Cold Spring Harbor laboratory in New York. He soon became a leading expert in the field. In 1915, Katzen-Ellenbogen sailed for Europe, leaving his wife behind, and settled in Germany with a Russian woman named Olga. When Hitler came to power in 1933, and the Nuremberg Laws were passed in 1935, he found himself classified as a Jew because of his Jewish ancestry, despite his having been raised as a Catholic. To escape persecution, he left Germany and traveled to Czechoslovakia, then Italy, then finally to France. In 1943, three years after the Germans invaded and conquered France, Katzen-Ellenbogen was taken into custody.

In his book, *War Against the Weak*, Black wrote, "Katzen-Ellenbogen discounted his Jewish ancestry, considering himself a eugenicist first and foremost. This made him different, and almost appealing to the Gestapo.... The war-stretched Nazis needed doctors, especially in occupied lands. As a distinguished physician and psychiatrist who spoke German [as well as English, French, and

Russian] and also enjoyed American citizenship, Katzen-Ellenbogen became very useful to both the Gestapo and the Wehrmacht."

Although technically a prisoner, Katzen-Ellenbogen found himself employed to treat psychiatric patients in the German army. But then, in September 1943, he was unexpectedly transported from France to Buchenwald. Rather than being repulsed by the savagery he saw at Buchenwald, Katzen-Ellenbogen was fascinated. "I was really amazed about the efficiency and quickness about everything that happened there," he said later at his war-crimes trial. "We were treated not badly there." Indeed, Katzen-Ellenbogen's reputation springing from his helpfulness to the Gestapo in France quickly earned him privileged-inmate status. He was assigned to run the infirmary in Buchenwald's Little Camp, where he had his own, semi-private room and dined on plentiful helpings of fresh meats and vegetables that only the SS enjoyed at Buchenwald. He was even allowed to wear a finely tailored three-piece suit while his fellow inmates went around in tattered, feces-stained striped uniforms.

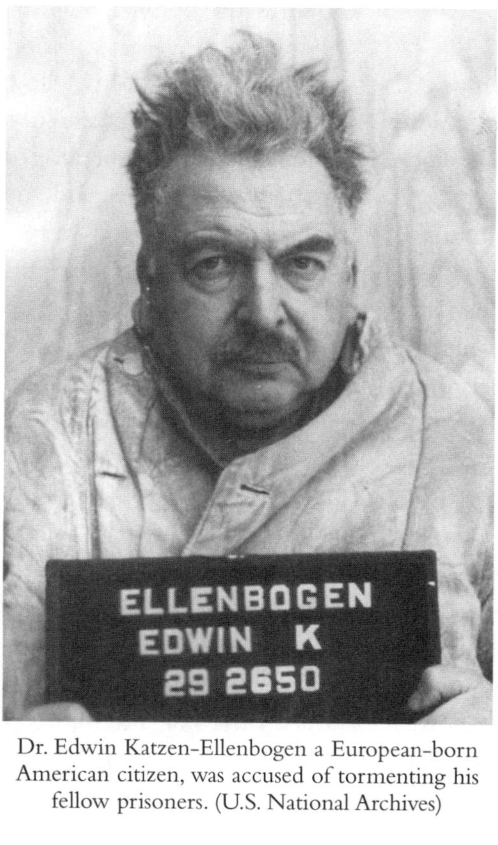

Dr. Edwin Katzen-Ellenbogen a European-born American citizen, was accused of tormenting his fellow prisoners. (U.S. National Archives)

It wasn't long before Katzen-Ellenbogen's reputation as a psychiatrist and skill as a hypnotist garnered even more trust from the camp staff and he began assisting the camp's Nazi doctors. One day Dr. Gerhard Schiedlausky, Buchenwald's then-chief physician, who had been unable to sleep for quite some time due to the depravity with which he was daily confronted (and in which he engaged), summoned Katzen-Ellenbogen and ordered the American to help him. Katzen-Ellenbogen replied, "I can help you only, Doctor, if you will forget that I am a prisoner and you are the SS doctor." Schiedlausky replied, "Naturally."

Katzen-Ellenbogen analyzed Schiedlausky's fitful dreams and

came to the obvious conclusion that Schiedlausky was troubled by a great, unstated burden. The psychiatrist told the camp's chief medical officer that unless he was willing to discuss those emotional burdens, "no further treatment would be of value." Schiedlausky reportedly answered, "You're right, but I can't tell you."

Katzen-Ellenbogen later saw Schiedlausky sobbing and tried to console him. Incredibly, Schiedlausky was apparently so impressed with Katzen-Ellenbogen's powers to comfort him that he recommended other camp officers, wracked by guilt over their crimes and unable to sleep, see the American for counseling. Black wrote, "Even though Katzen-Ellenbogen was a prisoner, the Nazis opened up to him."

One of the other SS men, the brutal Austrian named Dumböck, told Katzen-Ellenbogen that he had trouble sleeping because he continually saw images—the ghosts of at least forty men he had personally killed. Through Katzen-Ellenbogen's psychotherapy, Dumböck realized that it was the memory of the murders that plagued him. (It is not known if the epiphany caused Dumböck to change his ways.)

While Katzen-Ellenbogen was gaining the trust of the SS staff, his fellow inmates were viewing him with fear, enmity, and suspicion. And he returned their hate many-fold—especially the French communists. Katzen-Ellenbogen felt that they were the filthiest of the filthy at Buchenwald, bringing to the camp with them diseases such as diphtheria, scarlet fever, and various throat infections. He refused to waste his limited supply of medicines, human compassion, or bed space on them. As far as he was concerned, they could continue to work and suffer until they died. As a eugenicist, he believed in the "survival of the fittest," and felt it entirely appropriate that "natural selection" would kill off those too weak to survive the harsh environment at Buchenwald.

Katzen-Ellenbogen also had the power to decide who would be admitted to the hospital. According to Black, "He forced Frenchmen to exercise in the frigid outdoors without their scarves and often without their shirts—this to 'cure' infected throats. He smuggled in needed medicines through the SS medics but then sold them for money or favors. Such extortions allowed him to deposit some 50,000 francs into a camp bank account. He also cached large quantities of Danish food, medicines and cigarettes in his bedroom, mainly pilfered from the Danish Red Cross packets turned over by the sick and injured."

It was said at his war-crimes trial that Katzen-Ellenbogen personally administered at least a thousand lethal injections of phenol, but no witnesses at the

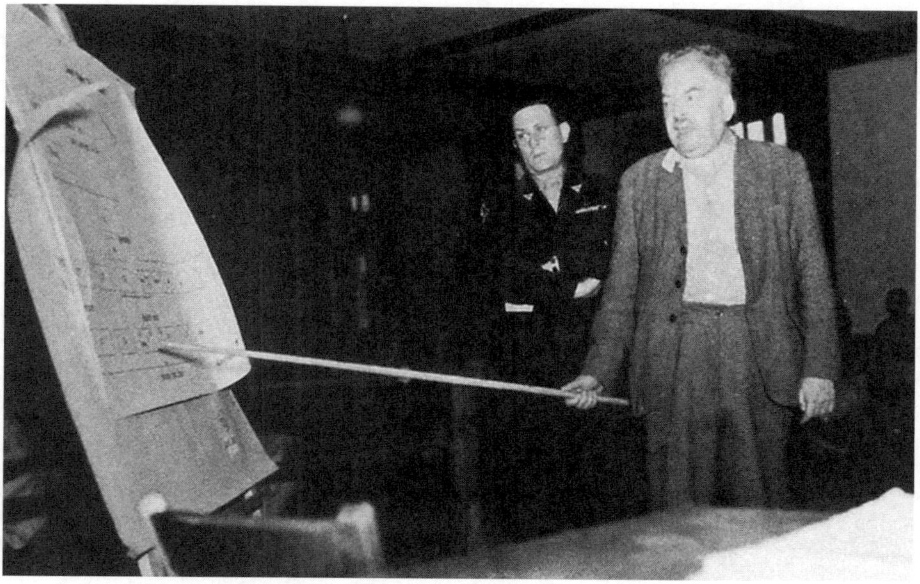

Dr. Katzen-Ellenbogen, testifies at his war-crimes trial held at Dachau in 1947.
(U.S. Army Military History Institute)

trial could conclusively prove that the doctor was one of those who applied the syringes.

On rare occasions, Katzen-Ellenbogen's expertise in eugenics actually helped save lives. Because of ongoing research into the ancestral and genetic backgrounds of Buchenwald prisoners, it was discovered that some Poles were of German ancestry. As such, when Polish children incarcerated at the camp were "discovered" by Katzen-Ellenbogen to have "Aryan blood," they were removed and given to German families to be raised as Germans.[2]

This accounting of some of the cruelest practices by Nazi doctors and their henchmen is only the barest tip of a much larger iceberg.* As Eugen Kogon summed it up, "Apart from the gruesome deaths, there were no practical results from these experiments."[3]

---

* If one has the stomach for it, more detailed studies of the medical-experiment atrocities can be found in several books, including *Doctors From Hell* by Vivien Spitz, and *The Nazi Doctors* by Dr. Robert J. Lifton.

8
SUPER WEAPONS

"I realized that any attempt of reasoning on humane grounds would be utterly futile."

Wernher von Braun
German rocket scientist

DURING THE FIRST half of 1943, the global war rolled inexorably onward, and the news for the Germans was invariably bad. The Nazi triumphs of the early years were being eclipsed by one costly setback after another. The Americans and British were slowly pushing German and Italian forces in North Africa back toward the sea. Germany's naval code was broken, and Allied warships at last began taking a toll on the U-boats that had been sinking so many cargo-laden ships bound from the U.S. for Britain and the Soviet Union. British and American bomber crews were also doing their best to ravage German cities and industrial installations by night and day.

In the Soviet Union, German *Generalfeldmarschall* Friedrich von Paulus's beleaguered Sixth Army was trapped in Stalingrad, and efforts by the Germans to rescue it were thrown back with heavy casualties; von Paulus surrendered what was left of his army on January 31. As Josef Goebbel's biographers wrote, "Goebbels did not hesitate to make the flesh of Germany creep at this dire news; muffled drums preceded the announcements on the radio, and the newspapers the following day were edged with the black bands of mourning." So devastating was the defeat that plans to celebrate the tenth anniversary of Hitler's ascendancy to the chancellorship were abandoned.[1]

So secure had Western North Africa become that in January 1943 President Roosevelt flew to Casablanca, Morocco, to confer there with British Prime Minister Churchill. At the "Casablanca Conference," the decision to invade Sicily was made and the broad strategy concerning a cross-Channel invasion from England to France was hammered out. Done with playing defense, Britain and America were about to go on the offense in Europe.

In the Pacific, too, American forces had ceased being the punching bag for the Japanese and were about to deliver some blows of their own. After absorbing attacks against their installations at Pearl Harbor and the Philippines, the Americans began flexing their own considerable military muscles and planning ways to take back the Pacific—all the way to Tokyo.

On February 18, 1943, despite the horrendous casualties the German armed forces were suffering in Russia, the looming defeat in North Africa, and the pulverizing of German cities and factories from the air, Joseph Goebbels whipped a huge gathering of faithful Nazis in Berlin into a frenzy, shouting to the massed throng: "Do you want total war?"

The crowd screamed back fervently: "*Ja!*"

Goebbels also continued beating the anti-Jewish drum: "The Jews are the root of evil in the world," he told the crowd. "They are the devil who pushes the West towards its downfall; they are the carrier of ruin and destruction within the body of Western civilization; they are the instigators of chaos in the world.... The crocodile tears shed abroad over the treatment of Jews in German-occupied territories will not deter Germany from carrying out its plans and ideas. On the contrary, Germany will pursue its course with more vigor, by lawful means if necessary, in order to implement its plan which provides for the total elimination of Jewry."

The audience went wild with fervent chants of "*Sieg heil!*"[2]

FOR MANY YEARS the Germans had been working on long-range missiles and rockets. Even before World War II began, Nazi Germany was at the forefront of weapons development; German scientists and engineers created tanks that were far superior to most of what the rest of the world was turning out, and they would be the first to come up with jet-powered combat aircraft; Hitler's physicists were even working hard to develop an atomic bomb. But it was the creation of the first practical missile that gave the Nazis hope that their wonder weapons would be their salvation in the event of a protracted war or likelihood of invasion.

The Treaty of Versailles had restricted or banned the types of weapons (tanks, aircraft, warships, etc.) that Germany was entitled to build but said nothing about rockets and missiles—mainly because the science of rocketry and missilery in 1919 was in its pre-infancy. In 1929, Lieutenant Colonel Karl Emil Becker, chief of the Research and Development Department of the German Army's Board of Ordnance, spearheaded a rocket program that was seen by members of the government as being of particular interest. What if, the ordnance men pondered, a rocket armed with high explosives or deadly chemicals could be developed that could hit a target hundreds, or even thousands, of miles

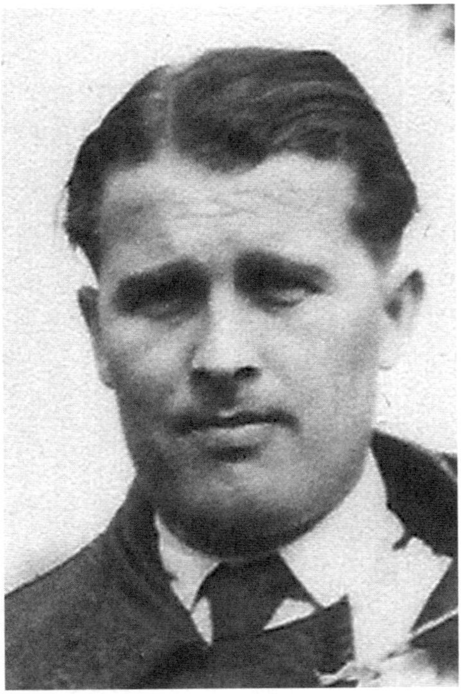

Rocket scientist Wernher von Braun, 1945
(U.S. National Archives)

away? What a tremendous advantage such a super weapon would give the German military! Of course, at that time, the late 1920s, Germany was still led by Hindenburg, not Hitler.

One of the early civilian rocket enthusiasts was a tall, blond, young man by the name of Wernher von Braun, born in 1912 to aristocratic Prussian parents in Berlin. Wernher was extraordinarily bright and was consumed by anything having to do with space. For his education, his affluent parents sent him to a private elementary school atop Weimar's Ettersberg hill in the similarly named village of Ettersburg. As a child, he devoured science-fiction stories about flights, tinkered with home-made rockets, and filled notebooks with designs for space craft. As a teenager in 1929, he became the leader of an amateur rocket group known as the *Verein für Raumschiffarht* (Space-Travel Club); his greatest dream was someday to be launched into outer space.

While launching experimental rockets from open fields on the outskirts of Berlin and working towards his doctorate at the Berlin-Charlottenburg Institute of Technology (today the Technical University of Berlin) von Braun in 1932 came to the attention of Colonel Becker, who invited him to go to work for the German army developing liquid-fuel ballistic missiles.[3] At first the army's rocketry program, which had been deemed to be of little practical value, existed on a miniscule budget, but once the Nazis came to power there was suddenly money and official, high-level interest. The young, idealistic von Braun later professed that he had no strong leanings one way or the other when it came to fascism or communism, but because of his nationalistic Prussian upbringing and his belief that Hitler was good for the country, he applied for membership in the Nazi Party in November 1933 and joined an SS cavalry unit. But his real passion remained rocketry.

Germany's rocket program was supposed to be *streng geheim*—top secret—but the Wehrmacht's test facility at Kummersdorf, about thirty miles south of Berlin, wasn't secret or secluded enough to suit the military. In April 1936, the Nazi government authorized the army to move the rocket test facility, first to the island of Greifswalder Oie and then to Peenemünde, along the Baltic shore of the remote, wind-swept island of Usedom in extreme northeast Germany. That same year, Becker named the twenty-four-year-old von Braun the center's technical director.

From a distance, the complex at Peenemünde resembled just another military installation, but it was much more. By 1938 the *Heervesversuchsstelle Peenemünde* (or HVP, Army Research Center Peenemünde), had grown into scores of buildings—offices, drafting rooms, machine shops, barracks, garages, mess halls, living quarters for hundreds of scientists, workers, and military personnel, testing facilities (including a wind tunnel), an Aerodynamics Institute, fuel storage depot, launch pads, and huge hangars in which the experimental craft could be assembled. At the facility the scientists and engineers planned, built, and tested a number of various rocket and missile designs, including one inter-continental ballistic missile that was intended to hit the United States.*[4]

Although several types of "V" weapons (for *Vergeltungswaffen* or "vengeance weapons" as Propaganda Minister Josef Goebbels called them) were being designed and tested at Peenemünde, two would ultimately emerge as production models—the V-1** (originally known as the Fieseler FZG-76 and nicknamed the "Buzz Bomb" and "Doodlebug" by the British) and the V-2 (originally designated the A-4, for *Aggregat 4*).[5]

The V-2s were forty-six feet in length, weighed thirteen tons, carried an explosive payload of 2,200 pounds, possessed an operational range of 200 miles, and could climb to an altitude of over a hundred miles. Once at the apogee of its trajectory, the V-2 would fall silently from the sky at 3,600 miles per hour (the V-1's motor, by contrast, made a loud "buzzing" noise that abruptly ended,

---

* U.S. Army Chief of Staff General George C. Marshall wrote, "[Hermann] Goering stated after his capture that it was a certainty the eastern American cities would have been under rocket bombardment had Germany remained undefeated for two more years. The first attacks would have started much sooner." (Marshall, p. 210)

** The V-1 project came under the aegis of the Luftwaffe; von Braun, who worked for the army, was not involved in its concept or production. (Béon, p. XI) The V-1 went into testing at Peenemünde, with the rocket's first successful test taking place on December 24, 1942. Full production began in April 1944. More than 30,000 V-1s would be built by Mittelbau-Dora, the Henschel Locomotive Works, and Volkswagen AG. From June 13 until September 1944, nearly 9,000 V-1s would be fired at England, almost all of them at London, killing thousands of civilians. By September 1944, with the Allied capture of all the launch sites, the V-1 threat to England ended. (Neufeld, *Von Braun*, passim)

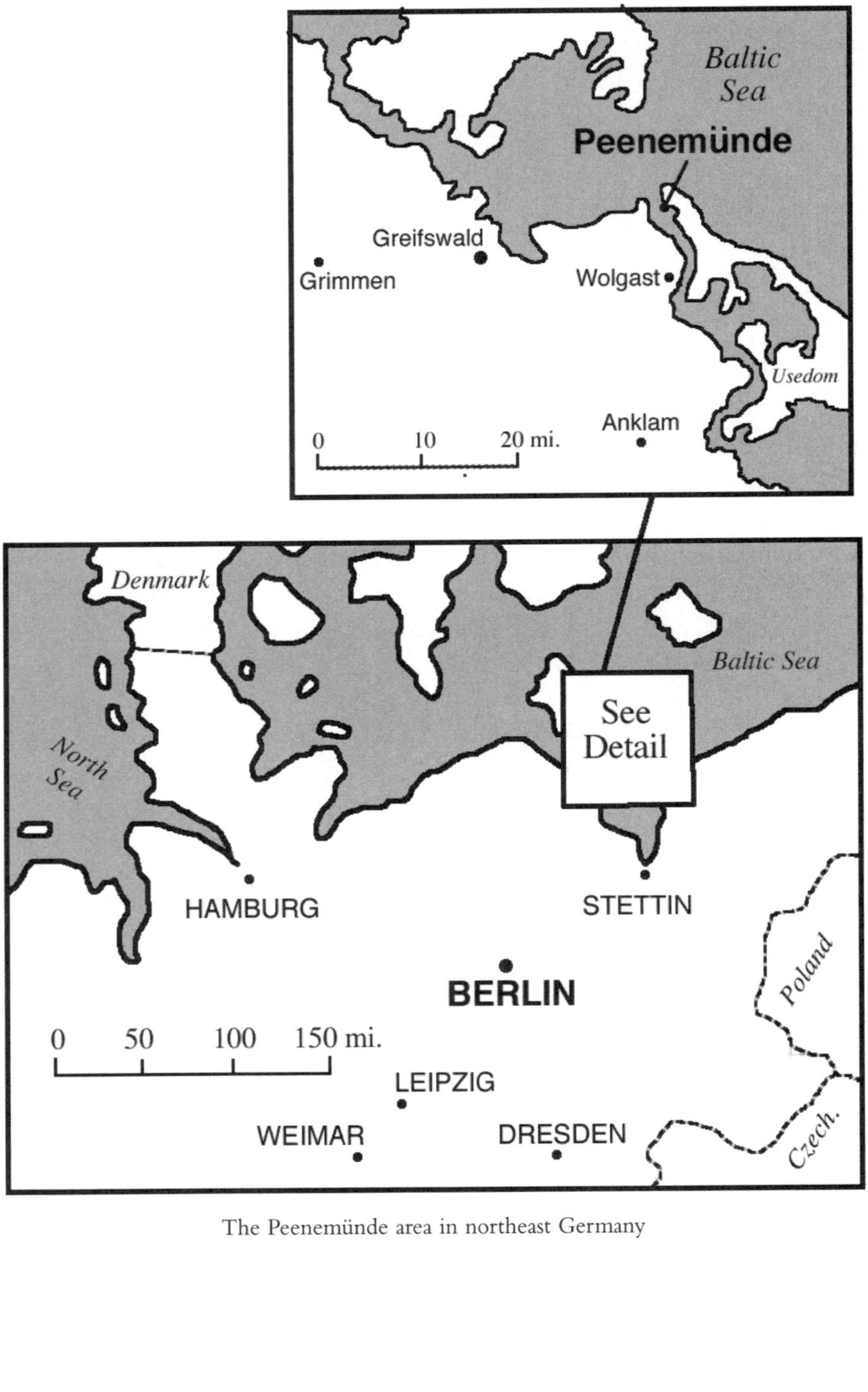

The Peenemünde area in northeast Germany

signaling the missile's plunge to earth), and cause great damage—both psychological and physical.* Heading up the A-4/V-2 portion of the Peenemünde facility was von Braun. Von Braun's baby was huge—and hugely complex. Built to deliver 55,000 pounds of thrust from its liquid-fuel engine, the V-2 was, in its day, the fastest machine ever created—and the world's first ballistic missile. And inmates from Buchenwald would play a major role in its manufacture.[6]

BECAUSE OF THE SS's involvement in Germany's weapons-building program, Weimar and Buchenwald received two DAW plants—one on Kromsdorfer Strasse in Weimar's industrial area on the northeast side of town (known as the Gustloff-Werk I,** plus the Fritz-Sauckel-Werk, a plant that manufactured rifles) and another DAW arms factory at Buchenwald proper that opened in 1940 near the clothing depot and employed up to 1,400 inmates.[7]

But small-caliber weapons weren't the only things on German minds. Beginning in July 1942, an army of inmates began cutting down another large swath of forest atop the Ettersberg. This effort was followed by inmates constructing a number of large industrial buildings in this clearing just beyond the eastern perimeter of Buchenwald's prisoner enclosure. It was a factory known as "Gustloff-Werk II," and its *raison d'être* was to manufacture precision components for the V-2 rockets.

One of the inmates on the construction detail was the Polish bricklayer Jacob Werber. In his memoirs, he explained that the project "was actually a complex of factories. In a relatively short period of time, we built an entire town from scratch with buildings, streets, and sidewalks." He tried to be conscientious in his work, fearing that a sloppy job would get him removed from the bricklaying *Kommando* and sent to the quarry, a true death sentence. He noted that the men doing a poor job of laying bricks would hide whenever the SS came around to inspect the work. "As a result, the SS saw only the good workers like me...and when they discovered the spilled mortar or crooked bricks that the others had left, we were blamed and punished with five or ten lashes."[8]

* Between June 13, 1944 and March 27, 1945, 5,475 British civilians would be killed by the V-1s—triple the number of those who would be killed by V-2s. (www. nationalarchives.gov.uk)

** Named for Wilhelm Gustloff, the German leader of the Swiss Nazi party who had been murdered on February 4, 1936, by David Frankfurter, a Jewish student in Switzerland. (Gilbert, *The Holocaust*, p. 51)

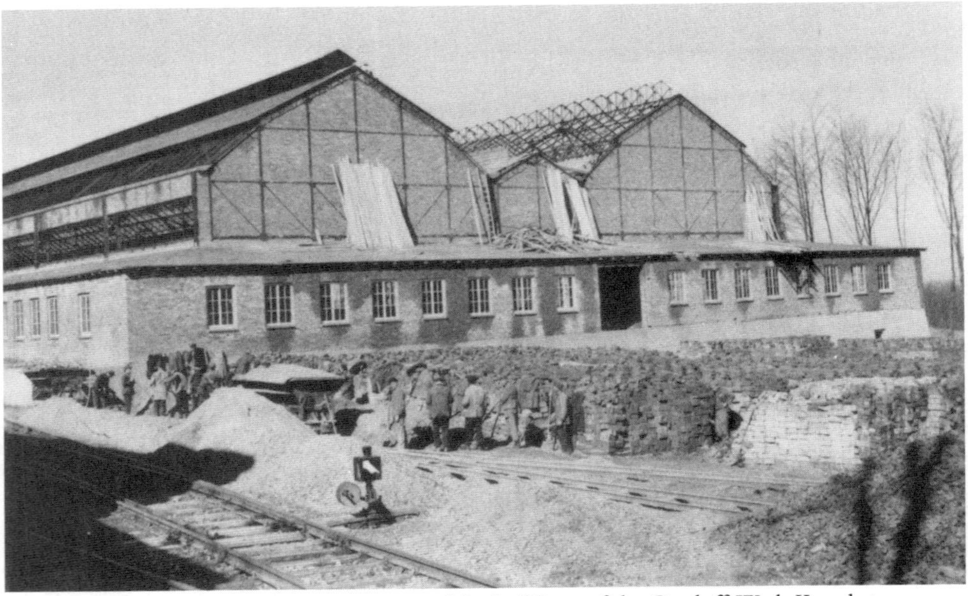

A work gang of prisoners constructs one of the buildings of the Gustloff-Werk II rocket-component factory adjacent to the concentration camp. (Buchenwald Memorial)

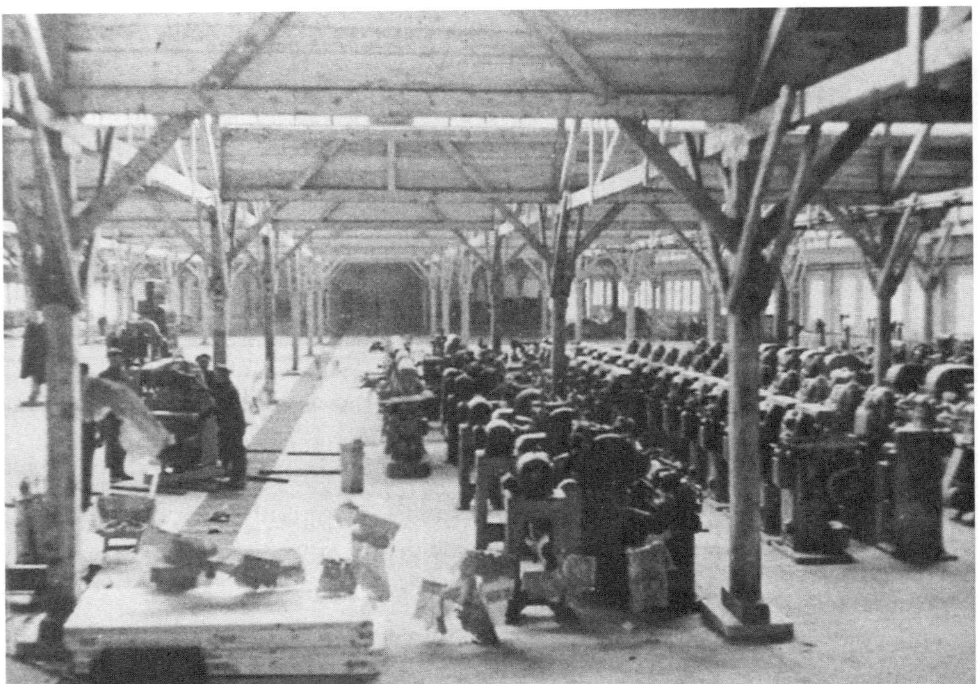

Interior of a factory building at Buchenwald's Gustloff-Werk II, 1943 (Buchenwald Memorial)

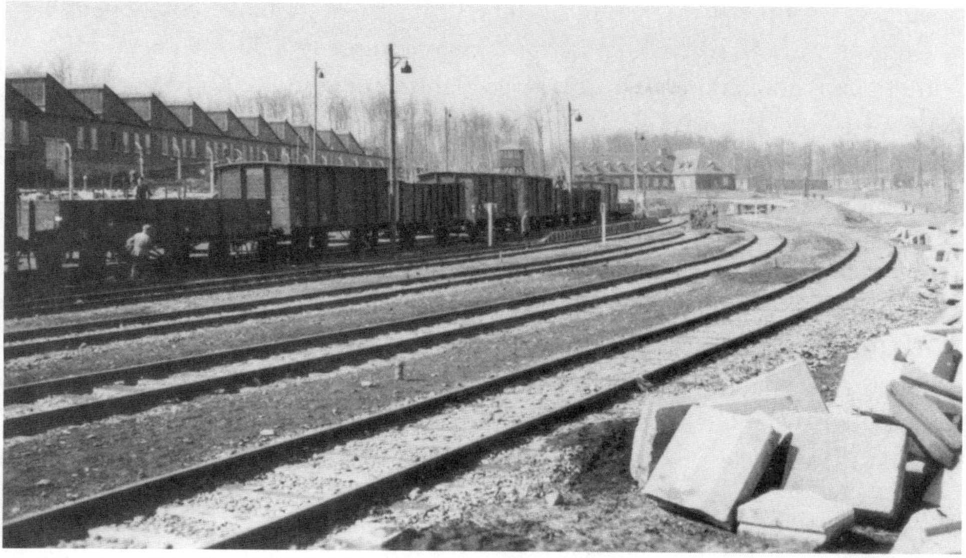

A portion of the Gustloff-Werk II rocket-component factory is visible behind the line of rail cars at left. (Buchenwald Memorial)

Throughout the fall and winter of 1942-43, the work went on without pause. When finished, it would be the workplace for about 4,500 inmates and would cover nearly as much acreage as the "protective custody" camp itself. The purpose of Gustloff-Werk II was still a mystery to the inmates assigned to construct it and eventually work in it. It wasn't until many months later that the inmates learned what the gadgets on which they so diligently worked were for.[9]

THE FIRST SUCCESSFUL test of the V-2 at Peenemünde did not take place until October 1942, for the V-2 was not an easy beast to tame. The program was plagued by engineering and construction problems from day one, and faulty engines and gyroscopes delayed the first launch of the missile. Von Braun faced another problem, one even more acute than the V-2's balky mechanics and electronics—with German industry and the armed forces absorbing nearly every able-bodied man, the production of V-2 missiles was seriously behind schedule. Arthur Rudolph,* one of von Braun's production engineers, had an idea: Since

---

* Rudolph, along with von Braun, was one of over 100 rocket scientists brought to the U.S. at the end of the war in what was termed "Operation Paperclip" to work on the American missile and space program. After the creation of NASA (National Aeronautical and Space Administration) in 1958, Rudolph was employed by that agency and became the project director of the Saturn V rocket program. Following an investigation into his Nazi past and his connection with the abuse and death of slave laborers, he gave up his U.S. citizenship and left the United States in 1984. (U.S. National Archives news release, January 29, 2000)

inmates at Buchenwald were already being used to build components at Gustloff-Werk II, why not conscript thousands more to help assemble the V-2s? In 1943, Rudolph's request to Oswald Pohl resulted in 1,200 prisoners being shipped from Buchenwald to Peenemünde, where they were housed in the nearby Trassenheide slave laborers' camp, built especially for them.[10]

Alex Baum, a French prisoner at Buchenwald, was one of those sent to the seaside rocket plant. "We had to work very, very hard," Baum recalled. "Constant running, *schnell, schnell*, but we had soup, and we had a decent facility where we could sleep." One day *Reichsführer-SS* Heinrich Himmler toured the Peenemünde facility, escorted by von Braun. Prisoner Baum, who was fluent in German, watched the visit. He said, "We [the prisoners] were not very close, but we could see them. I could hear von Braun talking [to Himmler] about the ultimate weapon that's going to destroy the United States and everything else."[11]

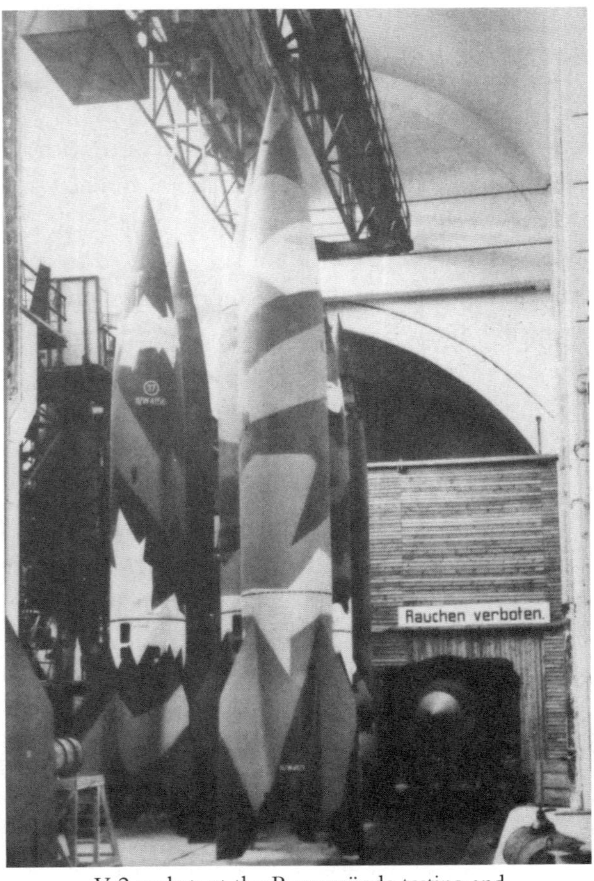

V-2 rockets at the Peenemünde testing and development center (U.S. National Archives)

The V-2 program's problems were not alleviated when the transferred Buchenwald inmates began assembling the missiles. If anything, the problems became worse, for many of the slaves were not interested in helping the Nazis build long-range weapons that could target Allied cities and troop concentrations, and they began performing small acts of sabotage that they hoped would set back the program. A loose bolt here, a bad connection there, perhaps a little foreign substance in a fuel line and—*boom*—the test firings would fail, the V-2s would veer off course, or explode on the launch pad. Of course, instant death awaited any slave caught, or even suspected of, committing sabotage.[12]

ON JULY 4, 1943, a few miles southwest of the major Russian railroad hub of Kursk, there stands a small, unremarkable town known as Prokhorovka. On that day, an event took place in the fields around Prokhorovka that profoundly changed the course of the war. That date marked the start of the biggest tank battle in history and, more than any other, the pivotal battle in terms of determining who would win the war in Europe. At Prokhorovka—in the center of the German front line that stretched from Leningrad on Finland's border all the way to the Black Sea—over 6,000 German and Soviet tanks faced off against each other, supported by 1.3 million Soviet soldiers and almost a million Wehrmacht and *Waffen*-SS soldiers. Nearly 5,000 aircraft also took part in the struggle, which has come to be known as the Battle of Kursk. Although the nearly two-month-long battle ended as a clear Soviet victory that would herald the eventual retreat by the Germans, the Russians paid heavily for it. Casualty numbers are conflicting, but even the most conservative are staggering: The warring armies lost a total of 350,000 men—most of them Soviets.[13]

The British historian Norman Davies wrote, "The significance of Kursk cannot be overrated. This was the decisive battle. The Wehrmacht's prime striking force was destroyed so completely that a major [German] offensive could never be launched again."[14] Although it would take nearly two more years of vicious fighting before the mortally wounded Nazi beast would keel over and die, Kursk was the dagger that delivered the fatal blow.

While the outcome of the Battle of Kursk was still in doubt, Albert Speer, Germany's Minister of Armaments, invited rocket scientists Wernher von Braun and Walter Dornberger to meet with Hitler on July 7 and make a presentation about the V-2 program, which included the showing of a film of a launching. Speer said that Hitler was very excited, calling the weapon "a measure that can decide the war," and looking ahead with gleeful anticipation to the devastation it could wreak upon Britain.

Speer said that Himmler offered the concentration camp inmates as "the simplest way to guarantee secrecy for this vital program. If the entire work force were concentration camp prisoners, all contact with the outside world would be eliminated. Such prisoners did not even have any mail, Himmler said. Along with this, he offered to provide all necessary technicians from the ranks of the prisoners. All industry would have to furnish would be the management and the engineers." Hitler approved the idea, and an additional 600 inmates from Buchenwald were transferred to the Peenemünde facility.[15]

VARIOUS OTHER FACTORIES throughout Germany were already engaged in turning out components for the V-2s—guidance systems, propulsion systems, warheads, etc.—which would then be shipped to the far-off Peenemünde installation for final assembly.

By March 1943, the fourteen-building complex was finished atop the Ettersberg, and the SS began assigning prisoners who had engineering, technical, or tool-making backgrounds to a new *Kommando*. One day this group of technically skilled prisoners, numbering about 4,000, was marched out the gate and into the factory. The prisoners were amazed—everything was new and pristine. Shiny, brand-new machine tools stood precisely aligned, just waiting to be used. The warm aroma of fresh-cut wood, paint, metal, and machine oil filled the weary nostrils of men whose noses had been assaulted by months of nothing but unclean clothing, decaying flesh, burning bodies, foul latrines, and rotten food.

A foreman stood before the assembled ranks of prisoners and told them they were assigned to Gustloff-Werk II and ticked off the rules: Everyone will be expected to work twelve hours a day; a half hour will be devoted to the midday meal. Following strict orders is of the utmost concern; anyone who does not follow orders will be punished, and anyone who tries to sabotage the operation will be immediately executed. It is forbidden to ask questions not directly related to the specific task to which each prisoner is assigned. One's eyes must be at all times focused on one's work; what someone is doing at another workbench is of no concern to them. Under no circumstances must anyone in the factory tell anyone outside the factory what type of work they are doing.

Once these orders were translated into the various languages of the factory workers, the group was broken down into smaller units and each person was given his assignment. Some prisoners were assigned to the drill presses, where they bored holes into pieces of metal. Others soldered wires onto contacts, or polished metal, or sandpapered burrs or rust patches, or bolted one piece of metal to another, or fitted electrical motors into housings, or packed and crated up the completed objects, having no idea what the end product was.

Prisoners possessing advanced specialty backgrounds were given more responsibility—which helped them gain slightly greater knowledge of the entire operation. It soon became clear to them that what Gustloff-Werk II was making were horizontal and vertical gyroscopes, electronic programming mechanisms, and wireless receiving sets for some sort of flying objects—aircraft or—or what?

The men continued to work diligently at their stations, obeying the orders that had been issued on the first day; no one wanted to be sent back to the quarry and its attendant dangers. Besides, here they were treated almost with courtesy and deference; there were few beatings and very little screaming.

Some forty finished devices were turned out at Gustloff-Werk II per day; simple math extrapolated the output to a thousand devices per month or 12,000 per year. The relatively low quality of the devices led some astute prisoners to conclude that the devices on which they were working were meant to be used only once. But why would a device that comprised sophisticated gyroscopes and radio receivers and programming mechanisms be used only once—unless the devices were meant to go into a single-use weapon, a weapon such as a pilotless aircraft or a guided missile?[16]

ANOTHER SIGNIFICANT MILITARY event also took place in July 1943. On the ninth, the largest combined amphibious and airborne assault up to that point of the war was unleashed upon the German-and-Italian-held island of Sicily. On that day, 180,000 American, British, and Canadian troops stormed ashore or were deposited by glider or parachute. The operation, known as Husky, would last just over a month, lead to Italy's capitulation, the overthrow of Mussolini, and the invasion of the Italian peninsula.

With the setbacks at Kursk and in the Mediterranean, Hitler's drive to maintain his dominance in Europe ground to an inglorious halt, and soon the tide would turn irretrievably in the Allies' favor. The only thing that stood a chance of saving Germany, believed Hitler, was its program of super weapons.[17]

IN THAT SUMMER of 1943, Allied spies reported—and recon flights confirmed with aerial photographs—that the Germans were building secret weapons at Peenemünde. The British decided to do something about it. A plan to destroy the rocket facility was personally approved by Churchill and his war cabinet on July 29, 1943, and a major mission, dubbed Operation Hydra, was scheduled for the night of August 17-18. On that night, Bomber Command sent a fleet of bombers to wipe Peenemünde off the map.[18]

Around midnight on August 17, the still night air at Peenemünde took on a new sound—the distant rumble of airplane engines, coming closer. The rumble grew louder and louder until 597 British Avro Lancaster bombers were 6,000 feet overhead. Air-raid sirens began to scream, and artificial fog generators, designed to hide the facility from enemy airmen, were switched on. Within seconds the sirens were drowned out by the whistle of bombs on their descent. While the German scientists and technicians began sprinting for the bomb shelters, only the Buchenwald slave workers in the Trassenheide barracks were prevented from seeking shelter.

The first wave of bombers managed to hit its primary target—the living quarters of the scientists* and German workers, but a mistake in marking the target resulted in about a third of the bombers striking instead the Trassenheide camp, two miles away.

The second wave of Lancasters then came in low and smashed the factory workshops. The bombs began detonating all over the facility, lighting up the night, ripping buildings apart, destroying the prototype rockets, and setting off huge explosions when the storage tanks holding millions of gallons of volatile rocket fuel were hit. A few minutes later, the third wave successfully struck the experimental station's laboratory and offices, but also accidentally dropped more ordnance on the shattered and smoldering Trassenheide camp. In all, nearly 800 people died in the raid, including most of the 600 slave laborers recently brought in from Buchenwald.

When the "all clear" sounded at about 1:00 A.M., von Braun and the other scientists rushed from the air-raid shelters into burning buildings to save what they could. Von Braun and the others were shocked by the devastation they saw all around them. The damage was extensive; everywhere were parts of buildings, parts of missiles, parts of test equipment, and parts of people. Years of incredibly difficult and precise work had just gone up in smoke and flame. Many of the precious plans and engineering drawings were nothing but ashes now. Yet von Braun knew that, somehow, it could—it *must*—all be built again. A nearly unlimited supply of slave labor was available to make certain the program could continue.

* Dr. Walter Thiel, von Braun's deputy and the man in charge of developing the V-2's engine, was killed, along with Thiel's family and hundreds of others.

The RAF lost forty aircraft and 270 airmen on the mission and, although Churchill and Bomber Command declared the raid to be a success, it came too late to stop the V-1 program, and only slowed down the V-2 program by two months. The V-1s would continue wreaking havoc on London and, soon, so would the V-2s.[19]

IMMEDIATELY FOLLOWING THE raid, Hitler, Himmler, and Speer met to discuss ways to protect the missile factory and program. Someone suggested moving the works underground, and various possible sites were discussed. One, a vast, abandoned gypsum mine, already existed inside Kohnstein Mountain, near Nordhausen in the Harz Mountains of Thuringia, not far from Weimar. However, it would need to be greatly expanded in order to accommodate the assembly lines and the thousands of prisoners from Buchenwald, as well as the guards, scientists, and civilian technicians who would work there. The order to expand the mine was given and work commenced.[20] On August 28, 1943, a truckload of 107 scared, sullen inmates from Buchenwald arrived at the site, code-named *Arbeitslager Dora* ("Work Camp Dora"), and were ordered to begin digging and blasting through the rock. Thousands more would follow, and those who survived would describe Dora as a "living hell."

As the prisoners jumped down from their trucks at the Dora site, they were handed picks, shovels, and pneumatic drills, and ordered into the tunnel. There they were informed that their job was to enlarge and improve the existing underground structure; no reason was given for their assignment. The men filed into the cavernous space, were told where to dig and drill, and were set to work. Immediately the truncheons came out as the guards and foremen whipped the workers into an unsustainable pace. Holes were bored into the rock walls, explosives inserted, and blasting caps detonated. Eardrum-breaking blasts rocked the enclosed space, and lethal fragments of stone were hurled everywhere. Men went down wounded and dead; the dead were dragged to the tunnel entrance and stacked in mounds while the injured were either forced to continue working without medical attention or, if too badly hurt, shot on the spot by their SS overseers.[21]

Alex Baum, who was moved from Peenemünde to Dora, recalled the brutal conditions: "We didn't have showers for maybe six to eight months. We had one cup of water to drink a day, and we had a cup of coffee, a piece of bread and soup, that's it. We lost a tremendous amount of people."[22]

The mortality rate at Dora was appalling. Eighteen slaves died in October 1943; 172 in November; 670 in December—and the death toll escalated exponentially from there. In addition to dying from malnutrition, exhaustion, beatings, and industrial accidents, the usual concentration-camp diseases such as dysentery, typhus, tuberculosis, and pneumonia claimed thousands of lives. From October 1943 through March 1944, some 6,000 prisoners expired at Dora, their corpses trucked back to Buchenwald for cremation.* During its twenty-one months of operation, it is estimated that some 60,000 prisoners worked at Dora and between 20,000-30,000 men died there. On September 30, 1944, a directive from WVHA made Dora an independent camp, and its name was officially changed to Mittelbau Concentration Camp ("Mibau"). Once full production was reached at the Mittelbau site, nine hundred V-2s were produced each month.[23]

The inmate-workers were not as dedicated to the rocketry program as were the German engineers, and some prisoners did their best to sabotage the project, even at the risk of death. For example, Albert Kuntz, a member of the German Communist Party and one of the Buchenwald inmates drafted into the V-2 assembly lines at Dora (he also supervised the construction of the camp), did his utmost, along with a number of others, to throw monkey wrenches into the works.[24]

NAZI ARMAMENTS MINISTER Albert Speer had grown disdainful of the V-2 rocket program, feeling that, at best, the rockets would amount to only an insignificant pinprick against the Allies, who were carpeting German cities and factories with an average of 3,000 tons of bombs a day. "From the end of July 1943," Speer grumbled, "our tremendous industrial capacity was diverted to the huge missile.... The whole notion was absurd.... Hitler wanted to retaliate with thirty rockets [a day] that would have carried twenty-four tons of explosives to England daily. That was the equivalent to the bomb load of only twelve Flying Fortresses."[25]

Under the eye of *SS-Brigadeführer* Hans Kammler, head of construction at Dora, the slaves were literally worked to death in the damp, dust-choked tunnels. After Tunnel B, over a mile long, was finished (along with dozens of side

* To handle the death load, a temporary crematorium was built at Dora in January 1944, and a permanent one in the following spring. (Béon, pp. XIV-XV)

chambers), Tunnel A was begun. For twelve or more hours a day, SS and civilian supervisors urged on their slaves with whips and electrical cables encased in rubber. Explosions resulted in toxic fumes, and the dust-laden atmosphere inside the tunnels also contributed to the illnesses and deaths of prisoners. The inmates slept on the hard ground of the tunnels, never seeing the light of day, while the blasting went on around the clock, robbing the slaves of precious sleep. There was no water for washing, very little for drinking, less than rudimentary medical care and, as far as sanitation was concerned, oil drums cut in half served as toilets for the slaves. As within the concentration camps, the slaves were kept on a starvation diet—certainly not enough to sustain strength and life for those who were performing heavy labor.[26]

One of those transported from Buchenwald to work in the tunnels of Dora was a Frenchman, Jean Michel. He painted a nightmare picture of life at the underground facility: "In the tunnels, cold and moisture were intense. The water which oozed off the walls caused a nauseating and permanent moistness; we had the impression that our emaciated bodies mildewed alive. Prisoners became insane, others had ransacked nerves as the installation progressed: the amazing din was one of the causes of these disordered states—noise of the machines, noise of the power picks, continual explosions, the whole resonant and reflected in echoes without end by the closed world of the tunnel. No heating, no ventilation, not the least vat in which to wash oneself. Death weighed on us by the cold, of the feelings of asphyxiation, a rot which impregnated us."

Michel also reiterated the familiar litany of complaints remembered by every concentration camp inmate: the continual harassment by guards and *Kapos*, the meager rations, the evil stench, the inadequate clothing, the abject sense of hopelessness and utter degradation. Not even when a man was relieving himself could he count on a few moments of peace. Michel recounted seeing men, while sitting on boards above the latrine, dumped into the foul mess by their guards: "Then, there were outbursts of joy [by the SS]. The joke was too funny. Irresistible! Never had these men laughed so much. The more so as all the deportees suffered from dysentery." Covered with excrement from head to foot, and without water with which to wash himself, the hapless slave was compelled to roll in the rock dust in a vain attempt to cleanse himself. Michel recounted that German pigs and cattle were better cared for than were the slaves of Dora.[27]

An abortive workers' revolt took place at Mittelbau-Dora on December 15, 1943. A group of Italian inmates who were detailed to dig tunnels protested the harsh living and working conditions, citing the 1929 Geneva Convention, the provisions of which specified that prisoners of war could not be forced to perform labor for their captors' war industries. The SS answered by shooting seven of the protesters.[28]

In spite of some workers braving death by sabotaging the V-2s, the work went on unceasingly, night and day, the clang and bang of the assembly line augmented by the thud and crack of truncheons and whips being applied to the heads and backs of the slave workers.

FOR THE GERMANS, the war news during the first few months of 1944 was almost unbearably bad. American and British bombers continued to pound the cities of the Reich into dust. Weimar itself suffered heavily on February 2, 1944, when Allied bombers clobbered the city center. The German National Theater building, which dated from 1908 and was where the constitution of the Weimar Republic had been written, had been converted into an armaments factory making rifles, vehicles, and 75mm and 88mm tank-gun barrels; it was destroyed.

A second devastating raid took place seven days later; the precision bombing once again hit the center of town, killing hundreds of residents, destroying Goethe's, Liszt's, and Schiller's homes that had been preserved as museums, as well as Anna Amalia's Wittums Palace, the market square, and all of the Baroque buildings dating from the fourteenth and fifteenth centuries that framed the square's north side.[29]

These raids were but a preamble to the "Big Week" over Germany, as the period of February 20-25, 1944, was called. The United States Strategic Air Forces launched Operation Argument, designed to achieve total air superiority over Europe by luring the Luftwaffe into a final, annihilating aerial battle. In addition to attempting to rid the sky of Hermann Göring's air force, the American and British air forces targeted the German aircraft industry as never before. By flying a nearly unending stream of heavily escorted missions against aircraft manufacturing and assembly plants deep inside Germany, as well as other targets in and around the cities of Schweinfurt, Gotha, Leipzig, Brunswick, Regensburg, Augsburg, Stuttgart, and Steyr, the Americans and British hoped to win the war through the application of sheer air power alone—or at least demonstrate air power's ability to utterly destroy and demoralize the enemy, thus softening him up for invasion. In six days, the England-based U.S. Eighth Air Force bombers flew more than 3,000 sorties, while the

U.S. Fifteenth Air Force, based in Italy, flew more than five hundred. Together they dropped 10,000 tons of bombs and seriously disrupted German fighter production, convincing Albert Speer to better disperse his aircraft and ball-bearing manufacturing facilities; many went into underground facilities. The Germans also lost more than 600 airborne fighters trying to stem the assaults.

Inflicting the damage had its cost, however; during the Big Week, the U.S. lost 226 heavy bombers and 28 fighters—and more than 2,000 airmen.[30]

SAFELY UNDERGROUND, BEYOND the reach of bombs, work at the Mittelbau-Dora V-2 facility rolled on. When finally completed in March 1944, the vast underground facility consisted of two parallel, S-shaped tunnels with forty-six traverse tunnels connecting them. The main galleries were ten meters high and eight meters wide. Overall, there were seven miles of underground factory space, with a million square feet, making Mittelbau-Dora the largest underground factory—and concentration camp—ever built.[31]

Von Braun, who was well aware of the wretched working conditions and the plight of the slave laborers, said he felt powerless to change them; after all, he was a scientist, not a general or a civilian with unchallengeable authority. He noted, "It is hellish. My spontaneous reaction was to talk to one of the SS guards, only to be told with unmistakable harshness that I should mind my own business, or find myself in the same striped fatigues!... I realized that any attempt of reasoning on humane grounds would be utterly futile."[32]

Von Braun could have, instead, appealed to Himmler and Speer on strictly practical grounds, and perhaps convinced them that by wasting the slave labor, the SS was thus hurting Hitler's V-2 super-weapon program. He even could have told them of his fears of SS reprisal against him personally, and pointed out how indispensable he was to the program, but he said nothing, did nothing.

9
OFFICIAL INDIFFERENCE

"It is a problem that belongs to humanity.
It is a challenge to the soul of man."

Jacob Ben-Ami
Broadway actor

IN EARLY 1943, as thousands of inmates from Buchenwald literally slaved away in the tunnels at Mittlebau-Dora, were worked to death in the Buchenwald quarry, or were tortured in medical experiments inside Block 46, it seemed to the prisoners that they had been forgotten and abandoned by the world.

In America, however, grass-roots efforts were springing up that the organizers hoped would finally convince the U.S. government to do something urgently to end the suffering in the camps. While Jewish leaders such as Rabbi Stephen S. Wise, head of the American Jewish Congress; Dr. Chaim Weizmann, president of the Jewish Agency for Palestine; and *New York Times* owner/publisher Arthur Sulzberger preferred to work quietly behind the scenes to inform Roosevelt and the State Department about the desperate plight of Europe's Jews, there were others who believed that a gentle nudge to the ribs was not enough to get the job done. They felt that nothing less than a two-by-four between the eyes would be effective.

The message was clear for anyone who cared to look—European Jewry was being systematically erased, expunged, eliminated, and exterminated. If the State Department refused to get the message, if Roosevelt privately voiced support for the Jews but publicly fell silent, if Jewish leaders and Jewish groups sought to tread lightly so as to not create waves and cause a backlash, others did not. One of the most outspoken was a Lithuanian immigrant named Hillel Kook, who called himself Peter H. Bergson.

Born in 1915, Bergson was an unabashedly militant Zionist. The son of a rabbi, Bergson had come to the U.S. in 1940 and formed an organization known as the Bergson Group with the mission of awakening America to the facts about the persecution of European Jews. He held news conferences and sent out press releases but soon realized that these were not enough to break through the wall of official indifference that had been building in America since 1933. If President Roosevelt was unwilling to issue directives to the State

Department to do everything possible to save the Jews, and if the State Department could not be budged from its position of non-intervention, then the only alternative Bergson saw was to create such a groundswell of awareness and protest that Roosevelt and Hull would be embarrassed and forced by a tide of public opinion into action.

Full of ideas on how to rescue the Jews (as well as establish a permanent Jewish homeland in Palestine), Bergson put together several committees and engineered several schemes, such as forming an organization in 1940 known as the "Jewish Army of Stateless and Palestinian Jews" whose purpose was to fight alongside the Allies.[1] On February 8, 1943, Bergson shocked New Yorkers with a full-page ad in the *New York Times* whose headline screamed, "Action—Not Pity—Can Save Millions Now!" Below an illustration of a soldier wearing a helmet with the Star of David on it, and holding a dying rabbi in one hand while defiantly brandishing a Thompson sub-machine gun in the other, the subhead rang out: "Extinction or Hope for the Remnants of European Jewry? It is for Us to Give the Answer." Bergson's voluminous text pulled no punches and detailed the situation: "Daily, hourly, the greatest crime of all time is being committed: a defenseless and innocent people is being slaughtered in a wholesale massacre of millions. What is more tragic—they are dying for no reason or purpose."

Calling on the nations fighting the Nazis to authorize the formation of a 200,000-man army* made up of "stateless and Palestinian Jews"—those living in North Africa and others who had managed to escape the Holocaust—the ad used rousing language to rally support: "Suicide squads of the Jewish Army would engage in desperate commando raids deep into the heart of Germany. Jewish pilots would bomb German cities in reprisal."[2]

Establishment Jewish leaders such as Rabbi Wise were horrified by Bergson's full-page call-to-arms and quickly condemned the whole idea as a terrible scheme that would do nothing but bring more Nazi hatred down upon the Jews and possibly even stir up trouble for Jews in the U.S.

As dramatic and shocking as the ads were, they weren't enough; Bergson needed something bigger, more dramatic, something so huge it could not be ignored. He and famed showman Billy Rose began collaborating on an idea that would produce heightened public awareness of the plight of European Jews—an idea that would turn New York upside down.

---

* Earlier, on December 4, 1941, Dr. Samuel Harden Church, president of the Carnegie Institute, proposed the same thing. He said a fighting force of 200,000 American Jews should be trained in Canada and, after they helped defeat the Nazis, they should be allowed to emigrate to Palestine. (Baker, p. 435)

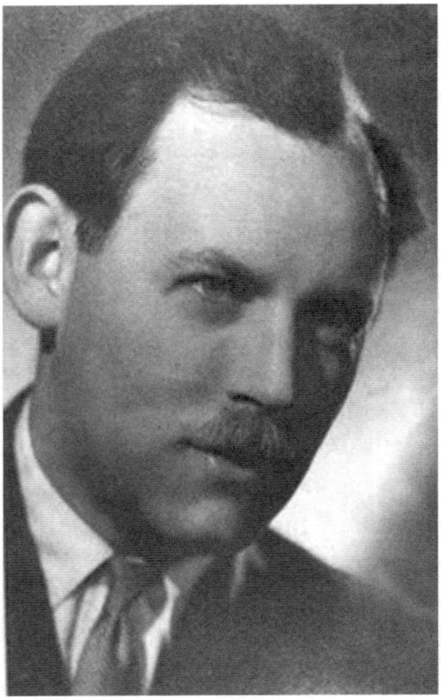

Peter Bergson (U.S. National Archives)

IN MARCH 1943, Rabbi Stephen Wise beat Bergson to the punch. Evermore aware that the fate of Europe's Jews was deteriorating by the day, Wise conceived of a ecumenical rally in which a stage full of both Christian and Jewish leaders would speak out forcibly against the Nazis. Wise gathered his American Jewish Congress, along with the Church Peace Union, the Free World Association, the American Federation of Labor (AFL), and the Congress of Industrial Organizations (CIO), and several other Jewish and Christian groups, and staged a "Stop Hitler Now" rally on March 1, 1943, at Madison Square Garden.

Flocking by bus, taxi, and subway to the arena were tens of thousands Christians and Jews—police estimated that a crowd of 75,000 had gathered outside the facility—all marching in solidarity with the persecuted people of Europe. While over 50,000 listened to loudspeakers set up outside the building, 21,000 crammed themselves inside the building to hear Rabbi Wise, along with Mayor Fiorella LaGuardia; Dr. Chaim Weizmann, president of the Jewish Agency for Palestine; 1933 Nobel Peace prize winner Sir Norman Angell; Bishop Henry St. George Tucker of the Episcopal Church of America; and dozens more read statements condemning the actions of the Nazis and urging actions to rescue the Jews. Numerous other notable leaders, including New York Governor Thomas Dewey; Great Britain's Chief Rabbi J.H. Hertz; the Archbishop of Canterbury; and Supreme Court Justice William O. Douglas spoke to the audience via radio hook-up. Statements and messages of sympathy were also read from the ambassadors of Belgium, Britain, Yugoslavia, and other nations. Republican presidential candidate Wendell Wilkie sent a message calling for "practical measures [to] be formulated and carried out immediately to save as many Jews as possible."

In introducing Rabbi Wise, Herman Shulman, chairman of the special committee of the American Jewish Congress on the European situation, remarked that months had gone by since the United Nations* had denounced the Nazis' crimes against the Jews and threatened to take action against Germany. But, said Shulman, no action had been taken.

At the rally, those in attendance adopted an eleven-point resolution—the concrete proposals which Roosevelt had requested during Wise's meeting with him on December 8, 1942. These points included that neutral agencies be called upon to pressure Germany into releasing Jewish victims from ghettoes, concentration camps, and death camps, and allowing them to emigrate to "havens of refuge as will be provided"; that the United Nations take immediate action to establish sanctuaries and safe havens in Allied or neutral nations for Jewish immigrants or escapees; that the U.S. State Department and Great Britain immediately loosen their restrictive immigration policies to allow for the entry of persecuted European Jews and other minorities; that Great Britain be urged to drastically increase the number of Jews allowed to emigrate to Palestine; that the United Nations urge South American countries to relax their immigration laws to allow for a temporary influx of refugees; that the United Nations guarantee to compensate neutral countries for the cost of housing, feeding, and caring for refugees that they allow in; and that in the event Nazi Germany refuses to allow refugees to emigrate, that the United Nations make arrangements for neutral agencies such as the Red Cross to distribute adequate food and medicine to Jews being held in ghettoes and concentration camps.

The final point made by the rally's organizers called for the collection of documentation regarding the atrocities being committed and the establishment of a tribunal to hold war-crimes trials of the Nazi perpetrators. To conclude the rally, several Jewish rabbis said prayers for the dead (*Kaddish*).[3]

The following day, an editorial in the *New York Times* repeated the calls for action that filled Madison Square Garden and requested that the United States "set a good example" by loosening its restrictive immigration laws. The message was clear: If the Allies did not act swiftly and decisively, there would be no Jews left to save.[4]

WHILE THE "STOP Hitler Now" rally was well-publicized and well-attended, Peter Bergson saw that it had one major flaw—it was all talk, talk, talk—one speech after another. Although the subject was emotional, he felt there was no

* The term "United Nations" was used generally to describe the Allied nations at war with the Axis powers. The formal organization known as the United Nations, which replaced the League of Nations, did not come into existence until June 1945 when representatives from fifty-one nations met in San Francisco to sign the United Nations Charter.

real emotion behind the presentation, nothing to wrench people's hearts and pull tears from their eyes. And it only played before New York audiences.

Bergson and showman Billy Rose met to put the finishing touches on something much bigger—a huge, dramatic presentation that could be taken on the road and stir passions wherever it played. On March 9, 1943, the pageant, titled "We Will Never Die," premiered at Madison Square Garden. Created in conjunction with Bergson's Committee for a Jewish Army and Billy Rose, "We Will Never Die" opened to a full house. So many people—20,000 of them—purchased advance tickets for the 8:45 P.M. showing that a second showing, at 11:45 P.M., had to be scheduled to accommodate another 20,000 spectators.

The moving, highly emotional pageant, which featured a cast of 200 rabbis, 200 cantors, 400 actors (including Paul Muni, Edward G. Robinson, Stella Adler, and Sylvia Sidney), 100 musicians of the NBC Symphony Orchestra, and a stage dominated by two towering tablets inscribed with the Ten Commandments, was written by Ben Hecht, directed by Moss Hart, with musical score by Kurt Weill. The production, financed by the Bergson Group, was billed as a memorial to the estimated two million Jews who had already perished at the hands of the Nazis. In the pageant's stirring final sequence, voices of the Jewish dead urged the audience to remember them.

The production's narrator, the distinguished Broadway actor Jacob Ben-Ami, ended the performance by reminding the audience that the mass killing of Europe's Jews was not solely a Jewish problem. "It is a problem," Ben-Ami intoned, "that belongs to humanity. It is a challenge to the soul of man."

The pageant was a sensation. Additional sold-out performances played in Boston, Chicago, Los Angeles, and Philadelphia, with Eleanor Roosevelt, six Supreme Court justices, and 300 Senators and Congressmen attending a performance in Washington, D.C. Mrs. Roosevelt described the performance as "one of the most impressive and moving pageants I have ever seen. No one who heard each group come forward and give the story of what had happened to it at the hands of a ruthless German military will ever forget those haunting words: 'Remember us.'"[5]

Not unexpectedly, the pageant ran into considerable opposition, but not by pro-Nazi groups. Rabbi Wise's American Jewish Congress and the Zionist Organization of America, still fearing that the pageant's message was too emotional and inflammatory, applied pressure on city officials in the steel city of Gary, Indiana, to cancel Bergson's plans to stage the production there. As Robert Beir wrote, "At a time when the unprecedented massacre in Europe continued 'unabated,' to use Roosevelt's word, Jewish leaders chose an internal struggle—disparaging the Bergson Group—over rescue.... Stephen Wise and Nahum Goldmann [president of the World Jewish Congress] denounced Bergson. They saw him as a threat to their establishment. They saw him as misrepresenting American Jewish opinion. They voiced concerns that his activities might stir up anti-Semitism, fearing that 'Bergson would bring pogroms to America.' Goldmann advised that the State Department either draft Bergson [into the military] or deport him."[6]

But Bergson was not intimidated. If anything, the criticism impelled him to think in even larger terms than a pageant. And what could be larger than creating new nation—a nation of, by, and for Jews? He began working on how to pull it off.

AT THE STATE Department, however, Assistant Secretary Breckinridge Long was unmoved by editorials, rallies, pageants, and the international cries for a change in America's immigration policies. President Roosevelt, although not unsympathetic to the plight of the Jews, could easily have called Long into the Oval Office and given him a blistering chewing out, demanding that the policies be changed. But he did not do so. Outside of the Jewish community, there was no groundswell of public support for such a change—but there were plenty of anti-Semites inside and outside of government determined to make the president's life miserable on the issue.

As early as 1940, Long had made his position clear: The mass of European Jewish refugees trying to enter the United States was deeply infiltrated with spies and saboteurs; to allow any of them in would seriously compromise national security.[7] The anti-immigrant Congress, too, seemed little interested in doing anything substantial or immediate to reverse the situation, and offered only vague reassurances that something would be done. In truth, almost nothing happened to aid the Jews or stop the Nazis from sending them marching to their deaths.[8]

It is likely that few if any of the inmates at Buchenwald during this time knew anything about the conflicting sentiments that were raging in the U.S. and elsewhere—everything from official indifference to desperate measures being demanded. All they knew was that their existence was becoming increasingly more difficult by the day, more of them were dying, and the rest of the world seemed to care nothing about their situation.

10
BUCHENWALD, INC.

"By acting in a polite, obedient, and submissive manner, it was our hope to be able to work in this almost civilized atmosphere for as long as possible."

Louis Gros
Buchenwald inmate

NOT ONLY WERE the concentration camps ideal places in which to conduct secret medical experiments, but the camps were also becoming tremendous profit centers for the SS. The only surprise is that it took the Nazis so long to figure it out.

After September 1939, as more and more able-bodied men were drafted into military service and the number of factory workers declined, numerous German companies had begun renting prisoners from the SS at a relatively small cost (about twenty cents per hour per worker at 2013 prices). Some of these companies are famous names today: BMW, Volkswagen, Daimler-Benz, Ford, Opel (a subsidiary of General Motors), Messerschmitt, Heinkel, Krupp Steel, I.G. Farben, Bayer, Siemens, Kodak, Hugo Boss, and scores of small, lesser-known firms such as Oskar Schindler's enamelware factory in Krakow, Poland.[1]

In December 1939, Himmler had announced, "The supervision of the economic matters of these institutions [concentration camps] and their application to work is the responsibility of...[*SS-Obergruppenführer* Oswald] Pohl."[2] The following year Pohl and Georg Lörner formed the *Deutsche Wirtschafts-Betriebe* (German Economic Enterprises) as a holding company, commonly known as the DWB Combine. This organization controlled many of the business enterprises run by the SS Administrative Department and at one time had a capitalization in excess of 46 million Reichsmarks.[3]

It was not until 1942, however, when manpower shortages at the front became critical, that the Nazi hierarchy finally grasped the importance of the tremendous workforce the concentration-camp prisoners represented—a resource that was not only being under-utilized but destroyed. As William Shirer observed in *The Rise and Fall of the Third Reich*, none of the Nazi leaders "understood at this time how valuable the millions of Jews might be to the Reich as slave labor."[4] It fell to the SS to convert this asset, languishing behind barbed wire, into manpower to benefit the Reich. While inmates had toiled in quarries and other make-work enterprises at the camps since the early days, it was Albert Speer, the Nazi Minister for Armaments, who urged Hitler to take full advantage of this resource and make the huge numbers of prisoners available to various industrial concerns. During the course of the war it is estimated that Nazi Germany squeezed the last ounce of productivity out of over 700,000 prisoners—the majority of whom were sent to their deaths when they ceased to be of value to the Third Reich.[5]

As previously mentioned, a special department of the SS—the WVHA, under Pohl—was established for the exclusive purpose of exploiting this abundance of free labor. As the war continued and German losses mounted and able-bodied factory workers were drafted into the military, concentration camp prisoners (male and female) were conscripted for factory work. If an armaments manufacturer needed laborers, they sent a request to the WVHA and soon had the requisite number of hands on the job site. As the SS charged a fee to the company for each slave laborer (from four to six Reichsmarks per worker per day),* the SS coffers quickly grew fat on the enterprise.

To compete with private industry. the SS established a number of factories under the aegis of *Deutsche Ausrüstungswerke* (DAW, or German Armament Works)—an SS defense contractor with factories and workshops inside various camps such as Auschwitz, Dachau, Sachsenhausen, and, of course, Buchenwald. Many of the rifles, *Panzerfaüste* (an anti-tank weapon similar to the U.S. bazooka), artillery pieces, cameras, binoculars, military uniforms, and footwear, were manufactured by slave laborers.[6]

Despite especially difficult conditions—the incessant bombing of the factories by the American and British air forces—German industry, manned by hundreds of thousands of slaves and under Speer's direction, began to do a remarkable job of turning out tanks, aircraft, ships, submarines, wheeled vehicles, munitions, artillery pieces, and the other instruments of war. And yet, even while these slave laborers were proving invaluable to the German war effort, millions more were still being herded into gas chambers.

Obviously, being forced to live the life of a slave is not an ideal existence, but at least the slave is alive. Even the antebellum American plantation owners knew that the economy of the South depended upon the productive output of slaves and did not slaughter them *en masse*; the Nazis, on the other hand, so single-mindedly driven to destroy the Jews of Europe, were slow to figure out that *their* slaves, if put to useful work in armaments plants and elsewhere, could have greatly improved the Reich's chance for survival—and possibly even victory.

* In World War II dollars, the SS would have received an average of $2.40 per worker per twelve-hour day.

Even Heinrich Himmler, the master of the SS, had a sudden epiphany and realized that a tremendous amount of "wastage" was taking place among the concentration camp inmates—wastage that must be stopped and inmates capable of working put to better use. Only in a few instances, and then only late in the war, were the inmates of the concentration camps, especially Buchenwald, consigned temporarily to factories instead of the ovens. Thus, on December 28, 1942, the SS Main Office of Economic Administration sent a most-startling letter to the camp doctors of all the concentration camps:

"The enclosed compilation of the current arrivals and departures in all the concentration camps is sent to you for your information. It discloses that out of 136,000 arrivals about 70,000 died. With such a high rate of death the number of the prisoners can never be brought up to the figure as has been ordered by the *Reichsführer* of the SS [Himmler].

"The camp doctors must use all means at their disposal to reduce essentially this death rate in the various camps. The best doctor in a concentration camp is not the one who believes that he must stand out for uncalled severity, but the one who by his supervision and exchange keeps the working capacity at the various labor commands at the highest possible level.

"The camp doctors must supervise more often than in the past the food of the prisoners and, with the approval of the administration, submit improvement proposals to the camp commandants. These, however, must not only appear on paper, but must be controlled regularly by the camp doctors. Furthermore, the camp doctors are to see to it that the working conditions at the various labor places are improved as much as possible.

"To this purpose it will be necessary that the camp doctors inspect the labor places on the ground and convince themselves about the conditions of work.

"The *Reichsführer-SS* has ordered that the death rate absolutely must be reduced. For this reason the aforementioned has been ordered and a monthly report on this matter is to be submitted to the Chief of the Department D III. The first report to be submitted on 1 February 1943.

[Signature illegible] Klueder [?]
SS Brigadeführer and Major General of the Arms Survey"[7]

IN MAY 1943, as a way of boosting production at the DAW and Gustloff-Werk

II, the SS instituted a bonus program at Buchenwald that rewarded exceptionally diligent inmates with "canteen coupons," the legal tender in the camp, that could be used in exchange for goods—cigarettes, food, and other products—at the prisoner canteen.

There was also another reward for diligence: In the spring of 1943 a brothel (known as the *Sonderbau*, or "special building") was established at Buchenwald (a number of other camps also had brothels*) that could be frequented by special prisoners as an incentive. On July 16, 1943, sixteen female inmates between the ages of twenty and thirty were brought in by the SS from the women's camp at Ravensbrück. The women had volunteered for the duty because they had been promised better rations, a quarter of the earnings (each visit cost two Reichsmarks, or eighty cents), and an early release from confinement. Harry Stein wrote, "Each of the women had to place herself at the disposal of an average of five men per day. Inmates of the Little Camp, Jews, Sinti, Romani [i.e. Gypsies], and Russians were prohibited from visiting the brothel. Others, primarily German, Austrian, Czech, and Polish inmates, could submit a written application for this privilege to the SS camp command by way of the officer in charge of their block. The authorizations were announced by the SS at the evening roll call."[8]

Jacob Werber said that he was one of those detailed to build the Sonderbau "for the Aryan prisoners at Buchenwald." He remembered that the women had come from Ravensbrück and were "treated like pets by the SS men. Each day they would take them out for walks. After a month or so the women were completely worn out. They would be killed and replaced by a fresh contingent from Ravensbrück. The political prisoners, because they didn't want to exploit other prisoners, and the Jehovah's Witnesses, for religious reasons, refused to participate in yet another example of barbarity."[9]

WILHELM GUSTLOFF-WERK II grew into a giant facility with various buildings, workshops, and warehouses, including two main halls each 120 meters in length. In order to more efficiently bring raw materials and components to the Gustloff-Werk II, and to ship the finished pieces out of Buchenwald, a railroad line was needed that would link the camp with Weimar. At the end of March 1943, hundreds of inmates were put to work building this

* According to an article in the January 15, 2007, issue of Germany's *Der Spiegel* magazine, these camps included Auschwitz, Buchenwald, Dachau, Sachsenhausen, and at least six more.

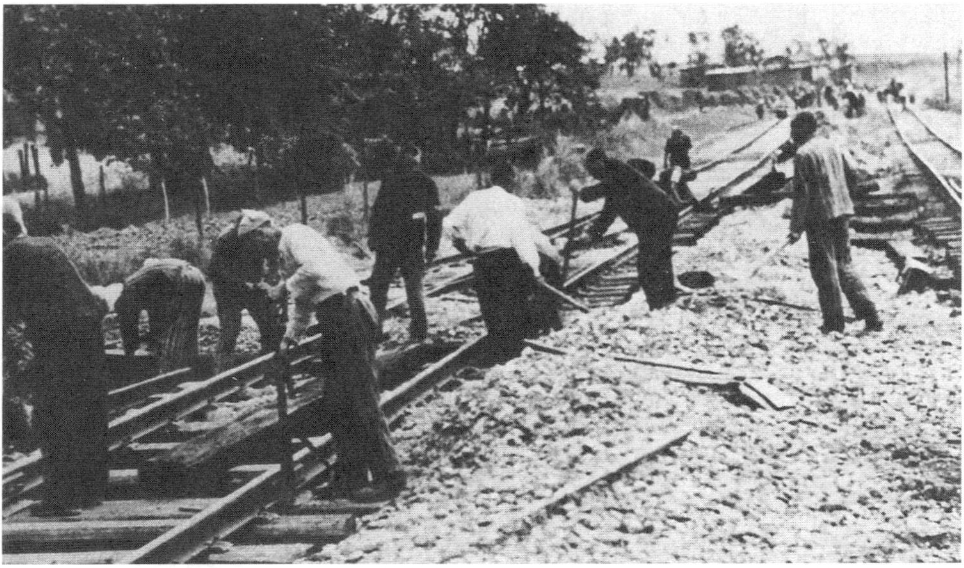

Buchenwald inmates working on the railroad line between Weimar and the camp. (Buchenwald Memorial)

line, which the SS demanded be finished in three months. Building such a line in such a short period of time would have been heavy, backbreaking work even for an army of strong, well-nourished workmen; for the living skeletons of Buchenwald, working on the railroad was akin to a death sentence.

First the planned rail line had to be cleared of trees—thousands of them—then the railroad bed had to be built up with packed earth and gravel. Next, the wooden ties needed to be set in place and the heavy steel rails staked down—all to the constant beat of the whip and rubber truncheon. Workers collapsed by the score, their hearts and lungs and will to live exhausted to the point of death. Whenever a man went down, another was conscripted from the camp to take his place, giving the whole merciless operation the appearance of a modern-day reenactment of the building of the Egyptian pyramids. Built at an unforgiving pace, the six-mile-long railroad line was inaugurated in June 1943, but it had so many faults and weaknesses that it was virtually unusable. More work needed to be done to stabilize the line—work that would take another year.[10]

To boost armament production to the maximum, Oswald Pohl, head of the WVHA, issued a directive to all concentration camps in November 1943 that read, in part, "In cases of extreme emergency the inmates are also to work on Sundays, but only in the morning. To a significant degree, the work which is relevant for the war and for victory is presently being carried out by inmates, and in view of this circumstance is it absolutely essential that daily working time amount to no less than eleven hours."[11]

AT THE BEGINNING of 1944, prisoners continued to arrive at Buchenwald by the thousands. A train full of 2,000 Frenchmen from Compiègne that pulled in on January 19, 1944, was just one of several that arrived each week. The journey had taken three days and the men huddled together in the cars had endured bitter cold as well as the usual lack of food, water, and sanitary facilities. Yet the ice-coated train sat in the Buchenwald rail yard for an hour while SS personnel greeted them with obscenities and hurled invectives at the men in the boxcars. "In Buchenwald, we don't have any sick," the guards yelled. "You are either healthy or you go to the crematorium!"[12]

The inmates sank into a collective depression; not even the news five months later that the Allies had finally captured, after months of heavy fighting, the German-held monastery at Monte Cassino on May 18, 1944, could cheer them. Monte Cassino was hundreds of miles away, in the center of Italy, of absolutely no direct help to them. Even the capture of Rome by the Americans on June 4, 1944, while pointing to an eventual Allied victory, did not elicit cheers of joy. At Buchenwald, the Gustloff-Werk II laborers knew that the devices they were assembling were going into unimaginable weapons that might somehow enable the Nazis to snatch victory from inevitable defeat.[13]

At dawn on June 6, 1944, the greatest, most important combined aerial and amphibious assault in the history of warfare unfolded along the northern coast of France. Operation Overlord, as it was called, deposited 175,000 American, British, and Canadian troops at five assault beaches across a sixty-mile stretch of Normandy coastline. Soldiers in gliders and suspended from parachutes were dropped farther inland to assist in the operation. Nearly everywhere the assault came off like clockwork; only at Omaha Beach, where the U.S. 1st and 29th Infantry Divisions landed, was the German resistance stronger than expected, and the carnage greater than feared. Yet, by noon, the Americans, with considerable loss of blood and life, had overcome the obstacles, climbed the bluff, taken their objectives, and were starting to move into the hedgerow country.[14]

By the time Hitler realized that the Normandy operation was "the real thing" and not the feint he believed it to be, it was too late for the Germans to repel it.[15] Now that the Western Allies had established a lodgment on the Continent, it was just a matter of time before the end of Nazi Germany—and the salvation of the hundreds of thousands of people in the concentration and death camps—was at hand.

The news of the D-Day landings buoyed the spirits of the inmates of Buchenwald gathered around clandestine radio sets. But no one expected that the Yanks would be crashing through the gates the next day—or even anytime soon. After all, Normandy was over 500 straight-line miles from Buchenwald, and there were millions of German soldiers between Normandy and Thuringia. Besides, Hitler would not suddenly panic and surrender just because the Allies had at last landed on European soil. Weeks, perhaps even months, would transpire before Buchenwald could be liberated—if the Germans didn't exterminate all of them first.

BY 1944, OVER 6,000 Buchenwald inmates were "employed" in Buchenwald's Gustloff-Werk II and DAW plants, usually in eleven-hour shifts, six days a week. One of those workers was Louis Gros, a teenager from France. After being arrested (along with his father) in November 1942 for delivering anti-Nazi propaganda leaflets around his hometown of Épinal, he was incarcerated in the transit camp of Compiègne, then endured a hot, week-long ride in a crammed-full boxcar without food or water or sanitation facilities to Buchenwald. Nearly crazed with thirst by the time they reached the camp, the nearly 2,000 men were released from their rolling prison and allowed to drink from large tubs of water set up inside the gate.

Gros recalled, "For now, Buchenwald is our oasis. This unexpected water of life is there for us in abundance, if only we can reach a tub." His father, with surprising calmness, removed a shoe, made his way through the frantic humanity struggling to reach the tubs, filled the shoe, drank, then refilled it again and brought it back for his son. "I drink, at length and without taking a breath, the best, the most beautiful, the most perfumed and the clearest of running water that it is possible to imagine, with the certainty that I will never again have the opportunity to appreciate the experience so much, since it seems impossible that I could ever be inflicted with such thirst again."

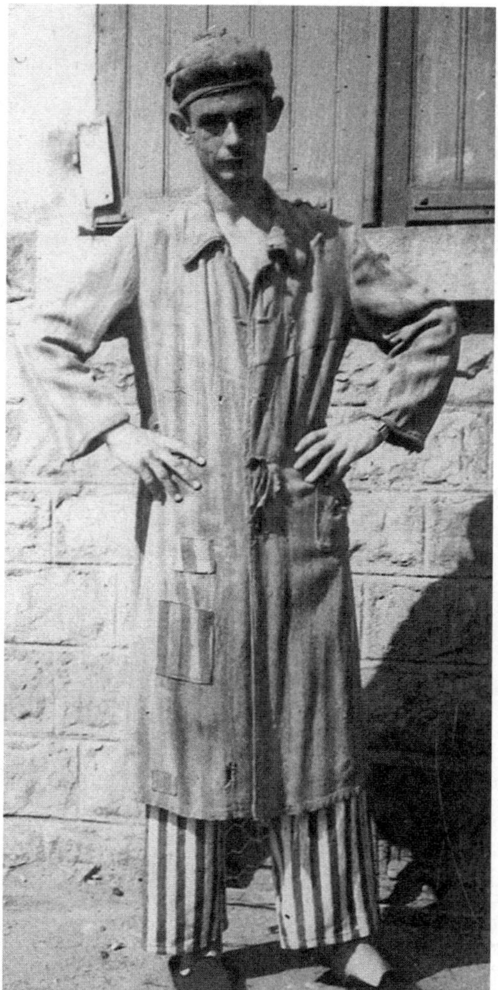

French inmate Louis Gros, photographed after his liberation in 1945. (Courtesy Louis Gros)

At that moment, a truck that Louis had seen earlier at the train station reappeared near the group at the water tubs. SS men began unloading corpses of men who had died on the rail journey, throwing them to the ground, treating them roughly as though they were nothing more than road-kill. The thirsty prisoners stopped to observe. Louis then noticed that two of the bodies—two men who had been executed during a failed escape from the train—were taken out and carefully placed behind the rear wheels of the truck. The SS driver then put the truck into reverse and backed over the two corpses, crushing them.

"We watched as the stomachs of the two men rupture under the weight of the wheels," said Louis, "an unbearable sight revealing the very particular ethics of these gentlemen in uniform. The truck then stops, engages forward gear, and drives off. We have no wish to see any more, and there is nothing more to see. We get the picture."[16]

A FEW WEEKS went by before Gros found himself at a work bench inside the Gustloff-Werk II factory. "Working in the factory," he said, "was considered a lucky assignment for any inmate; spared the backbreaking work in the quarry and other heavy construction jobs, the workers at either the DAW factory or

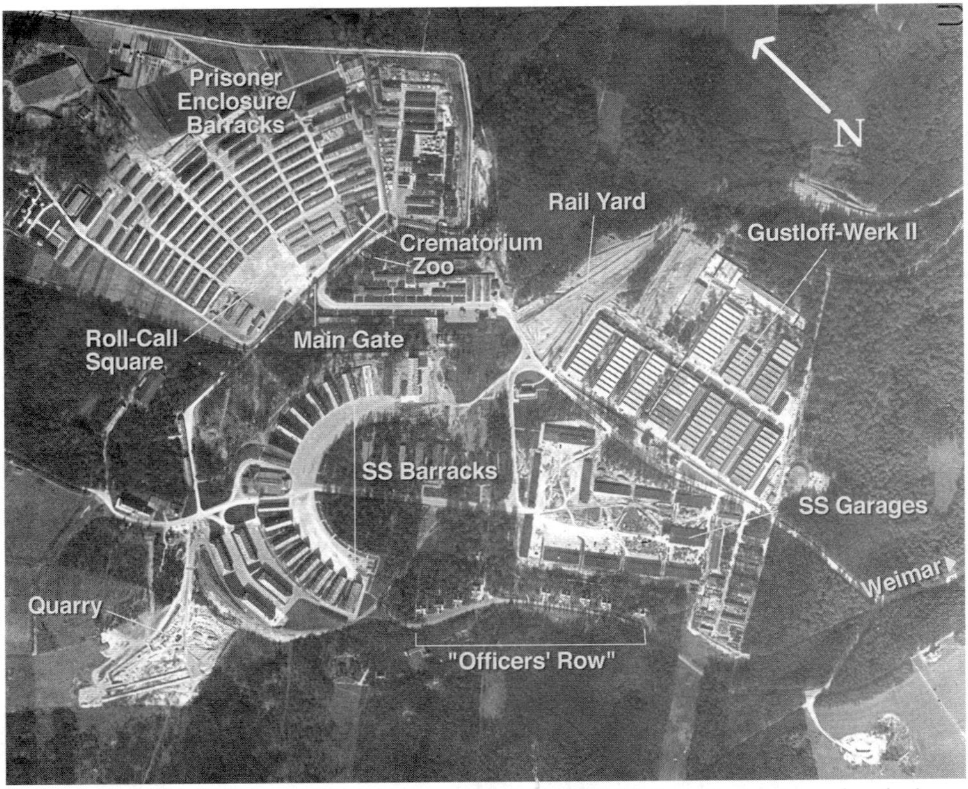

This aerial photo of KL Buchenwald was taken by the U.S. Air Force before it was bombed. (Buchenwald Memorial)

the Gustloff-Werk were able to work indoors and treated slightly more humanely than those who slaved under the weight of stones or felt the overseer's lash for not moving fast enough. Here, care and precision were regarded as being more important than speed." But he wasn't sure what he was working on; it wasn't until later that he learned that the factory was manufacturing precision components for von Braun's V-2 rockets.[17]

"It was forbidden for us to talk with one another or to move freely about the workplace," Gros said. "We were also forbidden to inquire about the project we were working on. We adopted a very 'Germanic-type discipline,' even to the point of requesting…our periodic need to use the toilet in the factory (a real pleasure compared to the foul latrines in the barracks; there was even hot water in the factory bathrooms). We even received an extra ration of soup! By acting in a polite, obedient, and submissive manner, it was our hope to be able to work in this almost civilized atmosphere for as long as possible."

The French teenager also noted, "I and a few others employed at our particular task sat at a large worktable. Our job was *Isolierer* ("insulator") or, in other words, making insulation for some of the [V-2 rocket] components. Using strips of kraft paper, our job was to take the paper from large bobbins and wind it around ring-shaped electrical reels. Someone—I don't know who—got the idea that a poorly wrapped reel was the Achilles heel of the rocket; if this reel failed, then the V-2 would fail. Therefore, it was in the best interests of Hitler's enemies to try and sabotage this project at its weakest point."[18]

GERMANY'S MALE POPULATION was being decimated in the summer of 1944 as more and more men were drafted, given rudimentary military training, and thrown into the gaping maw of battle in a futile effort to halt the tide of inevitable defeat. And the inmates from the concentration camps were taking their places in more and more factories of the Reich in ever-increasing numbers.

The requisitioning of slave laborers was all very bureaucratic and businesslike, as divorced from human empathy as the purchasing of office supplies or draft animals. To obtain workers from a concentration camp, a company would first submit a request in writing to the commandant of a nearby camp or directly to WVHA's *Amt D-II*; if a camp commandant received the request, he would forward it to *D-II*. (These requests came on an average of one a week.) If inmates were available (and they almost always were), *SS-Standartenführer* Gerhard Maurer, the director of *D-II*, and the camp commandant would visit the firm to determine the nature of the work. Maurer would then outline the prerequisites that the company must provide, such as security and housing. If the firm agreed to those prerequisites (and they almost always did), the *Amt D-II* director would forward the requisition to Oswald Pohl, the chief of administration of the *SS-Hauptamt* in Berlin. If Pohl approved the request (and he almost always did), the camp commander would be notified, arrangements to provide the workers were finalized, and the slaves were transported to the facility and put to work.[19]

Buchenwald did its best to contribute to the Nazi war effort. For example, in 1943, a sub-camp was established at Schönebeck, eleven miles southeast of Magdeburg, with the code name "Julius." Prisoners consigned to this camp worked at the Junkers aircraft factories there, known as *FZS* (*Flugzeug Zweigwerk Schönebeck*) and *MZS* (*Motor Zweigwerk Schönebeck*). Many other firms, such as Ford Motor Company's German subsidiary, Ford Werk AG, in Cologne, also benefitted from slave labor provided by Buchenwald.*[20]

DESPITE THE ALLIED invasion, the work at Buchenwald's Gustloff-Werk II factory continued through the summer of 1944, with more and more components being completed, crated, and shipped northward to Nordhausen each day. As they worked quietly at their assembly benches, the inmates began to have thoughts—thoughts of sabotage. It was obvious that the components on which they worked so diligently day after day were of great value to the Nazis' secret enterprise, perhaps even essential to victory.

Despite the relatively easier working conditions in the factory, some inmates had no desire to help the enemy. One inmate, Leon Weissmann, refused an order to report to the factory, a refusal that got him punished. "[SS sergeant] Jakobs screamed at me, beat me, and kicked me several times.... When I reported to him the next morning, everyone was sent away and Jakobs ordered me to jump into a pit of ice-cold water with all my clothes on. Three times I was forced to stay under water till I could no longer hold my breath. He threatened to kill me if I ever mentioned the occurrence to anyone. When I was finally permitted to climb out of the pit, Jakobs beat me and kicked me for another half hour." At least Weissmann was not murdered for his insubordination.[21]

In whispered conversations in the latrines, the only place inmates felt safe to discuss matters that might otherwise get them killed, methods of wrecking the assembly operations at the factory were discussed. Those thoughts of sabotage

* After the war Ford admitted that slave labor was used at the company's plant in Cologne, but claimed its U.S. head office had lost contact with its German subsidiary before America entered the war in December 1941, regaining control only seven years later. The favorable treatment accorded by Nazi Germany to Ford Motor Company/Ford Werke AG was attributed to a personal friendship between Henry Ford and Adolph Hitler. Henry Ford reportedly made annual birthday gifts of 50,000 Deutschmarks to Hitler; in return, on the automaker's 75th birthday in July 1938, Hitler awarded Henry Ford the Great Cross of the German Order of the Eagle.

No doubt much of Hitler's admiration for Henry Ford was because the automotive pioneer had written in the early 1920s a series of ninety-two anti-Semitic articles which were published in the *Dearborn Independent*—a newspaper owned by Ford—which blamed almost all the troubles facing America and the world on an "international Jewish cabal." These articles were later collected and published in a four-volume set of books entitled *The International Jew: The World's Foremost Problem*; the books were available at Ford dealerships (and can still be found on anti-Semitic websites). In 1927, Ford publicly apologized for writing the articles, but the apology apparently was ignored by Hitler. Following Ford's death in 1947, the Ford family and the Ford Motor Company disavowed the patriarch's anti-Semitism and have since donated considerable sums to Jewish charities. (www. jewishvirtuallibrary.org/jsource/anti-semitism/ford; *Bulldog News*, Fresno State, September 6, 1998; *The Daily Republican*, March 18, 1998).

were given voice and quickly discarded—German technicians checked every device before it was shipped out of the plant; any obvious signs of sloppy work or deliberate sabotage were sure to get the slave workers executed. Perhaps the factory, built mostly of wood, could be set on fire. That seemed possible, but the Germans had equipped the grounds and buildings with plenty of hydrants and fire hoses; any blaze would be extinguished in minutes and result in the execution of the arsonists. Perhaps, thought some inmates, improvised explosions could be used to destroy the plant. But obtaining enough explosive material was regarded as a sheer impossibility.

There was only one solution that seemed to offer any hope: Convince the Allies to bomb the factory. But how to contact the Allies? There were only two options: Carry a message to them or send a message by radio. The first was out of the question; no one, as far as the inmates knew, had ever escaped from Buchenwald. The second seemed more workable. A small, select group of inmates knew that radio receivers existed within the camp; perhaps it would not be all that hard to construct a workable transmitter. It was a matter of finding someone to do it.[22]

One of those with some knowledge of radios was Otto Roth, a German communist and staunch opponent of the Nazis, who had been at KL Buchenwald since September 1939. An electrician before being picked up by the Gestapo for anti-Nazi activities, he was given a red triangle to sew onto his uniform, indicating his status as a political prisoner, and assigned to the Electrician's Detachment. There he came into daily contact with other prisoners, all of whom had the skills, desire, and means to construct clandestine radio receivers with which they could learn about developments in the outside world.

One of the men Roth met at the camp was Armin Walther, a radio specialist, who noted, "My job in Buchenwald consisted of building and repairing [the SS's] communications equipment, transmitters, teletype machines, and signal apparatus." With their invaluable skills, Walther and Roth, along with as many as twenty other technicians—using parts pilfered from German radios and the electrical supply room—had already constructed seven clandestine wireless sets. With the right parts and the assembled brainpower, it would not be too difficult to build a transmitter. Walther and another electrician, Gwidon Damaszyn, put one together and installed it secretly in the camp theater.[23]

There was only one problem. Even if the inmates managed to build a transmitter powerful enough to reach the Allies and a message was sent that there was a factory at Buchenwald that was manufacturing components for some powerful secret weapon, who in their right mind would believe them? A campaign of disinformation had been waged by both sides since the beginning of the war—false messages, fake alarms, non-existent military units—all designed to confuse and confound the enemy. The Allies had, in fact, launched the greatest misinformation campaign in the history of warfare—the creation of a fake army around General George S. Patton, Jr., that convinced the Germans that the real invasion of France would come at the Pas de Calais instead of Normandy.* Why would London think that such a message from a "concentration camp" was genuine and not meant as some kind of trick?

Even worse, if the Germans instead of the Allies picked up the secret outgoing signals, they would swoop down on the camp, tear everything apart, and murder anyone suspected of even knowing about the clandestine radio transmitters. The idea of broadcasting a message was reluctantly abandoned. Somehow, though, despite everything, on those cold, dark nights in the Buchenwald barracks filled with hopelessness and fear, an idea began to hatch. No one knows where it first started—perhaps it was in the communist barracks—or who started it—perhaps some brave Spartacus-type of individual, a man who refused to be a slave any longer, someone whose will to fight back against his oppressors was not yet broken. The idea began to spread through the prisoner grapevine, one man at a time, until only the most trustworthy were talking about it in low tones: Somehow, some way, the men would stage a revolt, they would kill their captors, they would take over the camp, they would regain their freedom right there in the center of Nazi Germany, the belly of the beast, the most terrifying, pitiless nation on earth.

In a place where even the slightest disobedience to the rules would bring swift and painful punishment, such an idea was crazy. With the possibility that the man sitting on the commode next to you was a mole, a spy for the camp administration, even the merest hint or discussion of a revolt must have seemed like the first step toward suicide, yet men driven to the brink of desperation *did* discuss it.

Where will we get the weapons? the frightened-yet-curious ones must have asked. From the sympathetic guards, came the whispered reply; we will bribe them. And from the DAW armaments factory; we will steal the components one piece at a time and assemble them clandestinely in the barracks. *But where*

* Operation Fortitude is probably the war's best-known deception program. It was instituted by the Allies to disguise where the cross-Channel invasion would take place. By building a fictitious army around General George S. Patton, Jr., building a fake army camp in southeast England, and filling the airwaves with bogus radio messages, the Germans were fooled into concentrating the bulk of the coastal defense forces at the Pas de Calais instead of in Normandy. (Cruikshank, pp. 170-189)

will we hide such weapons? We will find places in the barracks. Or *under* the barracks. Or in places the guards will never think to look. *But how will we get past the electrified wire to overpower the guards?* Our numbers are far superior to theirs. We have tens of thousands to their hundreds. Yes, many of us will die in the attempt. If we take them by surprise, they can't kill us all. We have heard rumors of the revolts at Treblinka and Auschwitz-Birkenau and Sobibór and Janowska and the Warsaw Ghetto. It *can* be done. We *can* rise up and fight back. But unless we do it, *all* of us will die like sheep in the slaughterhouse. *None* of us will get out of here alive. *None* of us will be able to bear witness to what has been done to us.

Slowly, the fearful were converted to the brave. It seemed possible, just barely so, but possible nonetheless. Then came the ultimate question: *When will we do it?* Soon, very soon, my brother. The hidden radios are giving us news that the Americans are coming ever closer to us, pushing the ranks of German defenders back, day by day. And if not the Americans, there are always the British. And if not the British, then the Soviets will come from the east. The whole world is coming to our rescue, my brother. We must not lose hope. We *must* believe that it will happen. We *must* prepare for the day, whether it is a year or a month or a week away. We *must*!

The bravest of the brave were elected to be the leaders of the largest underground resistance group, which they called the "International Camp Committee," made up mostly of German communists. Others simply volunteered for the job, even though they knew that by so doing they would be signing their own death warrant if the SS ever found out.

Incredibly, the SS did not find out.[24]

And so, in 1944, secret committees of inmates, usually along national or political lines, formed with one goal in mind: To fight back when the time came. If the Allies weren't about to drive hell-bent-for-leather across the continent and deep into Germany for the express purpose of liberating KL Buchenwald (and it appeared that liberation, if it came at all, would be much too late to prevent a mass slaughter), the inmates would stage their own self-liberation.

French inmates organized the "*Comité des Intérêts Français,*" or CIF, followed by the "Polish Provisional Cooperative Committee," then a Dutch group formed, and an Italian committee (there were 200-300 Italians in the Main Camp) as well. For the most part, the national groups banded together to try and ease the suffering of their fellow countrymen and to ensure the fair distribution of goods, such as cigarettes that infrequently arrived from the Red Cross.

After a time, the groups became more militant. No longer was it enough to merely help members of one's own national group; preparing for armed defense or even insurrection became of paramount importance. The multi-national resistance leadership—men such as Walter Bartel, Ernst Busse, Harry Kuhn, Otto Roth (Germany), Otto Horn, Franz Schuster (Austria), Marcel Paul (France), Henri Glineur (Belgium), Domenico Ciufoli (Italy), Emil Hršel, Kvetoslav Innemann, Alois Neumann (Czechoslovakia), Jan Izydorczyk (Poland), Nikolaj Kjung, Ivan Smirnov, Nikolai Simakov (USSR), Rudi Supek (Yugoslavia), and others were planning for the day when they might need to revolt against their captors and so began to develop ways to obtain the means to do so.[25]

Obviously, for inmates to obtain weapons in a concentration camp was virtually impossible—and surely suicidal if the authorities found out. Yet, somehow, it was done. Some weapons were assembled from parts smuggled out of the DAW rifle factory, while a few others were obtained by bribing the few guards who seemed sympathetic to the inmates' plight.[26]

Prisoners working at Buchenwald's DAW and Gustloff-Werk II plants soon discovered that they could help the Allied war effort through little acts of sabotage—acts that could get them tortured or killed if their supervisors found out. Nothing major, just a bad soldering job here, a broken wire there, a little acid in the lubricating oil of an automatic rifle's mechanism—enough to get a severe chewing-out or a beating, but not enough to be hung at morning *Appell*.[27]

The problem was, little acts of sabotage designed to cause the V-2s to malfunction would not slow down or stop the manufacturing process of components going into some unknown weapon. Something truly catastrophic would have to happen to completely halt the work. Until that day arrived, the inmates working at Gustloff-Werk II continued to search for new ways to interrupt the process. They discovered, for instance, that if they dropped from a small height the vacuum tubes that went into the rockets' radio receivers, the shock was enough to loosen the electrodes inside and cause a malfunction—one that wasn't obvious to the Germans making a final inspection. If any of the managers suspected sabotage, the obvious retort was that the tubes must have arrived at Gustloff-Werk II in damaged condition.

It was a dangerous game, but it worked. Four months of painstaking work by the inmates went down the drain—and they could not have been happier.[28] It would not be long before Louis Gros's respite from backbreaking labor—and indeed the factory itself—would be shattered.

11
THE LITTLE CHILDREN SUFFER

"This was my new home."

Salek Orenstein
Teen-aged inmate at Buchenwald

BY THE SUMMER of 1944, not only were the Western Allies crossing France and battling through every town, village, and hedgerow toward Germany, but the Soviet armies were also inflicting massive casualties on Hitler's formations and pushing the Germans back. German factories and slave-labor camps in Poland—such as the Skarzysko-Kamienna slave-labor munitions camp, the Hortensja glass factory in Piotrkow, and the Czestochowianka munitions plant in Czestochowa, to name but a few—were being abandoned and the inmates evacuated in advance of the Soviet drive; many of the slave laborers who worked in those facilities were sent to Buchenwald.

Suddenly, there was also an influx of children at Buchenwald. Blocks 54 and 66 were turned into all-children's barracks, and they burgeoned with bewildered and frightened new arrivals. According to former inmate Jacob Werber, most of the children—about 700 boys—came to Buchenwald in August 1944 primarily from Skarzysko-Kamienna, a Polish town south of Warsaw. Remembering his own daughter who had been murdered earlier by the Nazis, and recalling a group of Gypsy children that had been taken out of Buchenwald when Koch was commandant, Werber enlisted other prisoners to do whatever possible to help save these children. Werber recalled, "It's incomprehensible that a small band of feeble inmates could keep such a deception from their oppressors. It just doesn't seem plausible that we could get away with housing, feeding, and protecting close to seven hundred children.... And yet we did."

With the war having turned badly for the Germans, the Buchenwald administrators and guards were thinking more about their own safety than they were about continuing to oppress the prisoners. As a consequence, fewer and fewer SS men roamed the prisoner enclosure, relying instead on the prisoners to police themselves. This created the perfect environment for Jewish members of the camp Underground to hide and care for the youngsters. "Our task was to save their lives," noted Werber, who played a major role in the operation, "and to give them hope for the future, even though we ourselves were often despairing."

The Underground realized that they needed extra rations in order to keep the boys alive and so other inmates, who were fortunate enough to receive packages of food from relatives, were persuaded to give up that food for the good of the children. Inmates who were working as clerks in the camp also cooperated by listing the ages of the boys in the personnel records as at least sixteen (officially, the camp was not supposed to have any prisoners below the age of sixteen), even though many were considerably younger than that.

To lessen the danger of all the children being found in a couple of barracks, a plan was devised to scatter them to many different barracks, including those in the Little Camp. "Elie [Eliezer] Wiesel,* Rabbi Ysrael Lau, the Chief Rabbi of Israel, and his brother, Naftali Lavi, who was [later] an Israeli diplomat, were also in this block [Number 66]," Werber related. "Of course, we had no idea at the time who they would become. They were simply part of a larger group of children whose lives we helped save."[1]

One of the new inhabitants, a sixteen-year-old youngster named Salek Orenstein from Opatow, Poland, who had toiled at Skarzysko-Kamienna, watched impassively as the corpses of the previous occupants of Block 66 were removed and piled outside the barrack. They had been dead for several days and had lain, untouched, in their own excrement and vomit.[2]

The boys were all quizzed by the mostly German camp prisoners who, under the aegis of the SS, were basically in charge of the internal operation of the camp. The men wanted to know if any of the Jewish policemen or *Kapo*s who accompanied the youths from Poland had treated them badly. When the boys informed on their tormentors, the camp's secret internal committee "took care" of them—killing them during the night.

Compared to what he had known, Orenstein looked upon Buchenwald as a sort of Garden of Eden. Here he was well fed, well treated, and had no fear of being murdered. The youngsters could even play games and sports, including soccer. The youngest children had no work to do in the camp, but the teenagers among them were put to work making V-2 missile parts at the Gustloff-Werk II. Many of the older inmates seemed to be genuinely interested in the well-being of the young prisoners and went out of their way to protect them from others who might want to bully or rob them of what few meager possessions they had.

On several occasions, a boy would be reunited with a relative in Buchenwald,

* Wiesel would grow up to become a distinguished writer, human-rights activist, and recipient of the 1986 Nobel Peace Prize. Another boy, the Hungarian Imre Kertész, who would win 2002 Nobel Prize in Literature, was also an inmate at Buchenwald.

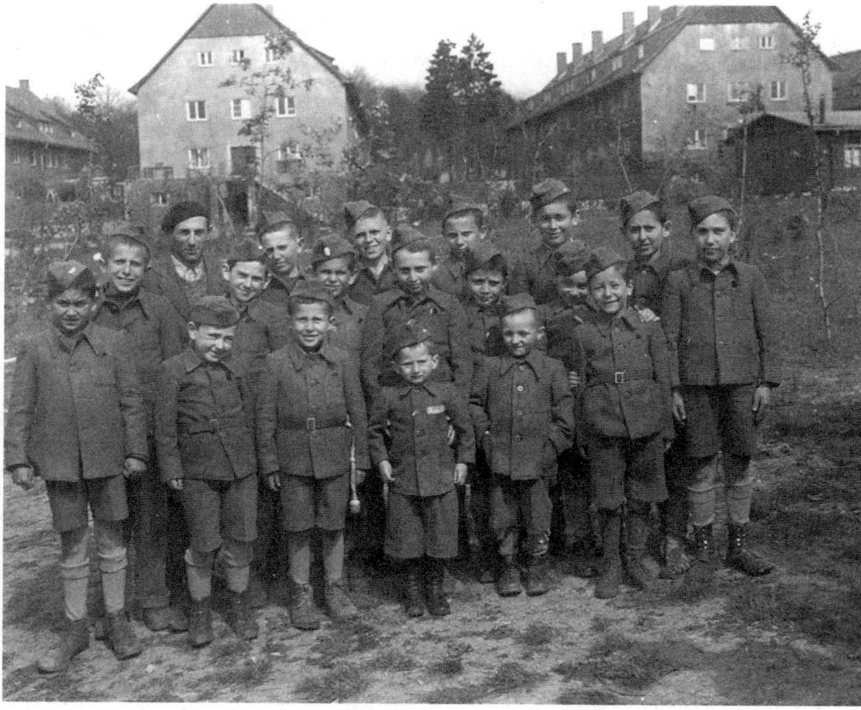

A group of children rescued from Buchenwald. The smallest boy in the center of the front row is Yisrael Meir Lau, who would become the Chief Rabbi of Israel. (Simon Wiesenthal Center, Harry Laugharn, Jr. Collection)

but not always with happy results. Sevek Finkelstein of Piotrkow, Poland, recalled that he was walking through the camp one day when his father, from another section of the camp, called out his name. "He was so happy to see me," said Sevek. "He embraced me and began to cry. He had a piece of bread which he gave to me. My father looked terrible. This powerful man, to whom I had so looked up, was a skeleton of his former self. He appeared beaten and powerless, and I was very uncomfortable being with him. I made excuses to him that I had to go back, and quickly left him standing there looking at me as I left. I could not allow myself to feel any love, concern, or care for my father whom I had so loved. He was a burden that I did not want to take on. He was no longer of any possible use to me." His cold-hearted treatment of his father would haunt Sevek for the rest of his life.

Another youngster, Moishe Nurtman, also found his father in Buchenwald. Although the elder man was on the verge of starving to death, his son tried to take care of him and restore him to health. But it was no use; beaten badly by some other inmates, the elder Nurtman, his strength gone, expired.[3]

Many inmates went out of their way to help. Werber even described one prisoner, a German communist, as "a saint." Others organized a school within the camp so the children could receive an education in history, music, Yiddish songs, and the Hebrew language. Werber said, "[Jack] Handelsman and I told them stories to give them hope, about how after the war we would all go to Palestine and grow oranges in a Jewish country." Other inmates acted as counselors and psychologists to help ease the children's trauma at being held in such a place of horror and hopelessness.

Whenever the SS got too close to a barracks where boys were hiding, they were scared off with false talk of disease, especially typhus, that was present in that barracks or area; the guards were deathly afraid of typhus.

Through the inmates' truly heroic efforts, hundreds of children survived Buchenwald—and lived to grow oranges in Palestine, a part of which, because of a United Nations mandate, became the new Jewish homeland, Israel. [4]

ON A BRIGHT, clear morning in the spring of 1944, before reporting for work at the Gustloff-Werk II, Louis Gros looked up and saw a lone airplane streaking a white contrail across the sky, meaning the air was dry—a good day for a photographic mission.

Gros' comrade, a man named Taillez, asked, "That one—do you think he's a tourist?"

"Yeah, reconnaissance at high altitude. That kind of tourist travels much and apparently finds pleasure in it."

The two men noted that the plane made several paths over the camp and the factory before disappearing to the west. They wondered if it presaged something important. Was the Gustloff-Werk II being singled out as a target?[5]

IN THE EARLY summer of 1944, Krupp AG, Germany's chief armaments manufacturer, sent executives to the concentration camp at Sachsenhausen-Oranienburg to meet with Oswald Pohl and discuss their need for two thousand prisoners to be used in Krupp's steel-rolling mill at the sprawling factory complex in Essen. Pohl approved the request in principle and told the Krupp officials to contact Pister at Buchenwald to work out the details.

For reasons probably related to not wanting to give up any of the male prisoners already "employed" at Buchenwald's on-site DAW and Gustloff-Werk plants, Commandant Pister said that only women—housed at the Buchenwald sub-camp of Gelsenkirchen—were available, even though they were currently being rented out to other firms. With Krupp possessing a higher priority for slave laborers, officials from the company traveled to Gelsenkirchen to inspect the women, ages fifteen to twenty-five, most of whom were Hungarian, Rumanian, and Czech.

The Krupp "recruiters" thought that the women appeared to be too weak and frail, but Pister simply shrugged with a "take it or leave it" attitude. During the negotiations that followed, Pister agreed to let the officials have 500 of the healthiest women, but only if the company could provide forty-five German women to act as guards. Krupp agreed to the conditions and the women were hauled off to Essen to begin their new careers as slaves in Krupp's steel-rolling mill and electrode shop.*[6]

But something big—very big—was literally in the air. The "tourist" that Louis Gros had seen flying over the camp a few weeks earlier was a portent of a major event that would change the lives of everyone at Buchenwald.

---

* In *Less Than Slaves*, Benjamin Ferencz noted, "The Krupp personnel office called for volunteers, and the forty-five guards were recruited from Krupp's German staff. Rubber truncheons and uniforms were provided by the SS." (Ferencz, pp. 94-95)

The jobs were interrupted a few weeks later when, on the night of October 23-24, 1944, a heavy British air raid severely damaged Krupp's Essen factory. On this mission, 1,055 RAF aircraft dropped 4,538 tons of bombs. Of this raid William Manchester wrote, "On one street two camps [for Krupp's slave laborers] stood side by side. When the tocsin of alarm sounded, Jewish girls took refuge in the remnants of a pulverized cellar behind the barbwire of their camp; Poles, in a ditch within theirs. During a...raid, a stray bomb fell in the ditch. Over a hundred Polish corpses were counted, and then the order came down—in the future the Jewesses would lie in the exposed ditch, the Poles in the safer cellar." (Manchester, p. 562)

Two days later, the barracks where the women were quartered were also hit and destroyed in another Allied air raid. Nor was this terrifying ordeal the end for the slaves. Their SS guards brutalized them with dog whips and kept them in a constant state of misery, even telling them that they would be killed if the Allies closed in on Essen.

As the end of the war approached, however, instead of killing the women, the SS decided to ship them back to Buchenwald. On March 17, 1945, 1,800 survivors were marched a few miles from Essen (whose rail facilities had been smashed flat) to Bochum and, along with 1500 male prisoners, placed on a train destined for Buchenwald. Pister, his camp full to bursting, refused to accept the shipment and sent the train away; it finally ended up at Bergen-Belsen. Enough women survived the nightmare to testify against Krupp during the war-crimes trials of German industrialists. (Ferencz, pp. 94-96)

12
THE END NEARS

"Sabotage is a duty."

Louis Gros
Buchenwald inmate

DESPITE THE INVASION of the Continent, Peter Bergson in New York could see no end to the ongoing, unceasing march of Jews toward the gas chambers—and America's refusal to do anything about it. By the time the Allied armies could reach the death camps—a drive that would probably take a year or more—the Jews of Europe would likely all be dead. He redoubled his efforts to shake America out of its collective complacency.

On the evening of June 19, 1944, during a "Rebirth of a Nation" rally in New York, sponsored by the American League for a Free Palestine (another of Bergson's political-action groups), he demanded that United States forces use poison gas against the Germans. Reminding his audience that both Roosevelt and Churchill had vowed to use gas on Germany if the Nazis used it against any member of the United Nations, and claiming that he had already declared a Jewish state into existence, Bergson stressed that a million Jews already had been gassed in the death camps and, because gas had been used against "the co-belligerent Hebrew nation," the U.S. and Britain would be justified in reciprocating in kind.

Although his audience cheered, others were stunned, and condemned what they felt was reckless and irresponsible language. But Bergson didn't care; he was fed up with official U.S. inaction. As far as he was concerned, the more provocative the language, the better, for it focused media attention on him, his group, and, most importantly, the plight of Europe's Jews.[1]

BETWEEN JUNE 1944 and March 1945, the thousands of V-1s that would be launched from European bases along the English Channel brought fear to Londoners and caused heavy casualties, but the pilotless V-1s were fairly easy to spot, track, and bring down with either aircraft or anti-aircraft artillery.

The slave workers at Gustloff-Werk II were horrified to learn from their gleeful foremen of the carnage being sown by these heretofore unknown V-1s. Was this the wonder weapon into which the devices they assembled were going? Were they, by their work, helping to kill British civilians and possibly bring about a Nazi victory? While the workers agonized over their role in the German missile offensive, a few of the French inmates were trying to figure out how to get a message to the outside world so that the Allies might finally take action and bomb the Gustloff-Werk II into oblivion.

With great danger to themselves, the French workers managed to smuggle out of the camp a note and map telling the Allies of the critical missile-component activities taking place atop the Ettersberg. Carried by a worker who had, incredibly, escaped from a work detail outside the camp, the message was on its way to France and—or so the workers hoped—into Allied hands. But even if it arrived, would the Allies believe it, or just cast it off as some amateurish Nazi trick?

Day after day, while on the way to and from their shifts in the factory, the workers glanced up at the sky in hopes of seeing a mighty aerial armada headed for Buchenwald. Day after day they were disappointed.

A few weeks after the prisoner escaped with the message and map, however, the inmates of Buchenwald got their first hint that the message actually may have made it safely to Allied lines: The Germans began installing anti-aircraft guns around Gustloff-Werk II.[2]

LOUIS GROS' PREVIOUS technical schooling (he had studied to be an architect) was recognized and he was assigned to work at Gustloff-Werk II. There his job was a boring one—wrapping insulation around the parts being manufactured. But being able simply to sit and perform mindless assembly-line work in a "semi-normal" environment—without being beaten or screamed at, without constantly having to view the wire fences and guard towers and the smoke belching from the crematorium's square chimney—was a respite from the deadly quarry and the general hell of the rest of the camp.

Not that the job was without its anxious moments. For twelve hours a day, the men wrapping insulation sat at a large workbench under the constant scrutiny of a German civilian *Meister* (master). Louis said, "Working with the Meister is an inmate foreman who speaks French and Spanish and whose role is to 'stimulate' the workers to work faster. The workers also have an interpreter whose name is René Klein. The workers are forbidden from speaking to one another, and also from moving; requests to go to the latrine must go through Klein and be approved by the Meister."

Louis noted that the work itself was not difficult. "It is not necessary to be endowed with great talent in order to wind insulation around the parts," he said. "Any grocer or schoolmaster is able to do that. We can do twelve or thirteen an hour, which means it's possible to do about fifty a day."

Somehow the workers learned through the grapevine that what they were working on so diligently was a vital part of a giant rocket-propelled weapon—the V-2. This filled the workers with alarm, for they realized that their work was helping the Nazis wreak destruction on the Allies—the V-2 might even turn the tide of war in Germany's favor. Therefore, the slaves working at Gustloff-Werk II realized they were on the horns of a dilemma; if they reduced their output, they might help the Allies defeat Hitler. But if they were caught deliberately slowing down or doing a shoddy job, they likely would be shot.

One of the French workers, a former professor named Lucien Delattre, whispered to Louis to slow down, work very carefully, and try not to finish more than three pieces per day. In on the sabotage game, Delattre also discretely suggested that the work not be done too well. Louis noted that Delattre told him, "Don't forget to give three turns more to one thread and three less to the other, but cut both to the same length. That way the reel will be declared good by the inspector but should not work properly when the V-2 is on its way to London."

Louis came to the conclusion: "Sabotage is a duty."

But the slow pace of production—wrapping, then unwrapping the insulation repeatedly to do a "better" job—soon brought the scrutiny and ire of the Meister. "The Meister is always very busy among us, looks perplexed, worried," said Louis. "He asks Klein if I am incapable or lazy. 'No, no,' answers Klein. 'Tomorrow he will do better, as soon as he is more familiar with the process. But look how well he works!' " The interpreter held up a perfectly wound device and admired the craftsmanship. The Meister looked skeptical but said nothing and walked away to evaluate the work being done at another bench.

The French workers quietly asked Klein, "Do you think he will dismiss us? Will he cut off our soup ration?"

Klein shook his head. "No, tomorrow you will do five reels and he will be happy. Besides, this is *his* hiding place, too; he fears being sent to the Eastern

Front.* He will not say anything to attract the attention of his superiors."

"Klein is both affirmative and cheerful," commented Louis. "His optimism is becoming contagious. We apply ourselves to our 'anti-work.'"

The next day, as promised, each man's production rose to five, but in the months they spent at the factory never rose above six per day.

Louis said, "The time I spent in the factory was my least-bad time at KL Buchenwald. I was seated, sheltered, and had extra soup! It's the extra soup which interests us. Envy is one of the seven deadly sins, everywhere except here, and that soup seems more precious than anything else in our world. No wealth could replace it—our survival depends on it!"

But Louis was worried about his father. The elder Gros was shipped from Buchenwald to work as a slave in the V-2 tunnels of Mittelbau-Dora—a place from which few, if any, ever returned.[3]

THE GERMAN ARMAMENT industry was furiously working to capacity but, by the summer of 1944, it still wasn't enough. Germany's economy was stretched to the breaking point due to a shortage of workers and raw materials. Aircraft, tanks, trucks, artillery pieces, warships, and all other sorts of military hardware were being destroyed at a record pace on the battlefields of France, Italy, and the Eastern Front, as well as on the North Atlantic. Industry, too, continued to be battered incessantly from the air, making it difficult for the Germans to make up the losses.

While British and American bombers continued to strike deep into Germany and pulverize German cities and factories, Allied armies marched onward toward the heart of Naziland. On June 22, 1944, two weeks after the successful American and British landings in Normandy, the Soviets launched a huge offensive on the Eastern Front—an operation known as "Bagration"—three years to the day after the Germans invaded the Soviet Union. Throwing four armies consisting of forty-eight divisions (2,400,000 men, 2,700 tanks, 5,300 aircraft, and 26,000 artillery pieces of various calibers) at the Germans along a 450-mile front, the Soviets unleashed their own version of Blitzkrieg. German losses were staggering, almost unimaginable (381,000 killed, another 160,000 missing or captured).[4] Historian Ian Kershaw noted,

* By this point in the war, the German army was suffering horrendous losses against the Red Army. With manpower shortages becoming greater by the day, tens of thousands of civilian workers were pulled out of their "essential" duties in the armaments factories, given a rifle, and shipped off to the front. (Kershaw, *The End*, p. 83)

"The disaster on the Eastern Front in summer 1944 was in terms of human loss by far the worst military catastrophe in German history, worse than the First World War slaughterhouse at Verdun, way beyond the losses at Stalingrad."[5]

Driving into Poland, the Soviets were the first to reach a major German concentration camp, coming across the smoldering remains of Majdanek, near Lublin, Poland, on July 24, 1944. Trying to hide evidence of their crimes, the Nazis, before fleeing, had tried to burn the camp down but were not totally successful. The world began to learn that the rumored evils of the Nazi regime were more than mere rumors.[6]

WHEN IT BECAME obvious to many officers in the German armed forces that Adolf Hitler was leading the nation to total destruction, a plot was hatched to assassinate him. On a hot summer day at his field headquarters at Rastenburg in East Prussia known as the *Wolfsschanze*, or Wolf's Lair, Hitler was receiving a briefing from his commanders and staff officers about the deteriorating conditions on the Eastern Front. At 12:42 P.M. on July 20, 1944, a terrific explosion blew apart the building in which Hitler and twenty others were meeting.

The bomb had been planted by Colonel Count Klaus Philip Schenk von Stauffenberg, the chief of staff to General Friedrich Fromm, head of the Home Army. Von Stauffenberg was the chief conspirator in the latest plot to kill the Führer—a plot that also involved a number of high-ranking German officers who were all convinced that the war was lost and that only by getting rid of Hitler could Germany be saved from utter ruin.[7] The bomb, although it mortally wounded four persons at the meeting, left Hitler with only slight injuries—and a thirst for revenge. All of the plotters, like von Stauffenberg, were hunted down and summarily executed.[8]

Within days, new transports arrived at KL Buchenwald and other camps as the Nazis corralled another few thousand people thought to be connected to the assassination plot or less than totally loyal to the regime (one of whom was *Generalfeldmarschal* Erwin Rommel, who was forced to commit suicide). At the end of July 1944, the prisoner count at Buchenwald stood at 66,609; by the end of August, after another roundup throughout the entire Reich known as Operation *Gitter*, the camp's population would balloon to 82,505. And still more were on the way.[9]

IN THE SUMMER of 1944, with aboveground factories being bombed without pause, German industry was forced into a troglodyte existence. Beneath the trees and shale rock of a mountain known as the Steinberg, in the small village of Berga located along the Elster River sixty-five miles southeast of Weimar, another massive underground industrial project got underway. A thousand Buchenwald inmates were put to work digging tunnels for a project code-named *Schwalbe Fünf* ("Swallow Five")—a bombproof underground factory for the manufacture of synthetic jet fuel.

Within months, the Buchenwald diggers at Berga would be joined by hundreds of American POWs who had been captured the previous winter during the Battle of the Bulge.[10]

13
NO PLACE FOR A PRINCESS

"The blackest carrion in the Italian royal house."

Adolf Hitler

FROM ALMOST THE very beginning, Buchenwald, like Dachau, was a vast holding pen for hundreds of politically important prisoners. A special prison-within-a-prison was reserved just for them—an area of the camp known as the *Fichtenhain* (English: spruce grove). Its adjacent isolation barrack located between the SS barracks and the Gustloff-Werk II also held a variety of men, women, and even children who were not allowed to mingle with the general concentration-camp population.

The special *Fichtenhain* facilities proved to be inadequate, and thus the Falconry, built as an elegant hunting lodge for Hermann Göring but never used by him, was turned into a place of confinement for "special inmates" from the spring of 1943 until April 1945.

French politicians, especially, were "guests" of the Nazis at Buchenwald. Léon Blum, the Jewish former Premier of the French Popular Front government from 1936 to 1938, was imprisoned at Buchenwald after the French Free Zone was occupied by the Germans in November 1942 following the Allied invasion of North Africa.* Other members of the French government held at KL Buchenwald included Édouard Daladier (Prime Minister in 1940); Georges Mandel (the last Minister of the Interior before the fall of France in 1940); and General Maurice Gamelin (Commander in Chief of French and British forces in 1940).

Also incarcerated atop the Ettersberg were an array of celebrities: Professor Alfred Balachowsky, Director of the Pasteur Institute; Paul Chandon-Moët, one of the owners of the Chandon et Moët champagne company; and Mssr. Clin, Director of the National Library of France. Paul Reynaud, the last prime minister before France fell, spent one day at Buchenwald before being jailed at Itter Castle in the Tyrol. Confined, too, at Buchenwald were Dr. Rudolph Breitscheid, former chairman of the German Social Democrat Party, and his wife.[1]

---

* Blum would be transferred to Dachau in April 1945, just days before Buchenwald was liberated. He survived the war.

KL Buchenwald did not discriminate when it came to the nationalities of its prisoners. In addition to Dr. Petr Zenkl, the former mayor of Prague, Buchenwald also held Anton Falkenberg, head of the Copenhagen police, and British Wing Commander Forest Yeo-Thomas. A former Prime Minister of Belgium, Paul-Emile Janson, died at Buchenwald in 1944.[2]

The Nazis were particularly hostile toward writers and intellectuals who refused to toe the Nazi Party line—even if they were foreigners. Leon Jouhaux, a French trade unionist and recipient of the Nobel Prize in Literature, was imprisoned at Buchenwald, as were other French writers, including Jean Améry and Robert Antelme. Held, too, were the German author Ernst Wiechert; the Austrian poet and dramatist Jura Soyfer; Ernst Thälmann, the leader of the KPD (German Communist Party); and Curt Herzstark, an Austrian and inventor of the pocket calculator. Konrad Adenauer, the former mayor of Cologne, was also jailed atop the Ettersberg; he would be the first post-war Chancellor of West Germany.

Other formerly prominent individuals who spent time at Buchenwald included steel-magnate-turned-Hitler-opponent Friedrich "Fritz" Thyssen (he and German treasurer Hjalmar Schacht had urged President Hindenburg to appoint Hitler chancellor) and his wife Amélie were also held at Sachsenhausen and Buchenwald before being transferred to Dachau in February 1945.

When the Nazis couldn't arrest their enemies, they often arrested the family members of their enemies. Ten members of the von Stauffenberg family were held in the *Fichtenhain* isolation barrack, as was the sister of anti-Hitler German diplomat Hans Bernd Gisevius, who was involved in the July 20 plot and who had fled Germany for Switzerland. Also included in custody was the wife of *Generaloberst* Franz Halder, Hitler's former Chief of the General Staff; Halder was accused of being involved in the July 20 plot. (Halder himself was arrested and later held at Flossenbürg and Dachau; he was freed when U.S. troops liberated the latter camp on April 29, 1945.)[3]

ANOTHER OF THE few woman held at Buchenwald was Princess Mafalda Maria Elisabetta Anna Romana of Savoy, one of the daughters of Italian King Victor Emmanuel III and his wife, Princess Elana of Montenegro.

The Italian composer, Giacomo Puccini, was so taken with the princess that in 1924 he dedicated his last opera, *Turandot,* to her. In 1925, against her parents' wishes (because she was an Italian Catholic and he a German Protestant),

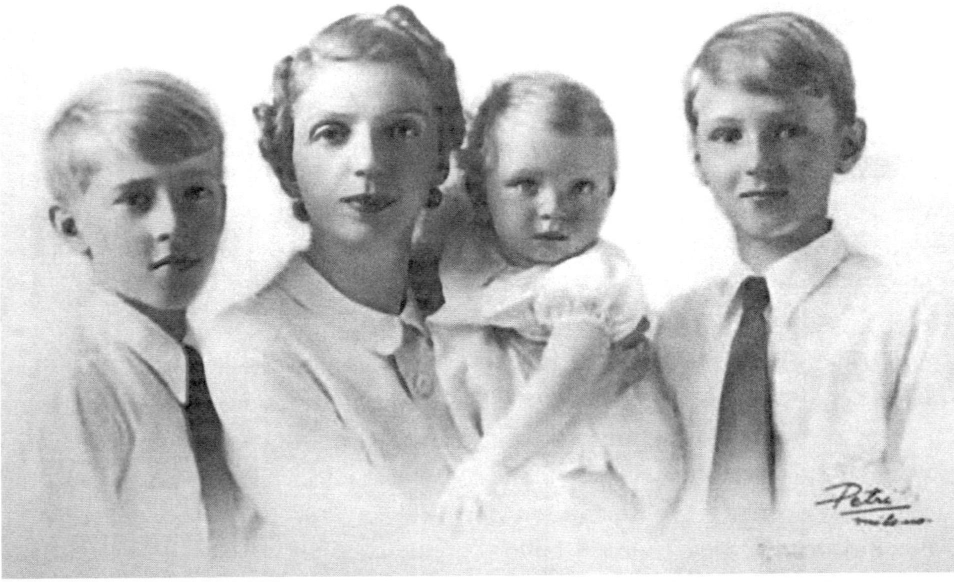

Princess Mafalda and her three sons: Enrico, Maurizio, and Ottone, ca. 1938
(Author's collection)

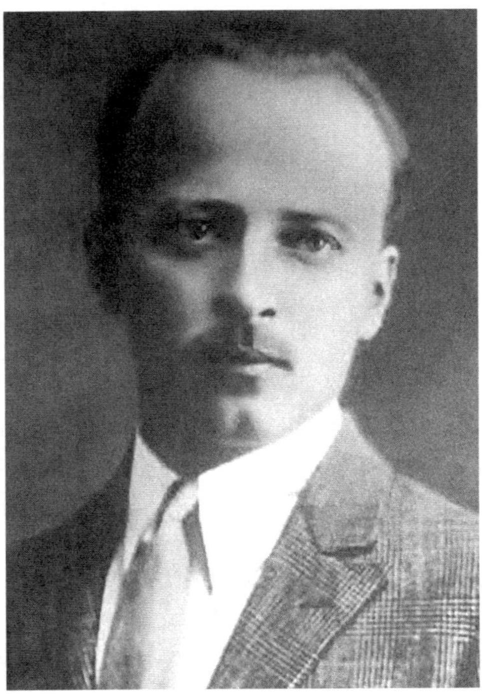

Prince Philipp of Hesse,
Princess Mafalda's husband
(Author's collection)

Princess Mafalda married Philipp of Hesse, Landgrave of Hesse-Kassel. In 1930 Philipp had joined the Nazi party; his marriage to the princess gained him a position as intermediary between the German and Italian fascist governments and also as Hitler's art agent in Italy, from which he obtained many masterworks. Philipp's brother Christoph was also part of the Nazi hierarchy and was married to Princess Sophie of Greece and Denmark, sister of Prince Philip, Duke of Edinburgh.[4]

Philipp and Mafalda had four children, who were known by both German and Italian names: Maurizio D'Assia (Moritz von Hessen-Kassel, born 1926); Enrico D'Assia (Heinrich von Hessen-Kassel, born in 1927); and Ottone D'Assia (Otto von Hessen-Kassel, born 1937. Their daughter was Elisabetta, born in 1940.)[5]

The Jews of Italy had enjoyed slightly better relations with Mussolini's fascist regime than the Jews had under Hitler and the Nazis. As Hitler pressured Mussolini to crack down on the Jews and ship them to the death camps in Poland, Mafalda became more vocal in her opposition to the Hitler regime, causing her husband to fall out of favor with the Nazis. A correspondent wrote that Philipp "denounced his wife as not enthusiastic enough over the Nazi regime," and so, to regain Hitler's trust, Philipp plotted to have her arrested. For his part, Hitler called Mafalda "the blackest carrion in the Italian royal house."[6]

To carry out the arrest, in early September 1943, as Allied armies were piling onto the beachheads of Italy at Salerno, Princess Mafalda's brother-in-law, King Boris III of Bulgaria, passed away (reports later surfaced that he was poisoned by Nazi agents), and she traveled to Sofia to attend the funeral.[7] While there, she learned that her father had capitulated to the Allies and ordered Mussolini arrested. She also learned that her husband had been picked up by the Gestapo and was being held in Flossenbürg Concentration Camp, while her four children were given sanctuary in the Vatican. Frightened, she decided to remain in Bulgaria. However, on September 23, 1943, she received a telephone call from the German embassy in Sofia, informing her that an important message from her husband was waiting for her there. When she arrived at the embassy, she was arrested by the Gestapo and charged with subversion. Princess Mafalda was then transported to Munich for questioning, then taken to Berlin. Finally, she was deported to Buchenwald. She would never leave there alive.[8]

14
FALLEN TO EARTH

"What lay ahead of us we dared not think."

Arthur G. Kinnis
Royal Canadian Air Force officer and prisoner at KL Buchenwald

IT WAS SHORTLY after midnight on July 8, 1944, a month since the D-Day landings in Normandy, when Lieutenant Arthur G. Kinnis, bombardier, was on a combat mission over France inside a four-engined Avro Lancaster belonging to the Royal Canadian Air Force. The formation came under intense ground fire and suddenly Kinnis' plane was ripped by fragments of an exploding flak shell.

One of the fragments severed a fuel line, causing the inner starboard engine to catch fire and begin spewing a trail of flames. The aircraft's skipper, Lieutenant Jeff Marchant, quickly assessed the situation and concluded that, in spite of the fire and damage, they could remain in formation and make it to the target. Two German fighter pilots, however, saw the flying torch and decided to pounce. Raking the craft with their cannon and machine guns, the Luftwaffe airmen managed to set the rest of the engines on fire and wound Kinnis in the legs.

With the Lancaster losing speed and altitude somewhere northwest of Chartres, Marchant ordered his crew to bail out. Bleeding and in pain, Kinnis did as ordered but, while drifting downward beneath his billowing canopy, a German Junkers Ju-88 G-1 night fighter made a pass at him; fortunately, the pilot held his fire.

Kinnis recalled, "It can never be put in words how grateful I was, and my first thought was a prayer of thanks and a prayer for those in my flaming, twirling plane. We were at 17,000 feet and it took ages to drop, for the night was pretty well windless."

While the stricken aircraft crashed and exploded some miles away, Kinnis landed softly in a wheat field. Cutting up his parachute for a bandage and tourniquet, he managed to hobble across the field to some woods near a village and fell asleep. The next morning, the injured airman attracted the attention of a passerby he hoped was trustworthy and asked, in his rudimentary French, for help in getting to friendly lines. The Frenchman indicated he would be glad to assist and returned shortly with food, drink, and civilian clothing.

Kinnis was then hidden under straw in a cart and taken to the village of

St-Ouen-Marchefroy, where he was given shelter in an attic. A local doctor soon came to dress Kinnis's wounds and give him an anti-tetanus injection.

For two weeks, Kinnis remained hidden in the attic, where he was well treated by the family—members of the Resistance—who owned the home. An infection did set in, however, and Kinnis became ill and unable to walk. Adding to Kinnis's gloom and fear was the news brought by villagers that three of his mates—Bill Hardcastle, Bill Gladstone, and Frank Patterson—had perished in the crash of the Lancaster; the three were buried by villagers in a solemn ceremony in nearby Oulins.

Fortunately, Kinnis's condition improved to the point that he could be moved to Paris and passed on to other Resistance members who promised to get him back to England. On July 22, 1944, Kinnis and another downed flyer, an American Marauder pilot named Donat ("Don") Dauteuil, whose father was French Canadian, were driven into Paris. Everything went smoothly for the pair; they were put up in a "safe house"—the Piccadilly Hotel—and told to wait for another contact who would get them out of the city.

Several days passed before their contact came for them. The Germans were watching the airfields around Paris, the contact told them, so they would be driven to Marseilles and then taken to Spain. Soon a car appeared for the two aviators and they were bundled into it. But instead of being taken to Marseilles, the pair was driven to Gestapo headquarters and arrested; the Resistance man turned out to be a double agent.

Taken by truck with other captured Allied airmen and arrested members of the Resistance to the notorious Fresnes prison, Kinnis and Dauteuil were thrown into a cell with thirty others to await their fate. After being fed, Kinnis and Dauteuil were moved to a two-man cell. For several days they were subjected to searches and interrogation, which sometimes bordered on torture. Two American POWs were added to their cell, then Frenchmen who may have been spies planted by the Gestapo; Kinnis and the Americans became very careful about what they said around the Frenchmen.

Kinnis later reflected, "One doesn't appreciate his freedom until it's gone. It's a hard lesson to learn, but we knew that if we ever managed to get out of here, we would quickly learn to see a much brighter side of life, and we knew that everything would be appreciated much more than ever before."

Like hungry men everywhere, the captives' conversations always seemed to come back to the subject of food. "Possibly it helped us to pass the time," said Kinnis, "but in any case it had the effect of letting us live, for a few minutes, in the past, making us realize more than ever before just how lucky we are to be [living] on the [North] American continent and free from the horrors and trouble that is war."

The days went by, then weeks. August arrived, and with it rumors that the Americans, advancing from the west, were closing in on Paris. Liberation was at hand!* During the evening of August 14, the jailers began clearing out the cell blocks and sending the prisoners to places unknown. At 4:00 A.M. on the 15th, the door to Kinnis's cell clanged open. He recalled, "Soon it was our turn and we, as had all prisoners before us, were led downstairs for a final roll call. It is interesting to note that after we left, the 532 inmates still in Fresnes were all released three days later."

Kinnis and the others—a total of 168 officers and enlisted men**—were crammed into trucks and taken to the railroad station, where they boarded filthy cattle cars. Eighty to ninety-five men were forced into each car, the dimensions of which Kinnis estimated at ten by twenty-five feet. "There was barely room to sit," he said, "providing all against the walls kept their knees up to allow those in the middle leg room. The doors were wired shut. We had no baggage, otherwise it would have been impossible." Kinnis learned later that this train was the last transport to leave Paris before the liberation and contained 1,650 men and 803 women.

The Canadian recalled, "There is no need for me to mention how limb-weary from lack of proper space we all were. The dirty and filthy conditions under which we found ourselves were so beyond our imaginations that we found it difficult to believe that this was happening to us. What lay ahead of us we dared not think for, if this was a sample of the new German culture, we wondered just what we would see and go through before our eventual release."

The captives all naturally assumed they were headed to a prisoner-of-war encampment, where they would sit out the rest of the war in diminished, but not life-threatening, circumstances. A week after departing Paris on a harrowing journey full of threats of death, however, the grimy, thirsty, and famished POWs reached Buchenwald—on August 21, 1944. Climbing the Ettersberg in reverse, the train backed into the railyard adjacent to the Gustloff-Werk II and the prisoners were ordered out, accompanied by shouts and the barking of

* Paris was liberated by French forces, assisted by the Americans, on August 25, 1944. (Gilbert, *The Second World War*, p. 580)

**The composition of the group was as follows: 82 from the USAAF, 48 from the RAF, 26 RCAF, 9 RAAF, 2 RNZAF, and 1 from Jamaica. (Kinnis, p. 20)

angry Alsatian guard dogs. As Kinnis and his sweating companions glanced at the nearby Gustloff-Werk II factory and wondered what sort of POW camp they had come to, "one American was hit for no apparent reason by a swaggering German officer. Our spirits were on the ebb."

Under armed guard, the group was marched down the Caracho Weg, past the zoo and crematorium, and made a right turn at the gatehouse. Once inside the electrified enclosure, Kinnis took stock of his surroundings—rows of barracks as far as the eye could see, watchtowers bristling with machine guns and manned by SS guards, and a building from whose tall, square chimney streamed a constant plume of foul-smelling, dirty-gray smoke.

The sightseeing quickly ended as the group of Allied airmen was hustled down to the de-lousing station and then had all their body hair shorn by a group of Polish "barbers." "It was done so fast that one didn't have time to question where those clippers had been before they were being used on you," Kinnis said.

Just as quickly the POWs, more hairless than newborn babes, were issued a striped shirt, pants, a brimless cap, but no shoes, and marched a few hundred yards across the rocky, uneven ground to Buchenwald's quarantine section—the dreaded Little Camp. Here Kinnis and his fellow POWs were aghast at the conditions they found: five big tents (a map of the camp shows four tents in this area, known as the *Zeltlager*, or tent camp) all crowded to capacity, fourteen permanent barracks (some of which were former horse stables), one small stone building used by the *Lagerältester* and his assistants, plus two foul-smelling latrine buildings. Scattered here and there around the Little Camp were stacks of corpses awaiting their turn in the crematorium. Kinnis estimated the number of prisoners in the Little Camp alone to be about ten thousand. Everyone received a prison number; Kinnis was assigned number 78391. The usual watery, lukewarm "soup" was ladled out to the new arrivals that night.

The arrival of the airmen created a sensation within the Little Camp, with everyone seemingly amazed that a group of Allied fighters had been suddenly thrust into their midst. Everyone wanted news of what was happening in the war and in the outside world; the Allied airmen gave their rapt audience as much information as they could about the D-Day invasion at Normandy, about the Allied push westward, and about the battles taking place across France. The confirmation that Paris had been liberated was especially exciting. When asked in broken English how much longer the Brits, Yanks, and Canucks thought the war might last, the airmen's answer—"one month"—caused considerable joy.

Smiles began to spread across faces that had long given up hope, that had long forgotten how to smile.

While their presence seemed to bolster the spirits of the other inmates, the fliers' spirits sank as they contemplated the conditions of their imprisonment. There were not enough tents to accommodate the new arrivals, so the Allied airmen were forced to sleep in the open without so much as a blanket. In spite of this, the exhausted POWs fell into a quick, deep sleep on the hard ground.

Before sunrise the next morning, the inmates of the Little Camp were all ordered to report for roll call. The *Appelle*, as previously noted, were twice-daily exercises in sadism and cruelty, like a college fraternity Hell Week run amok. Kinnis recalled seeing men beaten—not only by the SS but also by the *Kapos* and *Blockälteste* and their assistants—for the slightest infringement of the rules. It now sunk in to Kinnis and the other Allied airmen that instead of being in a relatively safe POW camp, as required by the laws of warfare, and guarded by Luftwaffe personnel, they were in the terrifying jaws of the Third Reich—their life or death totally at the whim of the SS. Designated *Terrorflieger* (terror-fliers), the airmen were denied access to the International Red Cross or recognition as official prisoners-of-war. Kinnis said, "We knew that our group must become very united and that we must make sure that the powers-that-be realize that we are all aircrew of the Allies, and that what is now happening to us is against the Geneva Convention." But how to accomplish the latter?

The airmen tried adjusting to their disgusting living conditions as well as they could. Luckily, the *Ältester* in their section of the Little Camp, a man with a wooden leg and a sense of humor, was decent to the airmen and tried to make their existence as bearable as possible. Because the Little Camp was already beyond overcrowded, nothing could be done immediately to get the airmen out of the elements at night, and so they continued to sleep on what they called "the rockpile."[1]

Another Canadian flier in Buchenwald was Carter Edwards, who, like Kinnis, had been betrayed by a French collaborator after he had parachuted from his stricken bomber. Shocked by the cruelty he saw daily at Buchenwald, Edwards was soon caught up in the callousness and disregard for human life. "The most humiliating experience was watching people on the ground crying, holding their hands up for you to help," he said, "and you would just step over them like you would step over a log. You just didn't have the capacity to help people, so you just closed your eyes and closed your ears."[2]

LIEUTENANT ARTHUR KINNIS and the other 167 Allied airmen were not the only Allied fighters imprisoned at Buchenwald. Shortly before the airmen arrived, thirty-seven British and French members of the SOE (Special Operations Executive—the British equivalent of the U.S. Office of Strategic Servcies, or OSS) were sent to Buchenwald and housed in Block 17 in the Main Camp.[3] The SOE was formed in July 1940 at the instigation of British Prime Minister Winston Churchill and Hugh Dalton, Britain's Minister of Economic Warfare. SOE's mission was to encourage and facilitate espionage and sabotage behind enemy lines and to serve as the core of a resistance movement in Britain itself in the event of a German invasion. SOE directly employed or controlled over 13,000 men and women, and it is estimated that the organization supported or supplied a million people worldwide. The SOE men sent to Buchenwald also became a source of outside information for the POWs.*[4]

One of the SOE men was Christopher A. G. Burney, who had been parachuted into France in May 1942 and arrested by the Gestapo. Burney said that it was the German communists, rather than the SS, who were the real authority in the camp. "They had absolute disciplinary powers over their fellow prisoners," he wrote, "backed by the SS and the threat of the crematorium. Anybody who savored of a capitalist or an intellectual was promptly marked down as a victim."[5]

Art Kinnis said that the SOE men "were accused of being spies, and had been in the camp just before our arrival and were awaiting an unknown future. They told us quite a bit about the camp and its surroundings." The airman was shocked when he learned that the SOE men had been called to the main gate, given a sham trial by the Gestapo, and sentenced to death. "According to a Pole working in the crematorium," he said, "some were quite badly beaten up and mauled before they were either shot or hung on meat hooks."[6]

Another inmate noted, "When seventeen [sic] of them were ordered to the gate one day, it was clear that this was a death sentence. I spoke to the English comrades and showed them how they could attack their murderers at the gate and at least put up a fight for their lives. They answered me more or less as follows: 'We have already given up our lives. If we attempt a mutiny now, there is the danger that the entire camp will suffer because of it, which is something we don't

* Besides its cloak-and-dagger operations in occupied France and elsewhere, SOE and its operatives took part in a series of raids against the Nazis' heavy-water plant at Rjukan in the Telemark region of Norway beginning in the winter of 1942 which destroyed the plant and wrecked Germany's plans to manufacture an atomic bomb. (M.R.D. Foote, passim) It is also believed that Ian Fleming, a former SOE member and author of the James Bond novels, based some of his characters on real-life SOE operatives. (Obituary: "Mr. Ian Fleming," *The Times* [London], October 14, 1975)

want. So we will not fight.' When the comrades were led to the crematorium, they requested that they at least be shot like honorable soldiers. Despite that, the Nazi beasts hanged them."*[7] Of the forty SOE agents who were brought to Buchenwald, only four—Burney, Maurice Southgate, and the Newton brothers, Henry and Alfred—survived.[8]

BARELY HAD THE Allied airmen settled into the Little Camp when an event of great significance literally struck Buchenwald—an event that would shake the camp to its very foundations and give every prisoner hope of liberation.

---

* This information was confirmed in the 1947 war-crimes trials: "On 10 September 1944, 16 Allied prisoners-of-war were called to the main gate of the camp and not seen again. The Polish underground intelligence service in the camp reported on 13 September 1944 that these 16 prisoners of war had been strangled to death on the night of 11-12 September 1944." A similar incident occurred at the end of September, when twelve Allied POWs were sent for by camp officials and never seen again. (U.S. vs. Waldeck, "Review and Recommendations," pp. 11-12)

15
MISSION 132

"The wild, inhuman, and devastating dance had begun. We were about to be liquefied by the conflagration from the bombs, tormented in hell."

Louis Gros
KL Buchenwald inmate

AT KL BUCHENWALD, a few of the inmates had either constructed or smuggled in a radio transmitter and, at the risk of their lives, began secretly sending to the outside world details about their precarious situation. There were also messages that contained information that the components for the guidance system of the V-2 rockets were being manufactured by slave labor at the Wilhelm Gustloff-Werk II adjacent to the concentration camp, as well as urgent requests for the Allies to bomb the factory.

No one in the camp knew whether or not the Allies had received the messages, or even if the Allies would act on them if they had. It was not until August 24, 1944—exactly five years after the first German bombs fell on London—that the inmates realized their messages had been received—and were about to be acted upon.

On that day, 129 B-17 "Flying Fortress" bombers of the 401st Bombardment Group lifted from their base at RAF Deenethorpe, 100 miles north of London, and headed toward their target, Gustloff-Werk II, 500 miles to the east. It was an operation known as Mission 132. Lieutenant Colonel Allison C. Brooks, the group's operations officer, told an interviewer later, "In the briefing on the Weimar mission, the intelligence officer stressed that there was presumed to be a concentration camp next to the factory and that we were to make every effort for precision bombing, right on the target and the confines of the target only."[1]

Joseph J. Geraldi, a crewman on one of the B-17s of the 613th Bomb Squadron, assigned to hit the target, said that he recalled no mention of a concentration camp during the briefing. "We were never told a concentration camp was there. Hitler was sending V-1 and V-2 rockets to England, so we were well aware of the V-1s and V-2s, and that was our target for the day. What we were told at briefing was, 'Today we are going to hit a V-2 factory at Weimar.'"[2] Indeed, in none of the 613th's official reports is there any mention of Buchenwald or a concentration camp; the target is simply designated as "a factory." Only in one document in the report file—a hand-written scrap of paper without the identity of the person who wrote it—is the word "concentration camp" even mentioned.[3]

Geraldi was worried about the mission to Weimar, as his group had attacked nearby Leipzig four days earlier: "Leipzig was terrible—we got shot up pretty bad." He expected that Mission 132 to Weimar/Buchenwald would be just as difficult—and it was. With his aircraft (No. 42-31591), piloted by Second Lieutenant Frank Carson, Jr., flying the "low box,"* they did not make it to the target. "One hundred fifty miles south of Berlin, we got hit by fighters," said Geraldi, who was serving as the plane's belly-turret gunner that day. "We had to jettison our bombs and return to Deenethorpe after receiving pretty severe damage. Three other planes were shot down on that mission."[4]

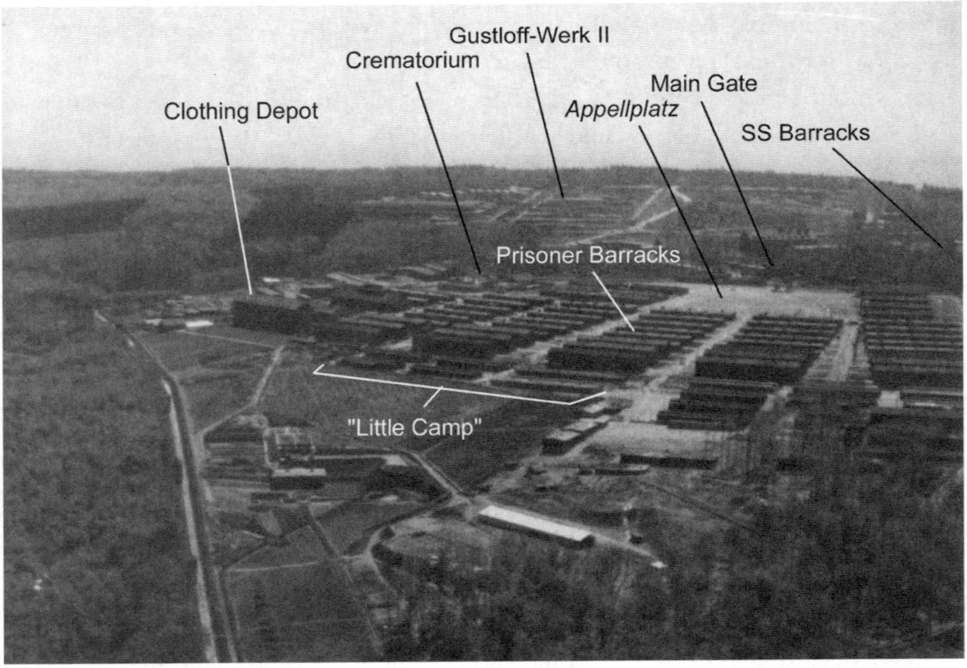

An oblique aerial photo of the camp taken before the raid of August 24, 1944. (U.S. National Archives)

* On most bombing missions, the planes were normally grouped into a tactical formation called the "Combat Box," consisting of three altitudes (designated high box, middle box, and low box), primarily to produce a tight bomb pattern on the target and also so that all the planes' machine guns would be mutually supporting.

AIR-RAID WARNINGS were a common occurrence at Buchenwald, but, until August 24, all had been false alarms; no bombs had previously fallen on or near the camp. Like children at a school fire drill, the prisoners at Buchenwald looked forward to the wailing of the air-raid sirens; it meant, for a short time at least, that they were granted a reprieve from beatings and their onerous chores.

Shortly after noon on August 24, the sirens screamed and camp personnel scrambled for the air-raid shelters, half-expecting that it was yet another false alarm. Many of the workers inside the factory, along with their German supervisors, began heading for the exits. The prisoners had no shelters; all they could do was flatten themselves on the ground. Within minutes, the deep-throated growl of hundreds of Pratt and Whitney engines pulsated the air molecules and assaulted the eardrums. The lookouts could see, off to the north, a dark cloud looming ever larger. No one could be sure if the air armada was headed for Buchenwald or for Weimar, just beyond, or for some other target.

The Canadian airman Arthur Kinnis had been enjoying an idle, sunny day in the Little Camp when he spotted the formation of B-17s heading his way. "Being at 22,000-25,000 feet," he said, "their appearance in perfect formation was a lovely sight, a remark that was passed by many of us. Just as the leading ship was directly over us, we saw a white smoke puff go down. The Americans and Bomb Aimers among us recognized this for was it was: the signal to drop their load."[5]

Louis Gros had been on the evening shift the previous night and was sleeping when the bombing began. Everyone piled out of their bunks, ran to the window, and watched the show. "We raised our heads and saw a quite extraordinary sight. The scene was terrifying both for its beauty and its extravagance. An immense square, straight as a die, had been drawn just overhead, forming a thick white carpet that covered the entire camp. The square hid the tracer planes from our view but beyond it we could see the white lines they had left in the sky. We never saw a single plane! But in the surreal décor we could hear the humming of the aircraft formations. It was clear we were in for an imminent deluge!

"'Do you think that is for us, all that stuff?' asked one of the Frenchmen nervously. Some men were more than nervous, not surprisingly. They guessed that this veil that had been drawn over our heads was to facilitate the task of the bombers, but they were not sure whether the purpose was to make a target for the bombs or to drop them around it.

"One of our crowd was more reassuring: 'No, no. Of course they are going to wipe out everything that is visible outside the square.' This seemed to make sense. In the same instant, the droning noise of a squadron drowned out the hum of the trace planes, which were probably already on the way back to their base.

"In the midst of the droning, which in seconds grew to a roar, the men became confused, each man dreading being caught up in the full tragedy and becoming a forced witness and possibly a victim of the imminent bombardment. No one doubted what was about to happen, but nobody knew, either, what to do. In a few minutes we would probably have to run from the bombs. But there was no shelter in the camp, no cellar, not even a hole, with the exception of the ditches filled with corpses in the Little Camp! And we had heard a lot of bad reports about the accuracy of American bombardiers and American bombs. Our camp was a trap, locked in as it was between blocks of factories, the sawmill, the barracks, and all kinds of other buildings....

"In the watchtowers, the SS remained vigilant, imperturbable. They were never going to quit their post, whatever the cataclysm. Their machine guns remained implacably trained on the camp, or to be more precise, on the inmates.... Suddenly, a piercing whistle tore the air and grew louder. It was not the same sound that I heard for the first time above my town of Épinal in June 1940. Then, there were only a few seconds between the little bombs being released by low-flying Heinkel IIIs and the explosions on the ground: hardly the time to hear a faint squeak or even take flight. And what is more, they missed the target, which was the railway station; they were not even anywhere near!

"But now, in Buchenwald, the whistle we heard was loud, harsh, and upsetting. Not surprising: The aircraft were flying at a few thousand meters altitude and the bombs they were dropping were high caliber. You could hardly feel indifferent! We were just (or rather, unjustly) below the merry-go-round of terror. Even though some of us were full of jubilation, recognizing the importance of what was happening (had not our American friends been reducing the major enemy arms centers to dust?), it was fear that was uppermost, grinding our guts and exposing raw nerves. Instinctively, from the opening of the window where I hung, I turned my gaze in the direction of the whistles, now so loud they drowned out the roar of the bombers.

"Thoughts and feelings flooded through me. A great flash of light and, like the knife on a guillotine, then I saw a wall of darkness descend beyond the beech woods that separated the quarry from the camp. The wild, inhuman, and devastating dance had begun. We were about to be liquefied by the conflagration from the bombs, tormented in hell.... The explosions of an unimaginable magnitude had just pulverized their point of impact. A second later, enormous columns of smoke and dust rose from behind the forest, taking with them tons of detritus and blending them with the white carpet that still hung above. It was fixed as if on hooks; no wind could blow it away; it seemed indestructible. But now the fragile satin veil was pierced by a hail of debris of all kinds and all sizes, tearing through the roofs, clapping on the ground, sending us flying in search of shelter, some protection, however meager."[6]

Within minutes the cloud of roaring aluminum was directly over the camp, and the noise of the engines was blotted out by the whistling sounds of incendiary and 500-pound bombs hurtling downward. The first salvo of bombs passed over the camp and struck the Luftwaffe airfield at Nohra. Kinnis recalled, "It was not over, for we soon spotted the main force, and this time, to our horror, the signal went down before they were directly above. Knowing how a bomb falls, we all knew that these were for us. Each chap endeavored to get lower than his mate and, outside of keeping our heads down, ostrich fashion, no cover was obtainable. I sincerely hope that I never hear the screech, thud, and rumble of dropping bombs again. It was far too close for comfort."[7]

The scream of falling bombs was replaced almost instantaneously by deafening explosions ripping apart the buildings of Gustloff-Werk II as though they were built of balsa wood. Trees were uprooted by the fiery blasts, and vehicles and railroad cars on the sidings were flipped into the air as if they were toys. From the ruins of the factory, men—supervisors and inmate workers alike—ran in panic, their clothes, hair, and skin on fire. Others were buried by falling debris and airborne mounds of earth and the trunks and branches of shredded trees.

Louis Gros noted, "A second array of bombs, this time out of my view, exploded somewhere to the left of the first. This time they must have hit the SS barracks! Good riddance! But what an infernal noise! A second deluge of stones, bits of wood and metal, etc., descended on our heads. I was astonished to see plates of soup on the refectory table still steaming and covered in plaster, dust, and bits of debris of all kinds. Some prisoners were still trying to eat this rather special brew, apparently unconcerned by the din outside....

"And it was not yet over! Panic set in everywhere. Normally there was hardly any movement in the camp during the day, save for the work *Kommandos*, but now it emptied of prisoners in a wild rush, the mad stampede of a herd of animals in flight towards the lower end of the camp and the purely theoretical protection of the forest, the point farthest away from the target zones.

"Further waves of bombers flew over, further explosions followed, now farther away from us, over by the factories. If you listened carefully, you could hear the squadrons of aircraft coming and going in the midst of the diabolical noise. The explosions were close and fast, immediately followed by enormous bursts of flames and smoke, creating a fantastic cloud that twisted painfully into the sky. This was the big fireworks show we had all been waiting for, and it was for free! But not, alas, in terms of human lives.

"A bomb exploded not far from us, the only one to reach the camp, apparently of low caliber. 'Did they mean to get the Krema?' But no, the Americans, as was well known, dropped their bombs from 4,000 meters altitude. It would be impossible from that height to aim with any precision at a rather small building, standing alone. It was just chance that it nearly hit this target. The crematorium would certainly not have been on their list of objectives to eliminate at any price.

"Now a shower of incendiary bombs came tumbling down. We were getting the whole works! They were invisible. They set fire to the sawmill adjoining the camp on the left, and to the washhouse down below. We could view the destruction from the front row.

"To close the first act of the show, we now had clouds of very fine aluminum strips descending from the sky, light as butterflies after so much steel and fire.* At last the white carpet up there was torn apart, as if to say, "The show is over!" Pamphlets, too, fluttered down and covered the ground. I picked one up, and cautious as ever, hid behind a tree to read part of it. It was a call from one Friedrich von Paulus, a German field marshal of whom we had never heard, mentioning the German defeat at Stalingrad and calling for the end of hostilities. Very interesting. But I dared never be found with this paper on me, so I buried it."[8]

One of the factory workers, Willi Gugig, who had been in Buchenwald since 1939, was hit by flying debris while taking cover in the woods and knocked unconscious. When he came to, he saw smoke and flames all around and some of his workmates dead, covered with roots and branches and upturned earth. He got up and began running to get away from the hellish scene and noticed a panic-stricken SS guard sprinting alongside him. Then Gugig expanded his vision and saw scores of inmates and guards all running for their lives in the direction of Weimar. (The prisoners' freedom did not last long; later that day, those who had escaped the bombing were rounded up and brought back to camp.)9

Sixteen-year-old Salek Orenstein, who worked in the factory but, on that

* The aluminum strips, called "chaff" and "window" by the Americans, were dropped in conjunction with bombing raids as a way of interfering with enemy radar by making it appear that more aircraft were in a particular location than actually were there.

fateful day, had not been at his work station recalled that there was nowhere to run or hide. Most of his co-workers died.[10]

Benedict D'Agostini, a crewman in B-17 #468, 615th Bomb Squadron, wrote this account of the raid from his perspective: "August 24, 1944—Target was Weimar, Germany, just west of Leipzig. Dropped 10 500# RDX* bombs on a factory manufacturing rockets and flying bombs. Three planes of the low element of the low box of the group lost to ME 109s. Enemy fighters attacked for 30 minutes. Group knocked down one ME 109. Light flak. Flying time was 8½ hours. Bombing altitude 23,700 [feet].... Enemy fighters i.e. 30-50 attacked in a pack."[11]

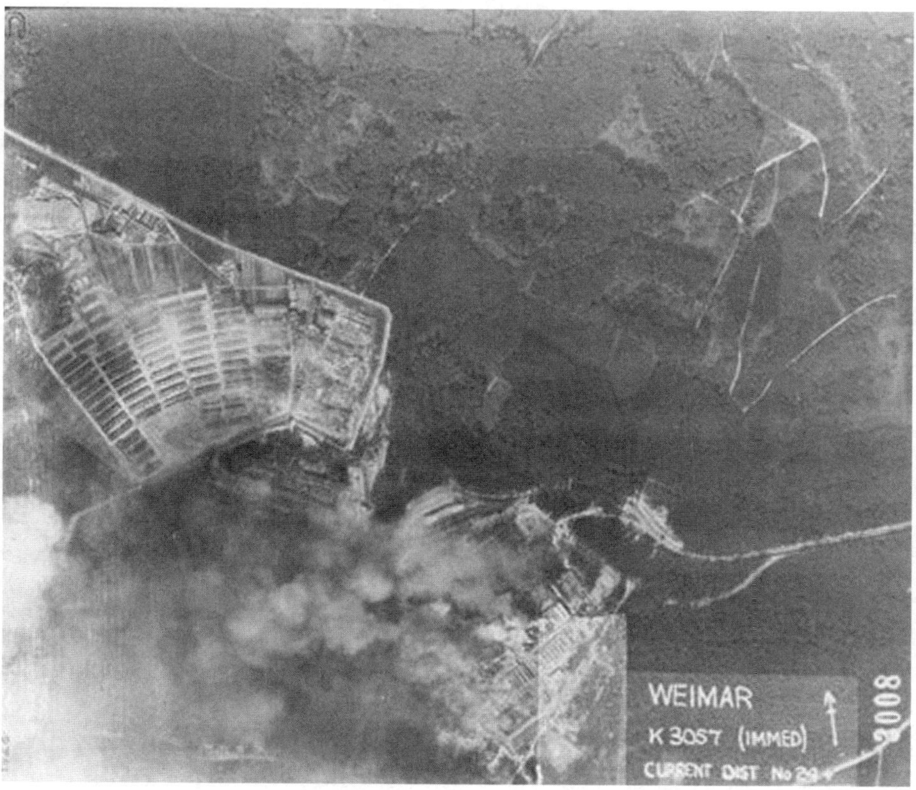

Post-bombing damage assessment photo shows smoke blanketing the Gustloff-Werk II V-2 rocket component factory at Buchenwald after the August 24, 1944, precision bombing raid by the Eighth U.S. Air Force. (U.S. Army Military History Institute)

* RDX is an acronym for Research Department Explosive, and is more powerful than TNT. It is also known as cyclonite, hexogen, and T4.

THE BOMBS AND their fragments did not totally spare the prisoner enclosure. Frank Salt, one of the twenty-six Canadian airmen in the Little Camp, was hit with a red-hot fragment of a bomb splinter that stuck out of his shoulder like a knife blade. One of the leaders in the Little Camp helped Salt get to the infirmary, which was overflowing with wounded and dying SS men and inmates. All was chaos. The dead and dying were carted away in horse-drawn wagons while civilian ambulances from Weimar came loaded with bandages and other medical supplies.[12]

In addition to the factory, which was almost completely obliterated and put out of commission for the rest of the war, bombs also fell on the SS garage area and the SS officers' housing area, smashing villas and killing officers' wives and children, along with inmates assigned to the homes as domestic servants.

Louis Gros again: "After the planes had gone and their hum had finally faded following those fifteen minutes of diabolical drama, we were back in the strange, almost uncomfortable calm that follows a fearful noise. Looking at all the debris blocking the alleys around the camp, we began to worry about the day-workers in the factory and the other camp *Kommandos*. For us it had taken about fifteen minutes when the alarm was sounded to run from the workshops to the woods beyond and below the train station. Had our comrades had the time to get to this summary refuge before the blind and deadly bombs hammered down?

"'God-almighty bombardment, eh, Jean?' I said to my friend Taillez, who was anxiously emerging from his bunk.

"'Yes, I thought we had all had it then,' he replied uncertainly. 'Amazing, you wouldn't believe....' He remarked on how accurate the bombs were, hitting their target without touching the camp as such.

"We learned after the liberation of the camp that, for this extremely special and delicate operation that we had just lived through, the U.S. Air Force had used its crack bombardiers and fighter pilots. They had sent us their elite to bomb an elite! Even if you hate war, even if you think that bombardment cannot be the work of an elite any more than an ordinary killer can belong to an elite, you have to admit that this bombardment was one of the most successful of the entire war, the exceptional means being used here unequalled anywhere else. Contrary to what happened at Buchenwald, the German cities, for example, came out badly, and the French cities, too, alas!

"Everyone around the periphery of the camp survived. It was the beginning of the end. Even the SS were disconcerted. Were they human after all? They appeared to have lost everything, even their arrogance. But still we had to take care, watch out! Up above, the sky now held only shreds of the muslin veil that had been so carefully drawn, witness to an event that had been both common and titanic. For a few last moments, we survivors could contemplate this ultimate décor!"[13]

It was a perfect strike, one of the most precise of the entire war. Jim Hastin, an American pilot imprisoned at Buchenwald, remembered that his countrymen "did a beautiful job of bombing. Then the Germans came down and said, 'All English and Americans out. Leave your stuff; you won't need it.' We thought that they were going to take us up and shoot us and then say that we had been killed in the bombing. People shook hands and said goodbye. We felt much better when they said to leave one man to watch our stuff. They took us up and had us fight the fires. I remember one Polish man who was walking along the road with an armful of incendiary bombs that hadn't gone off; he thought that he had a supply of wood! Steve Paxton [another POW] told him to gently put them down and get away from them."[14]

Art Kinnis noted that in order to keep the fires from spreading, the POWs were ordered to tear down with their bare hands all the buildings in the path of the flames. "It is surprising how fast this can be done with many hands working at top speed," he said.[15]

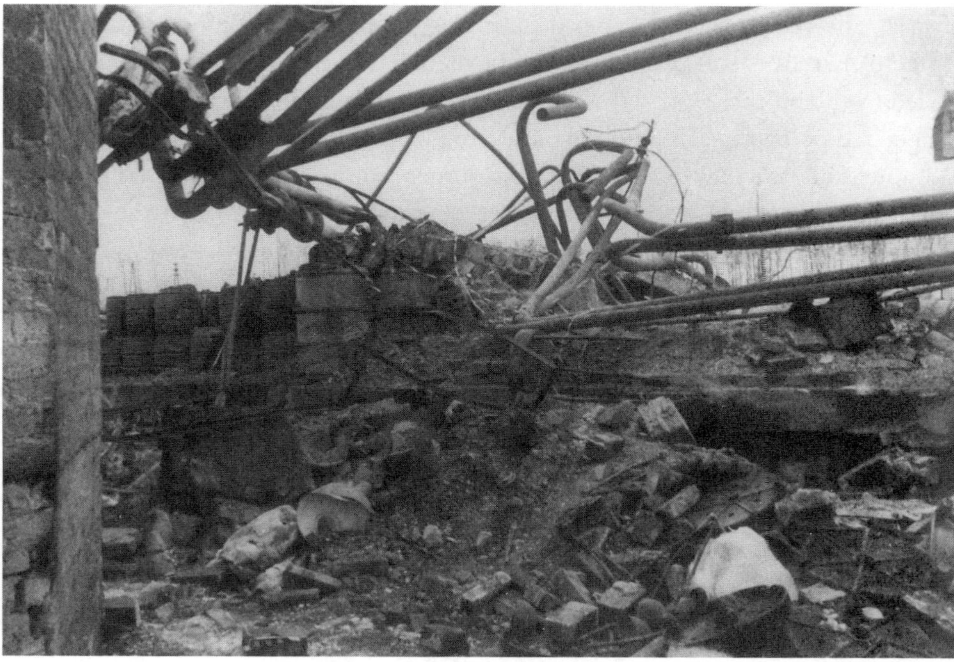

The ruins of part of the factory (Buchenwald Memorial)

Those who fought the blaze were neither thanked nor rewarded for their work. Myles A. King, an American fighter pilot incarcerated at Buchenwald, remembered that after the raid, "The SS sought their vengeance on us, the Allied airmen. Their reprisals took the form of brutal kicking, punching, pistol- or rifle-butting at any opportune moment."[16]

In an interesting twist, the air raid provided a new sense of security for those who were determined to not go down without a fight. In the chaos following the air raid, inmates removed as many weapons and grenades as possible from the SS replacement depot. These weapons were buried and otherwise concealed throughout the camp with the locations known to only a few. Now, they only needed to wait for the perfect time to put them into use.[17]

BOMBS DO NOT discriminate between friend and foe. When the ordnance came crashing down, at least one of the bombs exploded among the buildings in the *Fichtenhain* or "VIP section" of Buchenwald. One of those killed here was Dr. Rudolf Breitscheid, former chairman of the Social Democrats in the German Parliament, and a staunch Hitler opponent.[18]

Tragically, the building in which Princess Mafalda was jailed was also blown apart. She was buried up to her neck in debris from the collapsed building and one of her arms was badly torn and burned. It was reported that she was carried to the brothel, where the women working there cared for her. After being operated on by the camp doctors, a severe infection set in and her arm required amputation; she bled profusely during surgery and never regained consciousness. The forty-one-year-old daughter of the Italian king, once the ally of Germany, died during the night of August 26-27. Her body was removed from the camp and, instead of being incinerated in the crematorium, buried in grave #262 in a potters' field in Weimar. The grave marker listed her simply as *Unbekannt Frau*—"unknown woman."⋆[19]

⋆ After the war her body was recovered from the grave and buried in the small family cemetery at the Kronberg Castle in Taunus Frankfurt-Höchst, a suburb of Frankfurt-am-Main. (forum.alexanderpalace.org)

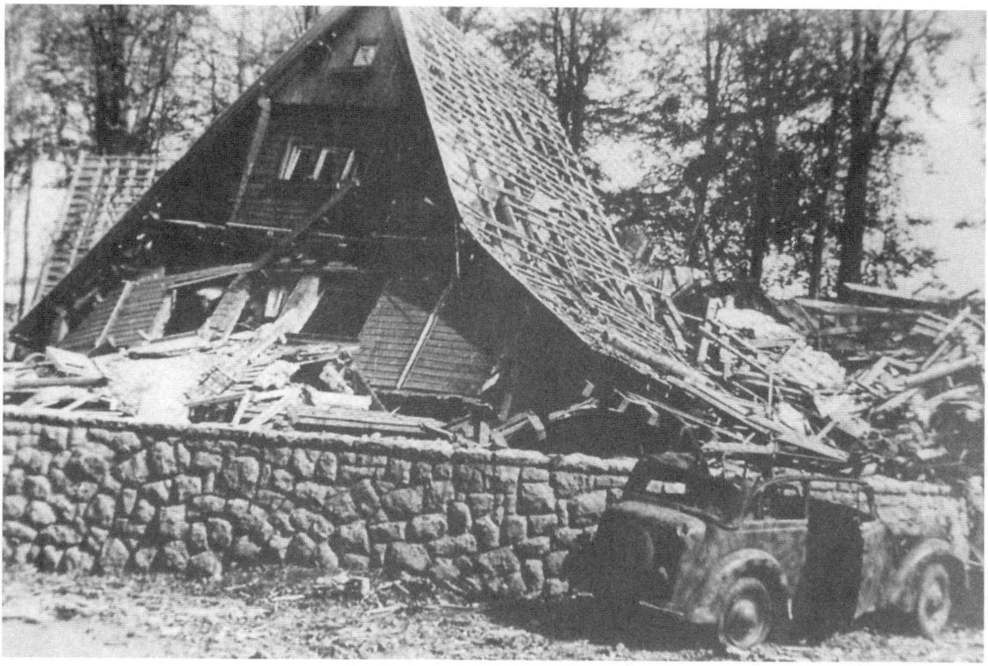

Wrecked homes on Officer's Row (Buchenwald Memorial)

WITHIN THE MAIN CAMP, the eastern edge—the section nearest the factory—suffered the most bomb damage. The laundry and disinfection buildings were wrecked, as were parts of the crematorium and clothing-storage depot. It is estimated that 388 inmates died in the raid, along with over 100 SS men, their families, and civilian supervisors at the factory.[21]

The bombing raid also smashed the homes along Officers' Row, including Haus Buchenwald—the one that had once been occupied by Karl and Ilse Koch, and which supposedly still housed the grisly objects the Kochs had once owned. Inmate Jacob Werber volunteered to help repair the damage there. "I was motivated by curiosity about Ilse Koch's home," he said. "I wanted to see the lampshade that had been made from Hans' skin....* Well, I got to see it with my own eyes. It was all the more shocking to look at since I had known the man it belonged to so well when he was alive. Underneath the lampshade was a stand made from pieces of human bone and, as a decorative item, a shrunken human skull. The parchment-like material [of the shade] looked like a Torah scroll. You could see the tiny holes where the hair once was.... To this day,

* Werber said Hans had been a friend of his. He recalled a day when Ilse Koch came by as the two of them were working bare-chested to build a gallows. She seemed to take a special interest in Hans' tattoos and wrote down his number. That evening, Hans was taken away and never seen again. (Werber, p. 75)

whenever I think about it, I close my eyes and the lampshade with Hans' tattoos is right there. It is a horrific vision that has always remained with me."[21]

A FEW DAYS after the air raid, the SS held a funeral service at the Weimar cemetery on Berkaer Strasse for the SS guards who had been killed during the bombing. A large gathering of relatives, townspeople, and fellow guards turned out to pay their respects.[22]

Perhaps the most symbolically important damage was done to the Goethe Oak. An incendiary bomb had set it alight; its charred remains were later cut down. An old German prophecy said that the nation would exist only as long as the Goethe Oak stood.[23]

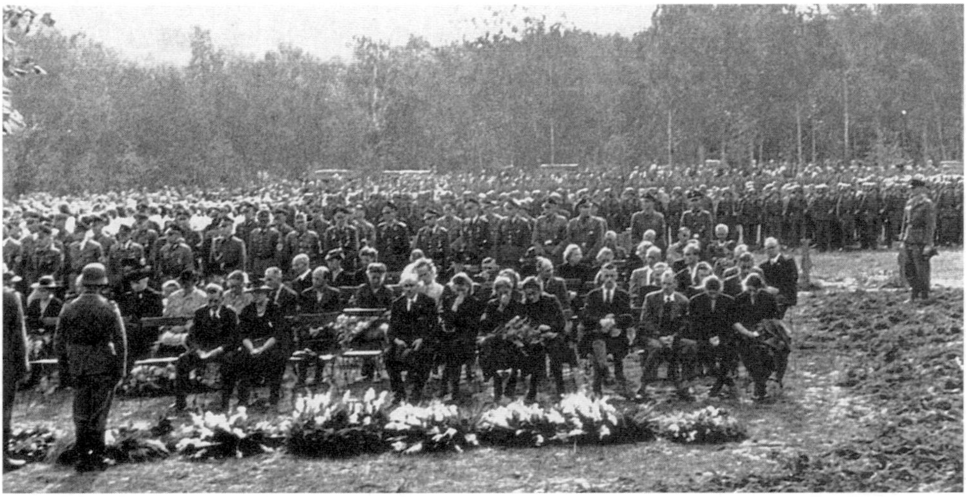

A large turnout of Weimar civilians and SS personnel at the funeral of the SS guards killed during the American air raid on the camp on August 24, 1944 (Buchenwald Memorial)

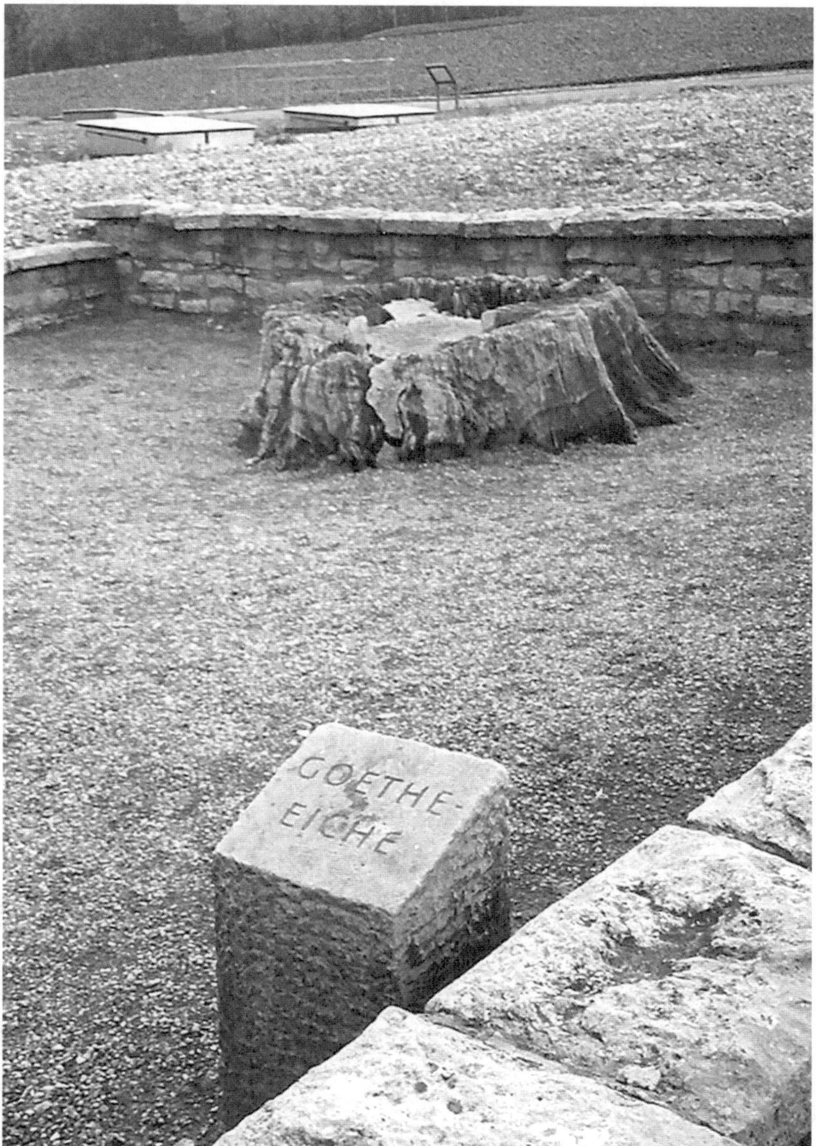

The stump of the "Goethe Oak"—all that remains after the U.S. Air Force bombing of the camp on August 24, 1944. (Author photo)

16
LIFE IN THE RUINS

"Work, whatever it might be, was the internee's only chance of survival. As soon as they were no longer of any possible use, they were done for."

Dr. Victor DuPont
Buchenwald inmate

AFTER THE RAID, Buchenwald returned to a semblance of normalcy. The roll call still took place twice a day, the daily beatings and torture sessions resumed, operations in the quarry and pathology lab went on as though nothing had happened, and those who died of disease, malnutrition, or other causes continued to be hauled to the quickly repaired crematorium for disposal.

But beneath the surface, a profound change had taken place, a change that had shaken the camp to its core. The knowledge that the Allies could mount such a precise aerial strike on the camp not only kept the guards and staff constantly scanning the sky, but the earlier confidence that Buchenwald was beyond the reach of the Allies and therefore immune to attack was suddenly shattered. Any day now, worried Commandant Pister and his SS guards, the advancing Allied armies might appear over the horizon, head for the camp atop the Ettersberg, discover what had taken place there, and exact retribution on the perpetrators; plans were finalized for the liquidation of the camp and its inmates.[1]

Besides the Nazis' formerly unshakable confidence, the factory was also gone; the total destruction of Gustloff-Werk II was a serious blow to the Nazis' V-2 rocket program, for it drastically curtailed the manufacture of the gyroscopes and other components. The equipment from the factory that was salvageable was moved to a deserted salt mine in Billroda in Sachsen-Anhalt, about thirty kilometers north of Weimar.* Here, 600 meters below the surface, the Germans tried to resume production, but the output of V-2 components was only a fraction of what it had been.[2]

* The workers would remain at Billroda until April 9, 1945, when they were marched back to Buchenwald. (www. vcalc.net/cu-bckup)

AT THE BEGINNING of September 1944, the salvo of first V-2 missiles, assembled by the slave laborers at Mittelbau-Dora, forty miles northwest of Buchenwald, were unleashed upon Britain from mobile launching sites 200 miles east of London near The Hague and Walcheren in the Netherlands. Hitler had once wanted a massed aerial armada of 5,000 V-2s to descend on England in a single salvo but, with the launching sites along the Channel coast of France now overrun by the Allies, only twenty-five of the tall missiles were ready for launch, and then only over a period of ten days. Sporadic launches, from The Hague and another Dutch site, Hellendoorn, would take place through March 1945. Although hundreds of civilians would be killed by the V-2s, they were, as an effective weapon of war, a failure.[3]

UNLIKE THE POLITICAL prisoners of Buchenwald, most of the Allied airmen were spared the deadly, dangerous work in the quarry. Most idled away their days sitting around the Little Camp, talking about their two favorite subjects: home and food. Others were assigned to odd jobs, while several were forced to perform repairs on the railway line leading from Weimar to the camp.[4]

Ed Carter Edwards, a Canadian aviator hospitalized at Buchenwald with malnutrition and disease, recalled that he was discharged from the infirmary and put to work twelve to fourteen hours a day repairing the railroad track that led down to Weimar—strenuous work that nearly killed him. "When a guard came up to you," he said, "you had to stand to attention with your hands palms up. If you made anything resembling a fist, you got either a rifle butt in the face or a bullet in the stomach." A friendly fellow prisoner, a former member of the Dutch underground and in charge of maintaining a list of prisoners who had died, told Edwards that he was putting the Canadian's name on the list of dead prisoners; it was an act that got Edwards removed from work details and undoubtedly saved his life.[5]

AT SOME POINT that autumn, the Police Commissioner from Weimar paid the Allied airmen a visit at their *al fresco* home on the Little Camp's rockpile. Arthur Kinnis recalled, "He said he deplored our being here, said that our presence here was all a mistake, and that immediate steps would be made to get us out, and in the meantime our conditions would be improved."

Nothing happened for about ten days and then, one day, the *Lagerältester* ordered the airmen to gather their belongings and follow him to one of the Little Camp barracks, known as Block 58. Hundreds of Gypsy children were moved out of the barracks, and the Allied airmen were moved in. Counting the 168 fliers, 232 Poles, and 400 Gypsy youngsters aged eight to fourteen, Block 58 now held 925 persons—along with several million lice and bedbugs.

"Our relief [at moving indoors] was very great," Kinnis related. "And the fact that we were going to be very crowded did not matter." That was before he noticed the vermin problem. "We thought the bedbugs were bad in Fresnes, but it was readily apparent that they were just an advance guard. These pests were to be found in every conceivable spot and it took us many days of scrubbing before we finally partly conquered this menace."

With little else to occupy their time, the airmen spent hours each day searching the seams of their striped suits for the tiny creatures and squashing them with their fingers. "In spite of this," Kinnis recalled, "those crawling, fast-moving blood suckers were soon back again. Our arms, legs, and bodies became covered with small red marks which in some cases merged to cover the whole area. There was no relief, for they made their presence felt the whole twenty-four hours, and scratching would result in open wounds." Even the daily, repeated scrubbings with a strong solution of lime and water failed to halt the infestation.

As the autumn of 1944 settled in on top of the Ettersberg, turning the beech leaves bright colors, Kinnis also noted that, once indoors, the treatment of the Allied POWs also improved, but only by degrees. They were allowed to toast the black, sawdust-laced pieces of bread over stoves in the barracks, and also to cook outside. Work details remained light: gathering coal and firewood, collecting barrels of soup from the mess and carrying it to the barracks. But trying to sleep on the wooden "shelves" proved to be an impossibility. "Many of the POWs slept on the floor, tables and benches," said Kinnis, "for we found it impossible to fit the five men required into the five-foot space. Three in this small space could move, four barely, if on their sides, and five was absolutely impossible."

Although the Allied airmen were, for the most part, spared the torture that was meted out at regular intervals to Buchenwald's political prisoners, they nevertheless were exposed to stories of some of the most egregious forms of abuse. A political prisoner named Karl told Kinnis chilling tales of men being whipped until their backs were a mass of open wounds, then being dunked in a tank of salt water; of twigs being jammed beneath fingernails and set on fire; of prisoners having all the hair burned off their bodies; of inmates being forced to stone at least one prisoner, half buried in the ground, to death.

The airmen also learned that someone in the Little Camp had an illegal radio receiver that could pick up broadcasts from the BBC. As a result, the prisoners were able to keep well informed about the progress of the war—at least until the SS found the radio and had its owner and six companions hanged.

But for Arthur Kinnis and his fellow POWs, the worst torture was the mental anguish—the uncertainty of their future, the growing mounds of corpses that seemed to presage their own demise, the vile smoke billowing from the crematorium, the sounds of gunshots emanating from the woods and different parts of the camp that indicated someone was being murdered by the SS—and the realization that their loved ones back home had no idea where they were, or even if they were dead or alive. Then there was the unspeakable foulness of the latrines and the gut-wrenching dysentery and other diseases from which nearly every man suffered. Going to the camp infirmary, Kinnis knew, was like committing suicide; very few ever returned.[6]

"A doctor who claimed that he was an American* had immediately made himself known to us," said Kinnis, "and offered to help us. He could speak several languages and must have been exceedingly clever. However, the old timers of the camp warned us against him, telling us he was high in Gestapo esteem, having sent several dozen men to the Great Beyond. On further examination of him, we could see how he could utterly disregard another human being. As might be well imagined, this man was never in our confidence and we were always on the lookout when he was in our vicinity."[7]

ARTHUR KINNIS NOTED that several hundred medical students from the University of Oslo were in Buchenwald during the time he and the other Allied airmen were there. "It was from these that we received a very pleasant surprise," he said. "They sent us a barrel of macaroni, meat, and potatoes, which in our state of perpetual hunger was a positive godsend. What a pleasure it was to have a solid meal, our first since capture. This was to be repeated at regular intervals, but was stopped by the SS."**[8]

* This undoubtedly refers Dr. Edwin Katzen-Ellenbogen, whose life was detailed in Chapter 7.

** According to *Buchenwald Concentration Camp 1937-1945*, some 1,250 University of Oslo students were arrested in 1944 and imprisoned in Norway; 348 were transferred to Buchenwald, where they quickly made friends by sharing the contents of their Red Cross packages. Harry Stein wrote, "The Norwegian students left Buchenwald between July 1944 and March 1945. On their odyssey through various camps, seventeen died, some of them in Buchenwald." (Stein, p. 175)

The airmen were also befriended by a group of 1,953 Danish policemen housed next door in Block 57 of the Little Camp. The Danish police, who had bitterly opposed the German occupation of Denmark in 1940, had been recently rounded up and shipped to Buchenwald via Neuengamme.★[9]

Arthur Kinnis noted that, as if by some miracle, the Danes received food parcels from the Danish Red Cross and shared them with the Allied fliers. Kinnis said, "In October 1944, permission was given to bring the supplies into the camps by Danish Red Cross trucks, which was extraordinary, as no other relief was allowed to be brought direct into the camps. We became very attached to this fine body of men, and over the many years that have passed we did not forget their many acts of kindness that took place at that time. We remembered the food that they obtained for us, their ability to help us in spite of their own problems, and how their entire group joined our party when we had a memorial service for P.D. Hemmens." ★★

The Canadian also recalled that life at Buchenwald wasn't all suffering. The one bright spot was music. Kinnis said that one of his most pleasant surprises was hearing the camp's symphony orchestra and jazz band playing English and American pieces. "Music is one language that requires no translator, and the evenings we spent listening to some very highly rated [European musicians] were exceedingly pleasant. The conductor had the reputation of playing before royalty, before his capture. How we loved to hear his rendering of *Tales from the Vienna Woods* or *Jesu, Joy of Man's Desiring,* and many other lovely creations. A Russian choir there was as good as you could hear anywhere. The mere fact that you could not understand one word drifted into the background, as one was carried into the world of music. This little haven of sound was possibly the only pleasant side of Buchenwald."[10]

WHILE MUSIC PROVIDED a brief interlude, the reality of death and suffering at Buchenwald was never far away. Dr. Victor Dupont, a Buchenwald prisoner,

---

★ A scarlet fever epidemic soon broke out in the Danish barracks and claimed scores of lives. Himmler, in mid-December, declared the Danish policemen prisoners-of-war and transferred them to a POW camp. (Stein, p. 175)

★★ Since 1984, the surviving Allied fliers imprisoned at Buchenwald have enjoyed a strong bond of friendship with their Danish counterparts. Both groups formed "Buchenwald clubs" and, with their wives, have visited each other in their respective homelands. Art Kinnis said, "We enjoy getting together to think back at what has happened and to renew our lasting friendship. We cherish that friendship that was forged so long ago." (Kinnis, p. 44)

noted that the inmates who were too ill or frail to work were sent to Auschwitz and gassed. But, during the autumn of 1944, the murder of these weak inmates was shifted back to Buchenwald. Block 61 was set aside ostensibly as a sick bay, but actually was used as a killing chamber. Dupont said, "The death toll varied daily from a minimum of ten to about 200 in Block 61. The execution was performed by injecting phenol into the heart in the most brutal manner. The ashes resulting from the cremations were thrown into the excrement pit and served to fertilize the fields around Buchenwald. I add this detail because it struck me vividly at the time.... Work, whatever it might be, was the internee's only chance of survival. As soon as they were no longer of any possible use, they were done for."[11]

ACROSS THE CONCENTRATION and death camp system, the victims of Nazism continued to rebel against their tormentors. On October 7, 1944, after learning they were about to be liquidated, prisoners working in Crematorium IV at Auschwitz-Birkenau revolted against their guards, killing three of them and using smuggled-in explosives to blow up the building and one of the gas chambers. As in previous revolts, the Germans acted swiftly and ruthlessly, killing hundreds of prisoners who had staged the uprising and hanging the Jewish women who had smuggled in the explosives from a nearby armaments factory.[12]

ON OCTOBER 18, 1944, after two months in KL Buchenwald, the Allied fliers were suddenly moved out. On that day, while Pister was absent, Luftwaffe Colonel Hannes Trautloft came to the camp and, upon seeing the American and Canadian fliers still there, ordered them moved by train from Buchenwald to *Stalag Luft III*, a POW camp for airmen, located 100 miles southeast of Berlin at Sagan, Poland—a two-day journey by rail.*[13]

The airmen spent their final evening in Buchenwald enjoying a relatively substantial meal, packing their meager belongings, saying goodbye to the friends they had made, and saying silent prayers for themselves and for the inmates who would not be leaving. Early the next morning, the 166 surviving Allied airmen (P.D. Hemmons had died and Lieutenant L.C. Beck was deathly ill in the infirmary and would not survive) were issued their old uniforms, taken

* *Stalag Luft III*, filled with captured airmen from various Allied nations, was immortalized in the book and film, *The Great Escape*, a spectacular breakout that took place in March 1944.

to the camp theater, given coffee, and told to board the cattle cars waiting for them at the railroad siding. This time it was a slightly less uncomfortable journey, for only thirty men shared each car.

At last they were leaving the hellhole of Buchenwald. For those inmates who remained behind, however, the fates would not be so kind.[14]

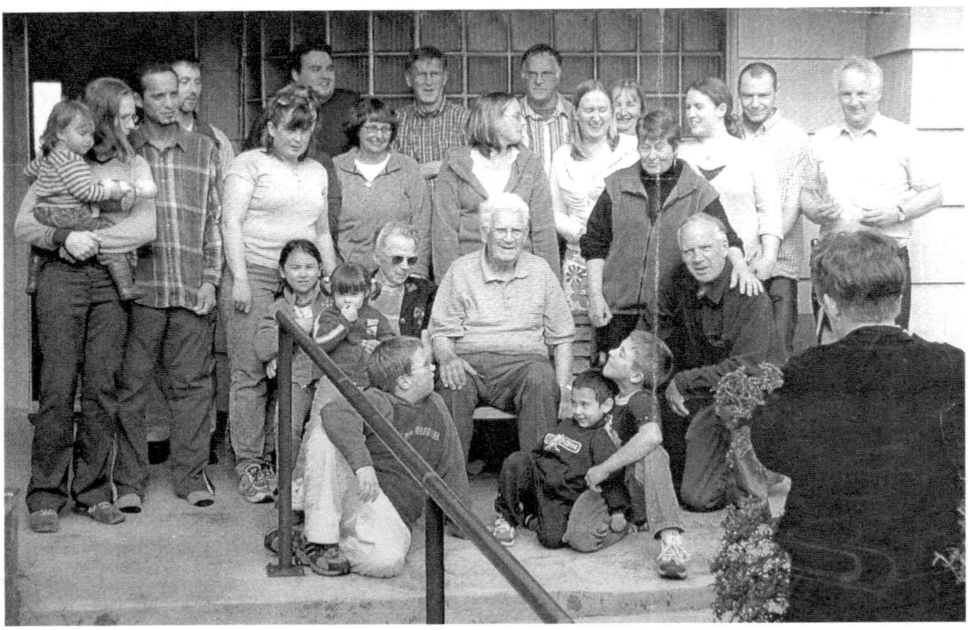

Arthur Kinnis (white hair, seated center) and his extended family being photographed in celebration of his 90th birthday, Calgary, Canada, 2005. (Courtesy Arthur Kinnis)

17
THE BEGINNING OF THE END

"Please take care of these Jews; they are my soundest capital investment."
Heinrich Himmler

EVER SINCE THE Allied landings in Normandy in June 1944, the British, Canadian, and American armies fought their way across France, driving eastward. This drive was combined with Operation Dragoon, the August 15, 1944, invasion of southern France. The two-pronged assault sent the Germans reeling, forcing them to fight a retrograde action as they pulled back to defend the western borders of their country. After Paris was liberated on August 25, the Allied armies pushed into Belgium and the Netherlands. In September 1944, a bold airborne operation—called Market Garden—designed to seize bridges in Holland and expedite a British thrust into northern Germany failed, but the setback was only temporary. Massive armies continued to build up along Germany's borders, and it was only a matter of time before the Allies would plunge into the heart of the Third Reich and put an end to Hitler's twisted dream of world conquest.[1]

As the Third Reich crumbled around him, as Germany's once-beautiful medieval cities were reduced to unrecognizable mountains of smoldering rubble, as Germany's once-invincible armies were destroyed on the battlefields in numbers not seen since the Great War or retreated deeper into the Fatherland, and as his god Adolf Hitler sank ever deeper into paranoia, *Reichsführer-SS* Heinrich Himmler began to see the hangman's noose dangling before his eyes.

Long suffering (not surprisingly) from nervous strain and debilitating stomach ailments,[2] the formerly devout Catholic Himmler wondered if there might not be some way he could atone for his sins. In the vain hope of being seen as a reasonable person, even a humanitarian, Himmler had already begun to make himself over as the savior of the Jews. For example, on July 26, 1944, he had issued a directive that halted the deportations of Hungarian Jews to Auschwitz. Two months later, he ordered Oswald Pohl and Dr. Ernst Kaltenbrunner (the latter Reinhard Heydrich's successor as head of the *Sicherheitsdienst*) to halt "any liquidation of Jews, and order that on the contrary, care should be given to weak and sick persons. I hold you personally responsible, even if this order should not be strictly adhered to by subordinate officers." In November 1944, Himmler astonishingly specified that "the crematoria in Auschwitz be dismantled [and] the Jews working in the Reich are to get normal Eastern rations. In the absence of Jewish hospitals, they may be treated with Aryan patients."

Himmler also allowed 2,700 Jews—after paying him a steep stipend—to find sanctuary in Switzerland. Behind the scenes, the *Reichsführer-SS* even tried to negotiate a secret truce with the Western Allies by going through contacts in Sweden, thinking that he might be made Germany's post-war Führer in a hoped-for American-Anglo-German war against the Soviets.[3]

FOR SEVERAL YEARS, pro-Jewish factions in the U.S. and Britain had been desperately urging the British and American governments do more to rescue the Jews from destruction in the death camps. *Why don't you bomb Auschwitz?* they wondered. *Why don't you bomb the rail lines leading to the death camps?*

Their pleas were, for the most part, ignored, the excuses for inaction ranging from the death camps being too far from the air bases, to the danger of killing and wounding the very people the raids would be designed to save, to the difficulty of pinpointing such a target as small as a set of railroad tracks.

However, as the pressure mounted, the decision was made that the I.G. Farben synthetic oil and rubber factory at Auschwitz-Birkenau—but not the death camp itself—should be bombed. On September 13, 1944, a fleet of B-24 "Liberator" bombers of the U.S. 464th Bombardment Group, flying out of Pantanella, Italy, hit the factory. Some of the bombs missed the Farben works but, by a stroke of luck, destroyed one of the gas chambers at Birkenau. The air strike, however, did not stop the killing operations there.[4]

This pinprick of an air strike prompted more thought and discussion about the possibility of disrupting the deadly work of the camps. On November 8, 1944, John W. Pehle, Director of the War Refugee Board, wrote to John J. McCloy, the Assistant Secretary of War. His letter contained two eyewitness reports about the conditions at Auschwitz-Birkenau and made reference to Operation Jericho—the RAF's precision, low-level bombing attack by nineteen Mosquito Mark VI aircraft on the prison in Amiens, France, on February 18, 1944, in which the walls were blown out, enabling hundreds of political prisoners held by the Gestapo to escape. Pehle suggested that a similar raid be made against the death camps.

The suggestion was rejected. McCloy responded that Auschwitz was beyond the range of the B-17 and B-24 heavy bombers, and pointed out, "At the present critical stage of the war in Europe, our strategic air forces are engaged in the destruction of industrial target systems vital to the dwindling war potential of the enemy, from which they should not be diverted. The positive solution to this problem is the earliest possible victory over Germany, to which end we should exert our entire means."[5]

Indeed, the inability of the Allies to develop a strategy for rescuing the prisoners of concentration and death camps was one of the great failures of the war. As McCloy noted, the range to the presumed targets from air bases in England, France, and Italy was extreme, putting aircrews in grave danger. Secondly, the term "precision bombing," so often used by the Americans, was anything but. Even with the much-vaunted Norden bombsight, bombs dropped from U.S. B-17s and B-24s rarely came close to their intended targets; the accurate strike in August on the Gustloff-Werk II at Buchenwald was an anomaly, a stroke of luck. Blowing up railroad tracks leading to the camps was even more unlikely. Not only was the chance of hitting the rails from several thousand feet slim, but the *Reichsbahn* workers were skilled at putting destroyed sections of rail back into operation within days, sometimes even hours.

Finally—and this was something that McCloy did not mention in his response—saturation bombing of the camps would no doubt have resulted in the deaths of the very people the air strikes were intended to save. McCloy's assertion that "the positive solution to this problem is the earliest possible victory over Germany, to which end we should exert our entire means" was, sadly for the incarcerated, correct.

No additional air strikes were mounted against Auschwitz or Buchenwald or any other camps, for that matter. If the millions of persons awaiting death at the hands of the Nazis were to be saved, they would either need to wait for the land armies to arrive and batter down the gates of their prisons—or liberate themselves.

IN THE AUTUMN of 1944, the Allies pushed into the Vosges Mountain region of eastern France. There, atop a 2,500-foot-high mountain thirty-one miles southwest of Strasbourg, near the border with Germany, French troops came across a former ski resort that had been transformed from a place of recreation in a spectacular alpine setting into a place of horror: the Natzweiler-Struthof

Concentration Camp, known in French as Le Struthof.

As the French approached, the Germans stayed one step ahead of them and evacuated the camp, marching the inmates hundreds of miles to Dachau; two thousand prisoners died along the way. When French troops reached the camp on November 23, 1944, all they found were empty buildings and mute evidence that horrible crimes had been committed there.

Natzweiler-Struthof and its fifty satellite camps once held 27,000 prisoners, mostly Jews, Gypsies, homosexuals, Jehovah's Witnesses, and criminals, who were put to work in the quarry. Captured by the Gestapo during the *Nacht-und-Nebel* ("Night and Fog") operations across France in the summer of 1944, members of the French Resistance had no chance to work for the Nazis; they were killed immediately upon arrival, their bodies burned in the camp crematorium, which had been completed in October 1943. Medical and scientific experiments (such as the effects of mustard gas) were also carried out on unwilling inmates at Natzweiler-Struthof by camp doctors and professors from the University of Strasbourg.[6]

A couple weeks later, a contingent of American soldiers arrived at Natzweiler-Struthof and were shocked. As this was the first camp discovered by the Western Allies, what the troops encountered was beyond comprehension. Milton Bracker, a war correspondent accompanying the troops, noted that once he had gone inside the electrified barbed wire he saw the crematorium, and the metal hooks protruding from a wall in the cellar of the building where men were hung by the wrists a few inches off the floor, and the pathology laboratory with its sparkling clean dissection table, and a room filled with red earthenware "flower pots" that were, in actuality, cremation urns. Bracker ended his report with statistics: Between October 1941 and July 1944, approximately 16,000 persons—Frenchmen, Belgians and anti-Nazi Germans—passed through Struthof. "Of these, they say, 4,000, including many women, ended in ashes."[7]

THE EXISTENCE OF the Auschwitz death camp finally came to the attention of the American public. Reports of atrocities rarely made the front page of the *New York Times*, but this time the news was too big to ignore. In a November 26, 1944, story headlined "U.S. Board Bares Atrocity Details Told by Witnesses at Polish Camps," noted that the report, based on the eyewitness testimony of two Slovak Jews and a non-Jewish Polish army major who had escaped from

Auschwitz-Birkenau, painted a truly frightening picture. The War Refugee Board's report said that three eyewitnesses provided irrefutable testimony that the Nazis were engaged in a widespread, systematic slaughter of Jews and others at the Auschwitz murder factory. The report noted that, while some 1,500,000 persons had been killed at the Maidanek (Lublin) camp over a period of three years, at least that number—and perhaps as many as 1,765,000—had been killed at Auschwitz between April 1942 and April 1944. No longer could the world look the other way and pretend that such atrocities were merely rumors or anti-German propaganda.

The rest of the nearly full-page article was devoted to quotes from the three escapees, in which they detailed the brutal treatment that Jews and other prisoners had received, including how thousands of victims per day were tricked into believing they were about to take group showers when, in fact, they were about to be gassed *en masse* with a poisonous substance known as Zyklon B.*

The article also included statements made during a news conference called by Peter Bergson, the flamboyant and controversial head of the pro-Zionist Bergson Group. He had particularly harsh words for the United Nations War Crimes Commission that had "refused to take into consideration any acts committed against persons other than nationals of the United Nations [i.e., stateless Jews]," and demanded that the Commission immediately issue a declaration stating that any atrocities committed against the "Hebrews of Europe" be regarded as a "war crime" and punished accordingly.[8]

After the publication of this article in the *Times* (and repeated elsewhere across the country), anyone who was not keenly aware of the persecutions and atrocities taking place under the Nazi banner simply was not paying attention.

OPERATION *WACHT-AM-Rhein,* which became known in the West as "the Battle of the Bulge," saw 290,000 German soldiers, 2,617 artillery pieces and rocket launchers, and 1,038 tanks and self-propelled guns hurl themselves at the Americans encamped along the German-Belgium-Luxembourg border on the night of December 15-16, 1944. It was Hitler's "last-gasp" offensive, one which he hoped would inflict such heavy casualties that the war-weary Western Allies

* "Zyklon B," is a mixture of liquid hydrocyanic (prussic) acid with chloride and bromide derivatives as catalytic agents and silica as a support. It was a powerful, commercial-grade pesticide originally created for the extermination of vermin. (Gilbert, *The Second World War*, p. 220)

would sue for peace and perhaps even join Germany in a campaign against the Soviet Union and Bolshevism.

Farther south, along the French border with Germany in Alsace-Lorraine, Operation *Nordwind*—the twin of *Wacht-am-Rhein*—got underway on December 31. It, too, scored some limited victories and made serious dents in the ranks of the American forces in the snowy region of the Vosges Mountains. Although initially successful in catching the Americans off-guard, Operations *Wacht-am-Rhein* and *Nordwind* both soon ground to a halt and ended in failure.[9] The Germans had very little left with which to hold off the Allies driving toward Berlin from east and west—and very little time left in which to hide the evidence of their efforts to annihilate the Jews.

THE YEAR 1944 ended with the prisoner population of Buchenwald and its sub-camps growing to 87,000, with 50,000 of them atop the Ettersberg, crowning it the bloated king of the concentration camps. Its *Totenbuch* also named 8,644 prisoners who had died during the year, making Buchenwald one of the deadliest of the non-death camps.[10] Throughout the Nazi empire, it is estimated that, by January 1945, at least 714,000 persons were still incarcerated in concentration and death camps.[11]

As he faced the dilemma of what to do with this huge number, Heinrich Himmler's stomach was in knots. At the beginning of 1945, with the Allies crushing Germany from all sides, the *Reichsführer-SS* realized that the prospects of him—and the Third Reich—surviving the onslaught were diminishing by the day. Could the evidence of the enormous crimes that the Nazis had perpetrated against humanity be destroyed before the regime collapsed in defeat? And would not the thousands of camp guards and administrators be more useful on the front lines than in continuing to watch over a sick and starving prison population?

Finally, to keep the inmates from falling into the hands of the advancing Allies, Himmler gave the order to abandon the camps; prisoners were to be removed and sent on evacuation marches. Already in mid-January 1945, Soviet forces were bearing down on Auschwitz-Birkenau, the Germans' principal extermination factory near Krakow, Poland. The camp was emptied and its 60,000 survivors forced to march through snow and bitter cold toward Wodzisław, thirty-five miles to the south. Anyone who fell behind was shot by the SS guards and left on the side of the road; over 15,000 never made it to

Wodzisław.[12] Those who did make it were then packed into boxcars and transported to Buchenwald, Bergen-Belsen, Dachau, Flossenbürg, Groß-Rosen, Neuengamme, Ravensbrück, and other camps inside Germany. With little or no food or water, and with the brutal winter weather taking its toll, thousands of evacuees died or were killed along their march to oblivion.[13]

An ice-coated transport carrying 2,000 inmates from Compiègne, France, pulled into the Buchenwald rail yard on January 19, 1945. Another train, this one from Auschwitz, which had pulled out in the face of the Soviet advance, had nearly 3,000 freezing inmates on board in open cattle cars, despite the fact that the temperature was well below zero. Although prisoners in each of the cars on the train from Auschwitz were dying from exposure, the train sat on the tracks at Buchenwald for five hours before the doors were unlocked and the prisoners admitted to the camp; many of the boxcars were full of frozen corpses.[14]

Louis Gros was working in the rail yard on the day that train from Auschwitz arrived. "The wood-fired locomotive wheezed its way up the hill," he said, "but on this winter day it seemed more arduous than usual, more abrupt, like it was tired. The other days it was just a *roulade* made of bass and sharp tones, of plaints and signs more or less perceived, according to the wind's humors and the vale's turns and detours. We usually no longer paid attention to it, for all it would bring to our mountaintop retreat was more misery, or, should I say, more miserable human beings....

"How many trains similar to this one had we seen arriving, full of men from the four corners of Europe, poor devils quickly made to detrain here in the legendary and hereafter awful Goethe's forest? But this one was somehow different. Today's train, which we later learned had come from Poland, was longer than usual and soon revealed itself as a genuine traveling nightmare. I stood back and looked at this long train, an entire convoy filled with people condemned to disappear for their lone crime of being born Jewish. It was a conducted tour to kill them all, slowly, surely, in the cruelest manner, like animals, or worse than animals, for animals do not know when they are about to die.

"It remained for the whole day in the rail yard, without apparent reason. We, the stevedores, who eight months before had known the anguish of such a journey in closed boxcars, had no difficulty in imagining the pangs, the physical and moral afflictions of these penned-up men, whom we tried occasionally, as they peeked their heads above the sides of the cars, to tell where they were. We could see their emaciated faces, with desperate, deep-set eyes. Somehow we could tell that they were all Jews. How long had they been locked up in this rat trap, we wondered. The tragic, the unbearable, were suddenly revealed to us, surpassing our own vision of past horrors.

"We heard horrendous tales from the survivors—that they had traveled without food or drink, at night when the temperature dropped to below twenty degrees [Fahrenheit], hardly protected from the elements by their striped, thin uniforms and maybe the fragment of a torn, shabby, rotten blanket.... During the next hour a thousand or perhaps two thousand cadavers, many of whom were frozen solid and adhering to the steel floors of the cars, were removed and thrown onto the ground of the station." These corpses were hauled off to the crematorium and quickly reduced to nothing more than smoke and ash. The survivors of the journey would soon follow them, killed by blows of a club in the basement of the crematorium.[15]

AT THE END of January 1945, Heinrich Müller, head of the Gestapo, issued a directive that instructed the camp commandants to identify, and then eliminate, potential troublemakers in their camps who might instigate uprisings in the event Allied forces approached.[16]

As Germany's battlefronts in the East and West crumbled in the face of unrelenting attacks, the rail transport essential for bringing desperately needed supplies and reinforcements to the front was requisitioned instead to carry Jews and political prisoners to their deaths. Donald McKale noted, "Despite the top priority given the Wehrmacht in the use of the trains for shipping troops and equipment to the battlefronts, the SS nearly always had the death trains it demanded. At least twice the deportations were apparently halted because of the intervention of the army, which requested the trains for its use.... In both instances, Himmler intervened successfully with the head of the Reich Transport Ministry to acquire the deportation trains....

"[Adolf] Eichmann's Gestapo office organized and scheduled the deportation trains. At the beginning of the deportations, each transport carried a thousand people. Later in the war, the trains frequently held two thousand or even five thousand people, as the SS attempted to kill as many Jews as possible before the conflict ended."[17]

There were also other ways of getting rid of the evidence. At Stutthof, for example, the concentration camp near Danzig in northern Poland, the Nazis herded 5,000 prisoners into the freezing waters of the Baltic Sea in early 1945 and machine-gunned them to death. The rest of the inmates, a group of nearly 50,000, was sent on an evacuation march into the countryside but were intercepted by advancing Soviet forces and turned back. Instead of freeing the prisoners or allowing them to be rescued by the Soviets, however, the accompanying German guards forced them to return to Stutthof. A combination of winter weather and the brutal treatment by the SS caused the deaths of thousands of prisoners on the return march.[18]

ON JANUARY 27, 1945, Soviet troops, driving deeply into Poland, entered the vast Auschwitz camp complex to discover over 648 corpses and 7,000 inmates clinging to life, along with gas chambers and evidence of mass murder. Yakov Vinnichenko, a nineteen-year-old Russian soldier, recalled recoiling from the sight and smell of so many filthy, scabrous individuals. "Some tried to kiss us, but it was uncomfortable, you didn't want to get infected," he said. "They were skin-and-bones, could hardly stand on their feet."[19]

Although having already endured the most pitiless war ever fought, the Soviets did not need any more reasons to wreak vengeance on the Nazis, but Auschwitz renewed their resolve.[20] In the U.S., however, the media underplayed Auschwitz and its attendant atrocities. Nor did the U.S. Army give its advancing forces any idea of what might lay ahead of them.

ON FEBRUARY 1, 1945, Berlin became a city under siege. As 180 Soviet divisions closed in for the kill, every Berliner capable of lifting a shovel was put to work turning the capital into a fortress, for they knew that hundreds of thousands of Soviet troops, burning with rage, were bearing down on them, ready to exact retribution for the terrible crimes that German forces had committed during the 1941 invasion of the Soviet Union.*

* The Americans and British, moving into and across Germany from the west, decided not to participate in the siege of Berlin. General Dwight D. Eisenhower explained in a letter to Army Chief of Staff George C. Marshall: "Berlin itself is no longer a particularly important objective. Its usefulness to the German has been largely destroyed and even his government is preparing to move to another area." (Eisenhower, *Crusade in Europe*, p. 401) For his part, Lieutenant General Omar Bradley, commander of the 12th U.S. Army Group, expanded on Ike's reluctance to expend American lives in a fight for Berlin: "I could see no justification for taking casualties in the capture of a city we would promptly hand over to the Russians [per an agreement arrived at by the Big Three at Yalta that established the post-war occupation zones of Germany]." (Bradley, p. 537)

Berlin's buildings were sandbagged, tank traps dug, streets barricaded with rubble, mines and booby traps installed, fighting positions carved into every nook and cranny. Slogans designed to instill fear and improve morale, such as *Sieg oder Siberien* ("Victory or Siberia"), were painted on what few walls still stood. Old men and young boys were handed a *Panzerfaust* or a couple of grenades or a bolt-action Mauser rifle and given a short course in how to use them. Hitler and his minions prepared to burrow into their bunker deep beneath the Chancellery and await a miracle, such as America and Britain suddenly falling out and going to war against the Soviets; it was Germany's only hope.[21]

That hope was dashed when, on February 4, the "Big Three"—Roosevelt, Churchill, and Stalin—met with relative amity at the Black Sea resort of Yalta to discuss the future of Germany and Europe after the war. Killing on a massive scale was still going on. Besides the huge, pitched battles on the Eastern Front, and the large German counter-offensive in the West, the start of 1945 saw heavy attacks by German V-2 missiles against English cities; 1,068 British civilians would be killed in the aerial assaults during January and February. Roosevelt and Churchill told Stalin at Yalta that they would step up their bombing campaign against German lines of communications in the Berlin-Leipzig-Dresden area.*[22]

IN EARLY FEBRUARY 1945, nearly two weeks after the liberation of Auschwitz, a train carrying some 14,000 evacuees that had been shunted from there to one destination after another showed up at Buchenwald, swelling the camp's prisoner population—including the satellite camps—to 112,000.[23] That same month—February—the bulging Groß-Rosen camp in Lower Silesia in southwest Poland was also emptied, with over 37,000 prisoners sent on forced marches; Buchenwald received 6,000 of its evacuees.

On the morning of February 9, 1945, another shipment of prisoners arrived at Buchenwald. Among the 1,400 men and boys on the train that had traveled from the Groß-Rosen camp was the French teenager Robert Max Widerman. Two-and-a-half years earlier, he and his family had been arrested in their Parisian apartment.[24] After spending nine months at the Blechhammer forced labor camp in Upper Silesia, and, with the Soviet army coming ever closer,

* Thus far unscathed, the baroque jewel of Dresden, through which German troops were being funneled to engage Soviet forces around Breslau on the Eastern front, would be essentially wiped off the map. (Kershaw, pp. 235-240)

Widerman was transferred again, this time marching along with thousands of other inmates for two weeks through deep snow to Groß-Rosen. Of the four thousand who began the journey, only half of them completed it.

The conditions at Groß-Rosen were appalling, even worse than Blechhammer. The weather was abominable, the barracks unfit for human habitation, and the guards cruel beyond belief. During their first three days at the camp, each new arrival received only one piece of bread per day. Fortunately, their stay at Groß-Rosen was brief; after only a few days there, Widerman and the Blechhammer group were on the move again—packed into cattle cars and shipped off to Buchenwald.[25]

On the same transport with Robert Max Widerman was Johannen Goldkranz, a twenty-four-year-old Jew from Bendzin, Poland. Like Widerman, Goldkranz, who later changed his name to John Ranz, had survived five other internments: the Bendzin ghetto, the Łódź ghetto, Cobelwitz, Groß-Rosen, and Blechhammer, where he worked in an I.G. Farben plant that made synthetic fuel.

Goldkranz, packed into an open-top gondola car, recalled that the train stopped briefly in Leipzig on a freezing day before continuing on to Weimar. "On the platform I saw men and women, elegantly dressed. They were aware of our presence but avoided looking at us.... Some of us dared to ask the civilians for water. 'No, it is forbidden,' came the answer. Some didn't even bother to respond. Above our heads German electricians were repairing the electric wires. They pretended not to see us. Were they really so cold and cruel? Even a stone would have been moved by our appearance.

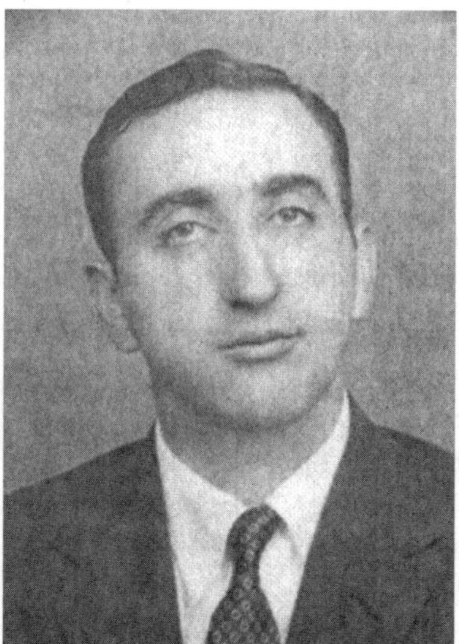

Johannen Goldkrantz (photographed in 1945), who changed his name to John Ranz after he came to America. (Courtesy John Ranz)

"Then I saw Red Cross sisters moving around the station, handing out coffee and rolls to the voyagers who were not prisoners. My eyes widened with excitement. Wasn't the Red Cross supposed to help all the needy? While a guard's attention was focused elsewhere, I asked a Red Cross sister, who passed near my car, for some water. She looked at me for a moment without expression, and kept walking. To the next passing sister, I extended my tin can, so it would be easier to put water or coffee into it. Again there was no reaction. Apparently I had been mistaken about the Red Cross.

"Then I heard groups of German civilians standing on the platform, pointing to us and saying, 'Jews, Jews.' During the hour or two we waited at the Leipzig rail station, we received not one morsel of food or water, despite our begging. I just couldn't comprehend it. The train finally left the station, ending our hope of getting something to drink. We had no other choice but to lick the snow from the surface of the railcar."[26] In minutes, however, getting a drink of water would be the least of Goldkranz's worries.

By February 1945, hundreds of Germany's cities and towns had been flattened by the British and American air forces. One of the few cities untouched up to that point was Weimar. Nearby Erfurt, Gera, Leipzig, and Jena had already been hit, and nervous Weimarers worried that it was only a matter of time before they, too, were targeted. Although Weimar had little in the way of industrial or military targets, and its classic old buildings, many dating from the 16th century, were considered some of Europe's most beautiful, it was on the Allies' list of cities to be bombed.

On that frigid morning of February 9, while Widerman's and Goldkrantz's train sat on the tracks at Weimar's train station, Mission 824, comprising 1,296 bombers and 871 fighter escorts of the U.S. Eighth Air Force, was taking off from bases in England and headed eastward for six targets. Of the 1,296 bombers, a group of 198 B-17s turned for Weimar.[27]

First Lieutenant Jack F. Stanley, one of the American pilots flying that day with the 487th Bomb Group, 837th Squadron, based at Lavenham, England, reported laconically on the February 9th mission in his journal: "We had two targets. One was Bollen [sic: Böhlen, a synthetic oil refinery at Merseberg] and secondary was Weimar (armament factory). I led the low squadron with Capt. Pete Riegal as Air Leader.

"Up at 3 A.M. and we took off at 8 A.M. Route was over North Sea across Belgium...into Germany. About 30 minutes from target we were jumped by 5 ME-262 jet-propelled E/A [enemy aircraft] that made a pass and came around in front. P-51s jumped that 262 and started firing. Dogfight over on our left was going on. I closed up my squadron with lead squadron and just then another jet came whipping by our Group. P-51s took after him. Some of the boys in our group took some shots, but didn't hit.

"We made I. P. [initial point—start of bombing run] and came in on our run. We bombed off Lead Squadron due to our mikey set [aircraft communication equipment] going out," Stanley noted. "Encountered light but very accurate flak. We dropped on Lead and target was visual. We got good results. Lt. Shepard, in the lead flying #5, was hit and seen to go down. Lt. Wertz, #13 in my squadron, lost an engine and his ship was badly hit.... Got boys home OK."[28]

At mid-morning, Widerman and Goldkrantz looked skyward as Weimar's air-raid warning sirens began to wail. As the wave of bombers approached the city, anti-aircraft batteries that ringed the city went into action. Most of the U.S. ordnance—250- and 500-lb. high-explosive bombs, plus incendiaries—came whistling down directly on top of Market Square, and the historic heart of the city was torn apart. Among the buildings smashed were the town hall, the Elephant Hotel, the adjacent Hotel zum Erbprinzen, and the Friedrich Schiller house that dated from 1777. The National Theater, where the German constitution had been written by the National Assembly on August 11, 1919, was badly damaged. Nearby apartment blocks, private homes, offices, churches, and pubs also disintegrated violently in the rain of bombs.

Gustloff-Werk I, the arms factory near downtown Weimar, was not spared by the Allied air raid. Eighteen hundred Buchenwald inmates who worked at the factory, and were housed nearby, were supposed to have been sealed in their barracks during the raid but, as the bombs began to fall, many escaped and dashed for the underground air-raid shelters. A bomb hit one of the shelters, killing from 230 to 280 of the slave workers and wounding many more; as many as ten SS guards were killed in the raid.[29] Three-hundred and thirty Weimar civilians also died.[30]

Locked into an open-top railcar at the train station, Robert Max Widerman felt he was a sitting duck for the attacking aircraft. "When we were ready to get off the train, we saw Allied bombers over us," he noted. "They were flying very low. The fliers must have been able to see our striped uniforms, our bodies crowded into the open cars, and the German soldiers guarding us. Yet, they started to drop bombs and then came in even lower to machine-gun us. In panic, we struggled to climb out of the cars, trying to jump down and hide under them. Fear of death triggered my adrenaline. Hoping that no bombs or bullets would hit me, I jumped as fast as I could and hid under the train. Two hundred of us died at the station that day at Allied hands. Most of us looked like corpses already."[31]

Johannen Goldkranz, too, was stunned by the raid. "We all looked up at the sky. The planes were like an orderly parade. In a minute a series of explosions ripped the air around us. Everything became dark, and clouds of dust and dirt covered the ground. I could only count the first few explosions, then I could no longer count, there were so many. The earth around me was moving up and down. I felt lifted up, with the railcar as well. I couldn't see. Everything around me was black.... After a while the explosions subsided. People started to come out, and we heard the cries of the injured, who called for help."

Goldkranz was woozy and slightly wounded from flying debris, but he was alive. Others were not so fortunate; the guards forced the survivors to collect the dead and pile them up. During this detail, Goldkranz managed to find a few heads of cabbage scattered about and he devoured a few pieces, stuffing the rest into his pockets; who knew when he might eat again?[32]

When at last the all-clear sounded in Weimar, the stunned civilians emerged from their shelters and began picking through the remains of their once-beautiful city. The streets were clogged with broken masonry, splintered timbers, shattered glass, shredded Nazi flags, and bits and pieces of furniture, crockery, silverware, bedding, draperies, carpets, framed artwork, and children's toys. The cobblestone streets were cratered. Firefighters made their way through the debris as best they could but, even when they reached a burning structure, there was little they could do, for the water mains had been ruptured. Dogs, cats, and the bleeding remnants of human bodies protruded from the wreckage. Cries and moans of the injured prompted the survivors to begin digging them out with their bare hands. Other survivors, less altruistic, came in to loot. The hospitals, mercifully spared by the bombs, soon overflowed with the wounded.[33]

THE BOMBING OF Weimar did not mean any reprieve for the survivors of the transport from Groß-Rosen. That afternoon another train arrived at the station and the new arrivals were hauled up the Ettersberg to their new home, Buchenwald, where they were stripped, shaved, immersed in delousing and disinfection solutions, and issued clean uniforms.

Hermann Pister's main prison and its sub-camps were now bursting at the seams, and there was no way the camp's resources could adequately house or feed them. The Little Camp was especially overcrowded; the pre-fabricated horse stables that had each housed 500-600 inmates when they were first installed now held three times that number.[34] One historian wrote, "The Little Camp was closed off and isolated from the rest of the camp. Hunger, disease, and death reigned there, and countless corpses lay sprawled between the barracks. The Jews who arrived from Auschwitz and Groß-Rosen...were thrown like discarded objects into a site that resembled a vast pigsty."[35]

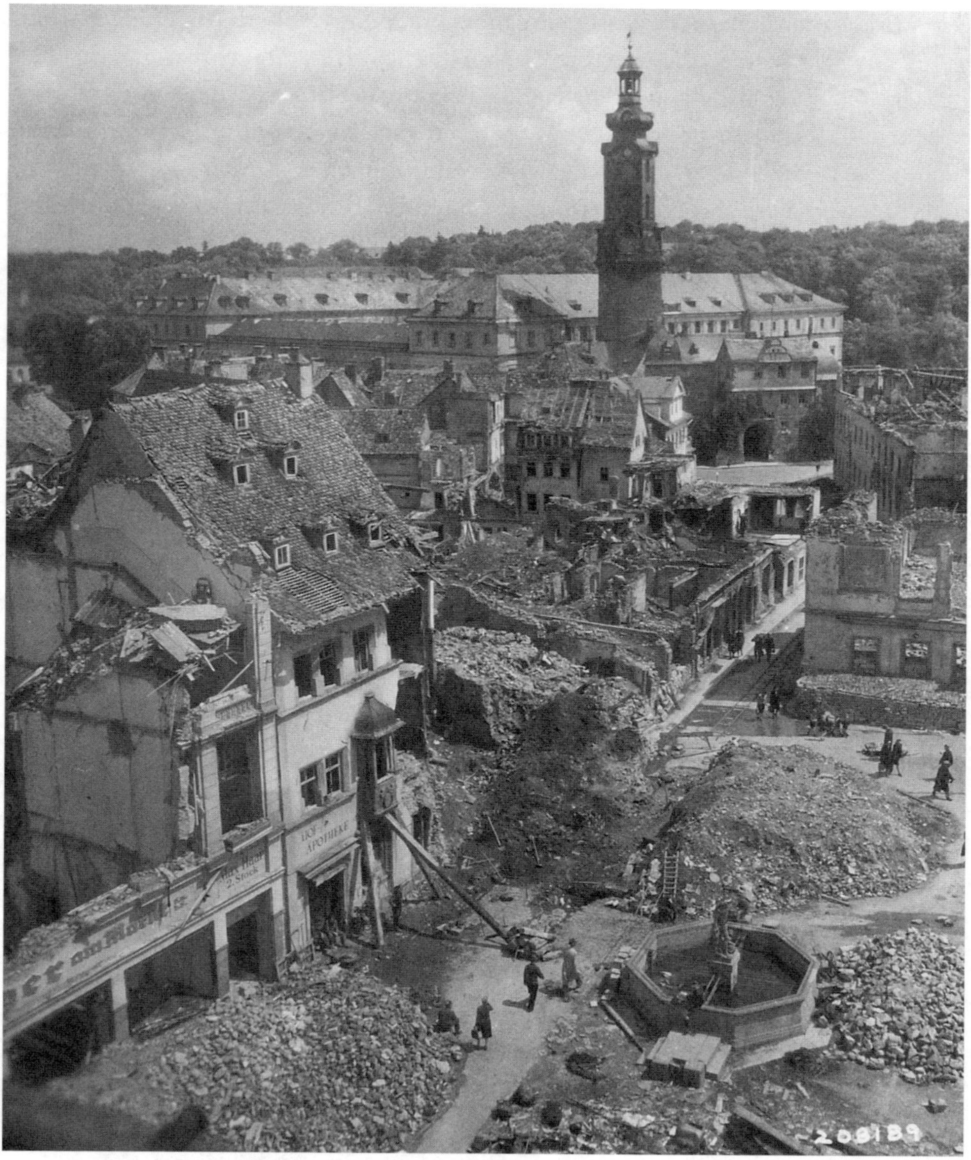

Despite the destruction of much of Weimar's Marktplatz, the tower of Weimar Castle, dating from the 16th century, still stands. (U.S. National Archives)

In less than 100 days, some 5,200 inmates had died in the Little Camp; between January and April 1945, more than 13,000 perished at Buchenwald. These grim statistics were repeated—or exceeded—at all of the remaining camps.[36]

But, compared to Groß-Rosen, thought young Robert Max Widerman, Buchenwald seemed like a resort camp. His exclusively French barracks in the Main Camp actually had clean beds, pillows, and blankets. There were tables, benches, lockers for personal items, and even a bathroom with sinks, toilets, and showers. Because he looked so small and young, the older inmates soon took him under their wing and "adopted" him, calling him *Bébé*, and providing him with nourishments such as sugar that most of the prisoners had not seen for years. He said, "I didn't have to fight for my life anymore. From that day on I was under their protection."

His many talents as a singer and dancer were noted, and he was enlisted by a small musical combo in the camp to visit the various barracks in the evening and perform—about the only thing that lifted the spirits of the inmates. During this period, Robert Max Widerman was convinced that, were he lucky enough to survive, he would make show business his life. From his friends at Buchenwald he would receive the stage name with which he would be forever linked: Robert Clary.*[37]

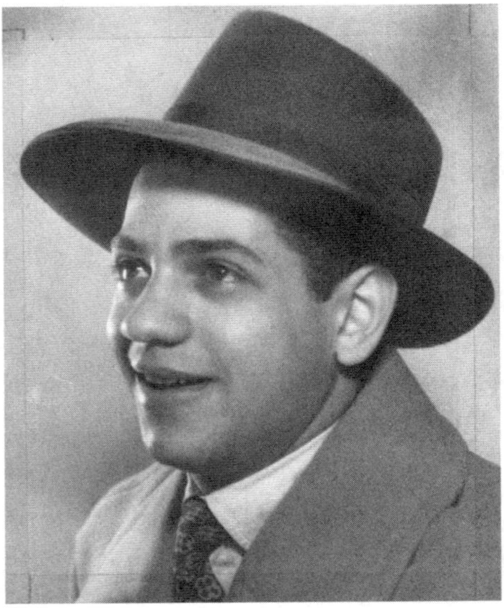

A publicity photo of the entertainer and Buchenwald survivor Robert Clary taken in 1948, shortly after he immigrated to the United States. (Courtesy Robert Clary)

* From 1965 until 1971, in a case of art imitating life, Clary played the role of Corporal Louis LeBeau, one of the prisoners-of-war being held in a German POW camp in the television comedy *Hogan's Heroes*.

BOYS INTERNED AT Buchenwald were recruited to clean up the bomb damage in downtown Weimar. One of them, Perec Zylberberg, recalled, "I was drafted along with most of my barrack inmates for that kind of work. We [were] taken by freight trains to the outskirts of the city and then distributed in smaller units to various parts of the city. Each group had a *Kapo* and a German guard."

It was on one of these wreckage-clearing missions that Zylberberg was struck by the ordinariness of life taking place outside of the camp, a life he had nearly totally forgotten. Despite the bomb damage, the burghers of Weimar seemed to be going about their daily business "in an unhurried manner," he noted. Once in a while, kindly German women might even sneak the filthy, ragged boys a potato or slice of bread.

Salek Orenstein was also on a rubble-clearing detail. He said that his group was put to work for a few days cleaning bombed-out houses. In the cellars of several houses, they found bodies—and food! Not caring if the food was spoiled or poisoned, they ate what they could. This unexpected sustenance helped them gain some of their energy and strength.

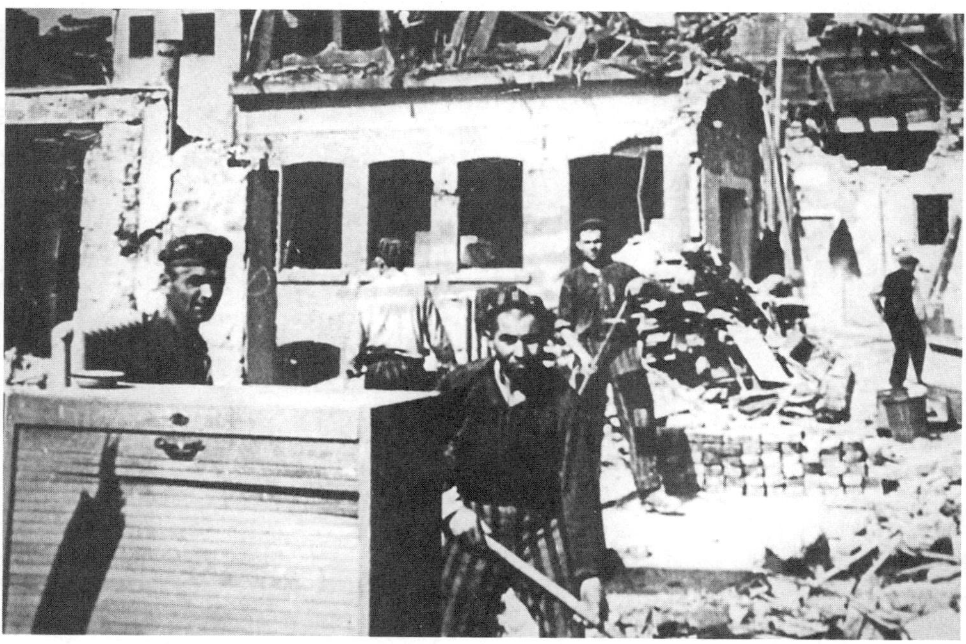

Buchenwald inmates cleaning up rubble after the bombing of Weimar, February 9, 1945. (Buchenwald Memorial)

Orenstein also felt a great deal of satisfaction and hope after seeing the destruction done to Weimar by the Allied planes, stating, "For the first time, I could see that the Germans were being squeezed, their lives and property damaged."[38]

New arrival Johannen Goldkrantz volunteered for clean-up detail. "In Weimar," he said, "the work detail cleaned up the rubbish of the bombed-out houses and dug under the ruins to find bodies.... At 9 A.M. our detail worked at removing bricks and cement slabs from the buildings and piling them into trucks.... I could see the civilian population, the stores, their life, and the streets. I hadn't seen these things in a long time. Although we were strictly forbidden to look and were constantly under the watchful eye of the guard, we managed to see."[39]

The bombing of Weimar, while it satisfied some deep-down longing on the part of the Buchenwald inmates to see death and destruction inflicted on the German civilians, did nothing to relieve them of their own suffering. The bombing did not end the war, nor did it signal that liberation for the prisoners was on the horizon.

Or did it?

18
THIRD ARMY TO THE RESCUE

"We pointed out that the only way to avoid casualties was to move fast."
Lt. Gen. George S. Patton, Jr.
Third U.S. Army commander

THE AIR ONSLAUGHT against Germany that followed the Yalta Conference was enormous and pitiless. Thousands of German civilians died in massive British and American air raids as part of Operation Argument, including at least 60,000 (and possibly more than double that number) in the February 13-15, 1945, aerial attack on Dresden; most of them burned to death in the firestorm that was created there.[1]

With Field Marshal Sir Bernard Law Montgomery's 21st Army Group firmly established along the northern Rhine, Lieutenant General Omar Bradley's 12th Army Group prepared to execute Operation Lumberjack—a plan that called for Courtney H. Hodges' First U.S. Army to attack southeastward toward the juncture of the Ahr and Rhine Rivers and then swing south to meet Patton, whose Third Army would simultaneously drive northeastward through the Eifel region. If successful, the operation would capture Cologne, Bonn, and Koblenz and bring the 12th Army Group to the Rhine along the entire area north of the Moselle River.

Bradley launched Lumberjack on March 1, 1945. On the northern flank, First Army established bridgeheads over the Erft River, entered Euskirchen on March 4 and Cologne the following day. Simultaneously, Patton's Third Army—consisting of Major General Troy H. Middleton's VIII Corps, Major General Manton S. Eddy's XII Corps, and Major General Walton H. Walker's XX Corps—swept all the way through the Eifel region to the banks of the Rhine.

The last natural barrier, the broad Rhine River, stood in the way—but not for long. On March 7, Combat Command B of the U.S. 9th Armored Division successfully captured the first intact bridge across the Rhine at a town called Remagen, south of Cologne. Even Hitler's use of V-2 rockets and jet aircraft against the Yanks crossing the bridge failed to halt the U.S. advance. Suddenly it seemed as if the entire American Army was pouring into Germany, with nothing to stop it.[2]

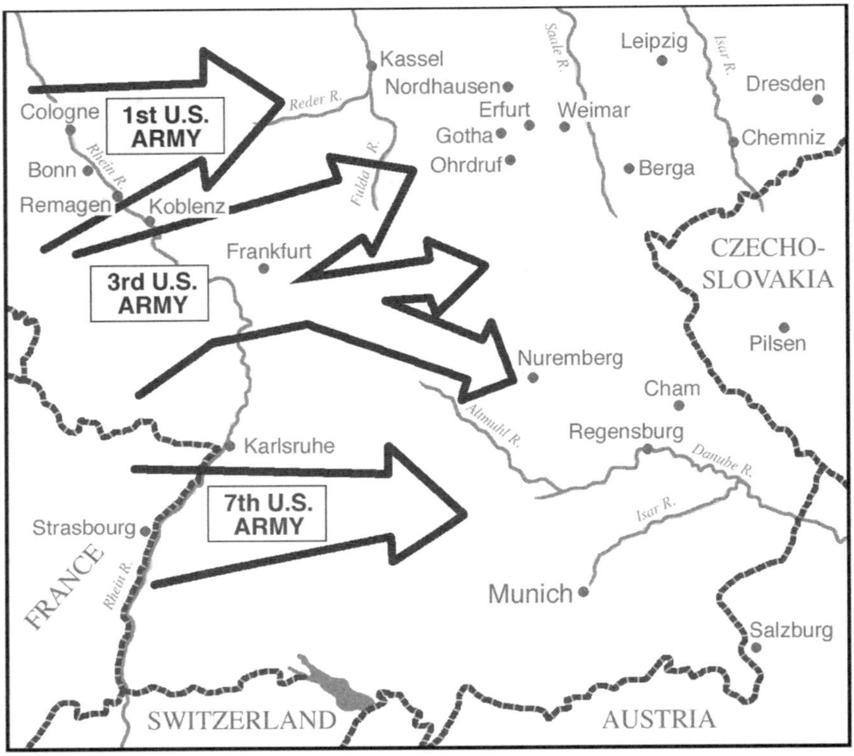

Driving deeply into Germany from the West in March 1945, the three American armies of the 12th U.S. Army Group are about to discover unimaginable scenes of horror—for which they are ill prepared. (Positions approximate)

AS HIS ARMIES defending Germany's borders disintegrated at an ever-increasing rate, Hitler in January 1945 had created a new force out of whole cloth—Army Group Vistula—and ordered it to halt the Soviets. Inexplicably, he appointed Heinrich Himmler, a complete military amateur, to be its commander-in-chief. To no one's surprise, Himmler failed miserably; after suffering staggering losses (including considerable desertions), he was fired in mid-March as head of Army Group Vistula.

To the stressed-out *Reichsführer-SS*, the sacking probably came as a relief, for now, as Nazi Germany's end seemed evermore certain, he could concentrate on his number-one priority—saving his own hide.[3] To accomplish this, Himmler had decided not to pass along Hitler's directive that the camps and anyone still in them must be destroyed before they could be liberated; the Jews, Hitler had insisted, "should not be permitted to rejoice at Germany's devastation." The Führer was particularly loath to abandon the Mittelbau-Dora facility, for it was the heart of his "wonder weapons" program; over 22,000 V-1 "buzz bombs" and more than 3,000 V-2 ballistic missiles had already been built in the tunnels there. Hitler wanted the technology and the 41,000 slave laborers who worked on the weapons relocated somewhere else, somewhere safer, somewhere where they could continue their work and create enough weapons to obliterate his enemies.[4]

American bombers, in mid-March, struck again, this time against the thorium ore processing plant at Oranienburg, which was part of the Nazis' atomic-bomb research program, dooming Germany's slim chances of developing a nuclear weapon in time to prevent total defeat. [5]

THE BLUE ARROWS on Patton's Third Army situation maps in his mobile headquarters trailer all pointed eastward. From the vicinity of Frankfurt-am-Main, Patton's three corps—Middleton's VIII, Eddy's XII, and Walker's XX—were plunging side-by-side over hills, across streams and fields, through woods, and into towns and villages, through barricades, road blocks, and mine-fields, destroying all efforts by the Germans to slow the advance. Since August 1944, the XII and XX Corps* had been the main striking arms of Patton's Third Army and, as such, had blazed a trail from the western coast of France, through Belgium, and into Germany.

The divisions that comprised Walker's XX Corps from the middle to the end of March 1945 were the 6th, 10th, 11th, and 12th Armored Divisions, and the 5th, 26th, 65th, 80th, and 94th Infantry Divisions. During that same period of time, making up Manton S. Eddy's XII Corps (which had been attached to Third Army on August 1, 1944), were the 4th Armored Division and 76th, 89th, and 90th Infantry Divisions. Middleton's VIII Corps, which had been added to Third Army on December 20, 1944, shortly before Middleton's units were mauled during the Battle of the Bulge, consisted only of the 87th and 89th Infantry Divisions. All told, the three corps that made up Patton's Third Army totaled some 203,000 men.[6]

---

* An army corps is the most fluid of military organizations, the number of divisions within it increasing or decreasing as the tactical situation demands. Each American armored division in World War II numbered approximately 12,600 men, while more than 14,000 men comprised a standard infantry division. (Stanton, pp. 15, 18)

By mid-March, Walker's XX Corps had taken Trier, Saarlautern, and Kaiserslautern. By March 21, Walker's advance elements had reached both the Rhine and the Main, then crossed both rivers and took Mainz, Wiesbaden, and Frankfurt.

Eddy's XII Corps, too, had progressed well, crossing the Mosel River on March 14, and capturing Bad Kreuznach on March 18 and Worms three days later. On the 22nd, XII Corps assaulted across the Rhine River at Oppenheim where it pummeled the German defenders. For six days—March 21-27—Eddy's units battled for and seized Mainz in conjunction with XX Corps. Middleton's VIII Corps followed behind the spearhead units and performed "mopping up" operations, i.e., eliminating pockets of resistance that were bypassed by the lead units in order to keep the advance from stalling.

By the end of March, the 4th and 6th Armored Divisions were seasoned, battle-hardened units. Highly regarded was the 4th, which had come ashore with VIII Corps at Utah Beach, Normandy, France, on July 11, 1944, and proceeded to cut a bloody swath through the Germans all across Western Europe. During the Battle of the Bulge in December 1944, 4th Armored was one of the key elements that made an historic winter march in record time to help break the siege on American forces at Bastogne, Belgium, thus earning the sobriquet "Patton's Best." So feared was the 4th that the Germans referred to the outfit as "Roosevelt's SS." Transferred from VIII Corps to XII Corps in January 1945, Major General William M. Hoge's 4th Armored was the tip of the spear for much of Patton's bold dash toward Germany—and into the history books.*

Major General Robert W. Grow's 6th Armored Division, too, had seen plenty of combat since arriving at Utah Beach eight days after the 4th Armored. Like the 4th, the 6th also took part in the action to relieve besieged Bastogne. The 6th crossed the Rhine on March 25, bulldozed its way through heavy opposition at Frankfurt-am-Main, and then headed in a northeast direction toward Kassel.[7]

On March 30, Grow's tankers saw firsthand the evidence of Nazi cruelty. The division's newspaper, *Armored Attacker*, reported that the 6th came across a

* The news wasn't always good; after crossing the Main River at Aschaffenburg on March 25, Hoge's 4th Armored Division, upon the instigation of Patton, sent a 293-man armored force known as Task Force Baum deep into enemy territory to *Oflag-III*—the POW camp at Hammelburg—in a failed attempt to rescue Patton's son-in-law, Lieutenant Colonel John K. Waters, who was being held there. The raiding party fought its way to and into the camp but was decimated in the effort. Waters was not rescued and only a handful of the raiders made it back to friendly lines. The failed raid was considered Patton's worst blunder of the war. (MacDonald, *The Last Offensive*, pp. 280-284)

camp of 900 Hungarian Jewish women near Homburg, a town about twenty-two miles southwest of Kassel:

"Most of the 900 had been working in munitions and poisonous-gas factories under incredibly hard slave labor conditions. For months they had received only one bowl of water-like soup and two pieces of bread per day, wore wooden shoes and burlap-like garments, and had no soap with which to wash. The women were under the strict control of SS troops, who shaved their heads....

"Most horrible part of the story concerned the treatment received by the women who became too ill to work. They were disrobed, thrown on trucks with the already dead and their fate then became unknown."[8]

Even this initial encounter with evil did not fully prepare the men of the division for what they would discover in just a fortnight.

THERE WAS STILL much confusion in Berlin as to what should be done with the bloated camps and their inmates; Himmler still dithered, continually suffering from second thoughts, changes of mind, and agonizing stomach cramps. On March 20, Oswald Pohl, head of the economic administration of the SS, visited Buchenwald and reiterated to the leadership Himmler's earlier order to spare Jewish prisoners, including giving them sufficient rations and providing all necessary medical care to keep them alive.[9]

On the night of March 23, the British and Canadians crossed the northern Rhine in Operation Plunder. Heinz Guderian, one of the last generals Hitler could trust, went to his Führer, tried to explain the rapidly deteriorating military situation, and pleaded with him to conclude an armistice with the Western Allies; Hitler fired him on the spot.[10]

The next day the largest and most successful airborne-and-glider operation of the war—Operation Varsity—took place in the vicinity of Wesel.[11] The inmates of Buchenwald, trying to get war news on their clandestine radios, no doubt cheered silently.

Three days later, from its last remaining launch site near The Hague, Germany fired its final salvo of V-2s; hundreds of the other sites had already been overrun or wiped out by aerial attacks.* Guderian's warnings proved to be true; before the month was out, Soviet troops were in Poland, Hungary, and Austria, and the Americans and British were about to encircle the Ruhr.[12]

* During the course of the V-1 and V-2 attacks on England between September 8, 1944, and March 27, 1945, 1,050 of the missiles killed 2,754 and wounded 6,523. (*New York Times*, April 27, 1945)

LIKE HIMMLER, PROPAGANDA Minister Josef Goebbels realized that the Allied discovery of the camps would mean death for the Nazi leadership if ever they were caught. In early April, he noted, "I fear that the concentration camps have grown a bit above Himmler's head. Just suppose that these camps should be overrun by the enemy in their present condition. What an outcry would be heard."[13]

Himmler knew he faced Hitler's wrath—or even more—by countermanding his Führer's orders, and his nervous condition grew worse, but this was a straw worth grasping. Himmler had begun secret negotiations with Count Folke Bernadotte, vice-president of the Swedish Red Cross, and arranged for the removal of Danish and Norwegian prisoners at Mittelbau-Dora, from which they would be transported to Neuengamme, where the Swedish Red Cross would look after them; other transports took sick inmates to Bergen-Belsen. Himmler got up the courage to tell the camp commandants to halt the evacuations and executions of prisoners and leave the camps intact for the Allies to liberate. It was an order that did not long remain in force, for American troops were coming dangerously close to the hell-holes of Mittelbau-Dora, Ohrdruf, and Buchenwald, and Himmler suddenly lost his nerve and decided not to countermand Hitler's wishes.[14]

Here the historical record gets confused. According to Himmler's biographers Roger Manvell and Heinrich Fraenkel, "[Ernst] Kaltenbrunner [the head of the RSHA, Reich Security Main Office] had ordered the wholesale evacuation of Buchenwald which began, probably without Himmler's knowledge, on 3 April; Himmler, says [Walter] Schellenberg, stopped the evacuation on 10 April as soon as he learned of it from the son of the Swiss President, Jean-Marie Musi, to whom on 7 April he had given his word that Buchenwald should be left intact for the Allied liberation, a promise intended to impress General Eisenhower in Himmler's favour."*[15] Schellenberg's intervention was, however, too late—the evacuation had already begun; thousands of prisoners were trudging the countryside on forced marches under armed guard.

* Harry Stein has different information. He wrote, "There is evidence that during the first days of April 1945 the SS command temporarily considered surrendering the camp to the Allies.... As late as April 3, Hermann Pister declared his intention to surrender the camp.... Himmler gave the order to evacuate the camp on April 6." (Stein, p. 227)

BEFORE THE BATTLE to take Mühlhausen began on April 4, General Grow said that XX Corps issued an order that changed his direction of advance. According to an interview he gave to Army historian Hollis Alpert, the 6th Armored was to advance "with all possible speed and take the cities of Weimar and Erfurt."[16] At this point in the war, it was Army doctrine to team an armored division with an infantry division for, without the support of foot troops, the tanks were exceedingly vulnerable to enemy fire. Accompanying 6th Armored, therefore, was the 80th Infantry Division, while the 76th Infantry Division was paired with 4th Armored.

Of the two infantry divisions assigned to accompany the tankers, only the 80th—made up of draftees from Pennsylvania, Maryland, Virginia, and West Virginia—could be considered an experienced outfit. Major General Horace L. McBride's "Blue Ridge" boys had entered Europe at Utah Beach in August 1944, then proceeded to fight their way eastward with barely a break in the action. Like the 4th and 6th Armored Divisions, the 80th was hurled against the German breakthrough during the Battle of the Bulge and contributed to restoring the shattered American front lines.

By contrast, the 76th Infantry Division, commanded by Major General William R. Schmidt, had been in combat only since early February 1945. Although it had seen a few skirmishes, the 76th was still relatively new to the rigors of combat and the horrors of war.

Assisting these units in a mop-up role were Major General Frank L. Culin, Jr.'s 87th "Golden Acorn" Infantry Division and Major General Thomas D. Finley's 89th Infantry Division. The 87th had not seen its first action until December 8, 1944, near Metz, France, but was in the thick of fighting at the end of December during the Battle of the Bulge. The division also was engaged in the U.S. Army's attempts to crack Germany's vaunted West Wall, the so-called "Siegfried Line."

The least experienced of Third Army's combat divisions heading eastward was the 89th Infantry Division. Although it did not arrive in Europe until January 1945 and did not receive its baptism of fire until March 11, the "Rolling W" Division, so named for its shoulder patch that depicted a "W" inside a circle, was champing at the bit, eager to roll over and crush the enemy.[17]

The American military machine was making good progress across Germany on its drive to link up with the Soviets at the Elbe River. But 12th Army Group commander Bradley considered slowing down or halting Patton's Third Army to prevent a salient from forming while, at the same time, pushing Hodges's First

Army to catch up with Patton's forward elements and straighten the front line. Patton reported, "We received instructions to move as rapidly as possible to the line of the Werra-Weser Rivers, and after that to move east on the Elbe River. It was suggested by Higher Headquarters that we make this move slowly. However, we pointed out that the only way to avoid casualties was to move fast...."

Patton was told to halt, but 12th Army Group then received intelligence obtained from a German officer deserter regarding a vast underground German communications center at Ohrdruf, a small, ancient city in the Harz Mountains about thirty miles west of Weimar. The details were sketchy but enticing and, when First Army reported that it would be unable to reach the line of Third Army's advance any time soon, Bradley gave Patton the go-ahead to push on to Ohrdruf.[18]

Patton recalled, "[Bradley] had a plan for the capture of the German communication center in the vicinity of Gotha, Erfurt, Weimar, and Ohrdruf, which, when he explained it to me, seemed full of promise.... We explained the idea of the rapid advance on the Weimar Quadrilateral—Eddy on the right, Walker on the left [and Middleton in reserve]. I told them they would have the greatest chance in history to make names for themselves, and to get moving."[19]

Apparently nothing, however, was then known about a possible slave-labor camp at Ohrdruf—a sub-camp of Buchenwald.

19
ORDEAL AT OHRDRUF

"The most strategic point in Germany at that time."

Leo Laufer
Ohrdruf inmate

THE OLD, ATTRACTIVE Thuringian town of Ohrdruf, founded in the eighth century by St. Boniface and situated in a scenic part of the Harz Mountains some twenty-eight miles west of Weimar and eight miles south of Gotha, is steeped in history. In 1625, the ten-year-old Johann Sebastian Bach came to live with his brother in Ohrdruf and compose music at the Church of St. Michael. During the 1800s, Ohrdruf became a center for the manufacture of toys, as well as the site of a military training ground (*Truppenübungsplatz*) that was created to prepare troops for the Franco-Prussian War of 1870-1871.[1]

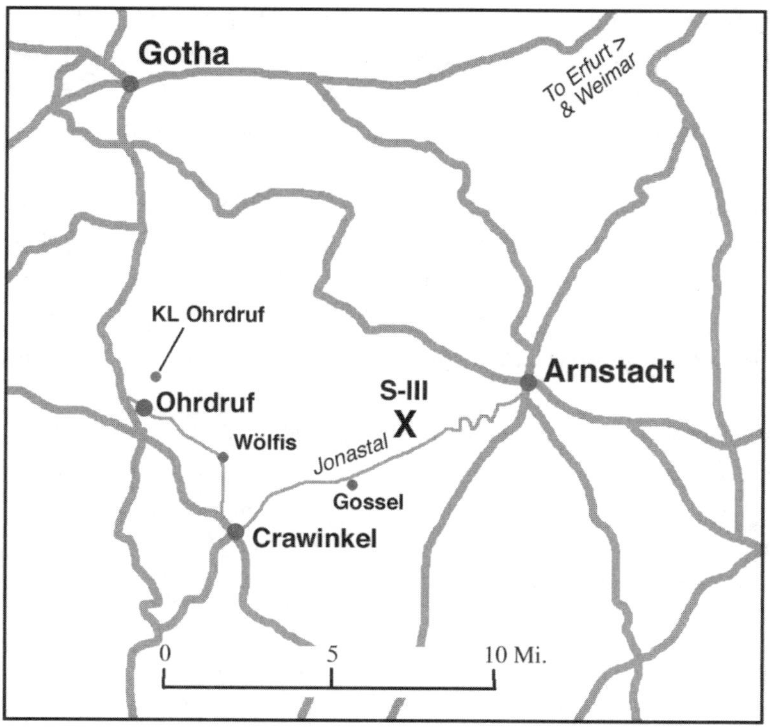

The Ohrdruf prisoners were put to work digging a massive headquarters and communications center known as S-III in the Jonastal area.

In the late 1930s the military facilities at Ohrdruf were home to a modest underground Wehrmacht communications center called *Amt 10* ("Office Ten"), which had been started but not completed some five-and-a-half miles east-southeast of Ohrdruf and a short distance north of the town of Gossel, between Crawinkel and Arnstadt, in the limestone cliffs of a valley known as the Jonastal. It became one of the Nazis' major underground construction projects—*Sonderbauvorhaben III*, or S-III. Owing to the severe aerial pounding that Berlin and other German cities were taking from American and British bombers, S-III was greatly expanded beginning in the summer of 1944. Doing the expanding and upgrading at the underground facility were a thousand slave laborers from Buchenwald.[2]

To house the slave work force, which would eventually grow to some 12,000 men, a labor camp on a plateau within the military post northeast of the town of Ohrdruf, the Buchenwald sub-camp officially known as *Ohrdruf-Nord Stalag III* was established in October 1944. The first transport of 778 Hungarian Jews arrived there from KL Sachsenhausen on November 19, 1944, followed five days later by fifty-five other Hungarian prisoners. On the 26th, a thousand Jews from the Stutthof camp arrived; another 2,498 prisoners reached Ohrdruf on December 13. By the end of January 1945, some 11,000 slave laborers were crammed into the small camp. Other prisoners were brought in from the Muna camp at Crawinkel and a tent camp at Espenfeld to assist in the secret, massive underground project.[3]

Prisoners were also transported in trucks, moving vans, and buses to the construction sites; later a small tram line was constructed and the workers either rode the train or were forced to walk; long after the war, elderly residents still recalled the sight of long columns of prisoners in their striped uniforms clattering through the streets in wooden shoes, accompanied by the barking of guard dogs.[4]

Given the severity of the work, brutal treatment at the hands of their guards, and their meager diet—not to mention work-site accidents—prisoners died in droves. The SS physician Dr. Werner Greunuß, previously at Buchenwald, was one of Ohrdruf's camp doctors. During his war-crimes trial, he testified that some 15-20 percent of the inmates died or were killed during his time at Ohrdruf.[5]

OTHER OMINOUS ACTIVITIES had also taken place near Ohrdruf during the last months of the war. In March 1945, a "small explosive device" of tremendous power was reported to have been tested at the Ohrdruf *Truppenübungsplatz*, and some reports say that twenty SS guards and 200 Ohrdruf inmates died as a result. Speculation is that this explosion was in connection with the rumored Nazi atomic bomb.* That same month, a huge rocket with enough range to hit American East Coast cities was reportedly test-fired from the area; residents told of seeing a long, fiery tail streaking into the night sky.[6]

Germany's respected weekly magazine, *Der Spiegel*, ran a story in 2005 that was skeptical of some claims of an atomic test but gave credibility to the account of one witness, an Ohrdruf resident named Clare Werner, who said that, on March 4, 1945, she saw something that was "as bright as hundreds of bolts of lightning, red on the inside and yellow on the outside, so bright you could've read the newspaper. It all happened so quickly, and then we couldn't see anything at all. We just noticed there was a powerful wind. . . ." The woman complained of "nosebleeds, headaches and pressure in the ears."

Another witness, Heinz Wachsmut, said that he was ordered by the SS to help build large pyres on which hundreds of horribly burned bodies of prisoners were to be cremated. The question remains: Was this the test of an atomic bomb?[7]

HIGHLY SECRET AND well-guarded, the S-III installation was designed to become a field headquarters for Hitler and the Nazi high command in the event they were forced to abandon Berlin. S-III had a multi-level tunnel system with some shafts more than a mile-and-a-half in length; the shaft entrances were disguised to look like chalets. Colonel Robert S. Allen, Patton's deputy intelligence officer, was amazed at extent of the underground headquarters: "This place also had paneled and carpeted offices, scores of large work and store rooms, tiled bathrooms with both tubs and showers, flush toilets, electrically equipped kitchens, decorated dining rooms and mess halls, giant refrigerators, extensive sleeping quarters, recreation rooms, separate bars for officers and enlisted personnel, a moving-picture theater, and air-conditioning and sewage systems. Begun in 1944, the installations had been completed but never occupied. Third Army's lightning advance through central Germany had blocked that."[8]

* In his 2005 book, *Hitler's Bombe*, German historian Rainer Karlsch claims that the Nazis detonated two atomic devices—one at Rügen Island (a few miles north of Peenemünde in the Baltic Sea) in October 1944 and the other at Ohrdruf in March 1945. Soviet spies reportedly informed Stalin of this terrible new weapon. (Karlsch, passim)

According to a report by General Hans Krebs, Chief of Staff of the German Army General Staff (OKH), *Generalfeldmarschall* Albert Kesselring and a large proportion of the OKH staff had transferred to the Ohrdruf area between February 12 and March 29, 1945, in anticipation that the facility would soon become operational.[9]

With the American front lines pushing ever closer, the SS leadership ordered the evacuation of Ohrdruf; three transports filled with a total of 2,900 inmates departed for Bergen-Belsen where, presumably, they were killed. At the beginning of April, several groups totaling nearly 10,000 prisoners were marched to Buchenwald. Those judged too sick or infirm to make the three-day, thirty-mile march were either killed with a bullet to the back of the neck or beaten to death by the guards and thrown into a large cremation pit made of railroad tracks and timbers; only a few hundred prisoners remained behind.[10]

HERMANN PISTER AND his staff at Buchenwald were indeed worried that if the Americans, British, or Soviets showed up before evidence of their crimes could be erased, every German associated with the camp would be summarily executed. Such an ending must not be allowed to happen. A roll-call taken on April 1 showed a total of 80,813 inmates assigned to the camp, with approximately 34,000 of that number working off-site at sub-camps and armaments works. Death certificates in the camp medical office told of 32,705 deaths that had taken place in Buchenwald since its opening in 1937. But there were far more—perhaps as many as another 20,000. The scale of the crime was huge.[11]

Pister did not know what to do. There was no way to disguise the horrors from the advancing Allies other than by utterly destroying the camp and killing the remaining inmates. Yet, such a tremendous undertaking was beyond the scope of his detachment of SS personnel. Besides, as the advancing Allies encroached upon the outlying sub-camps, transports full of prisoners evacuated from those camps continued to pull into Buchenwald, further straining its ability to house and feed them. The time had come to move them out, irrespective of the inmates' ability to stand such an evacuation.[12] As Ian Kershaw noted in *The End*, "The death marches were completely pointless, except as a means of inflicting still further enormous suffering on those designated as the regime's eternal enemies. But the commandants and the guards treating the prisoners on the marches with such sadistic brutality did not seek any rationale. Their system still functioned—after a fashion. They remained, even in its dissolution, set in the same mentality that had earlier seen them torture prisoners pointlessly or force them to carry out pointless backbreaking labour.

"Ultimately, by April 1945, the regime just did not know what to do with the hundreds of thousands of prisoners still in its domain. In the gathering chaos of the last weeks, the death marches reflected the futile flailing of a regime on the verge of its own destruction but retaining its murderous capacity to the very end."[13]

PERHAPS AS A way of keeping him at his post indefinitely, Heinrich Himmler promoted Hermann Pister to Inspector of Concentration Camps of the South,[14] much in the way Hitler had promoted General Friedrich von Paulus to General Field Marshal in hopes that the elevated rank would dissuade him from surrendering the Sixth Army at Stalingrad in January 1943. But, just as a promotion failed to work in von Paulus' case, it likewise did nothing to convince Pister to hold out until the end. Pister clearly realized that the Third Reich's—and maybe even his own—days were numbered. Perhaps, thought the commandant of Buchenwald, he could somehow make a deal, something to prove to the Allies that he wasn't an evil monster like Koch.

"There is evidence that during the first days of April 1945 the SS command temporarily considered surrendering the camp to the Allies," wrote Harry Stein. With that bright, dangling straw nearly within his grasp, Pister called a meeting on April 3 of German and Austrian inmate leaders in the camp's movie theater. There he floated the idea that he might indeed be willing to turn over the camp if the inmate leaders would put in a kind word for him with his captors. Four inmates—the Frenchman André Marie, the Belgian Eugène Soudan, the Dutchman Pieter Cool, and a British SOE officer, Captain Christopher Burney—replied to Pister's offer in a letter, promising to speak favorably in his behalf if Pister kept his word to hand over the camp intact—and the prisoners alive—to the Allies.[15]

Jacob Werber recalled being told by others who attended the meeting that Pister had said, "We know that you have ammunition. We know everything that you're doing. But don't provoke us. And if you don't revolt, I give you my word as a soldier to turn over the entire camp to the Americans at the end." Werber added, "Of course, we didn't trust them. We continued with our preparations and laid out earthenware white plates on a tar roof background, in a pattern spelling out the letters S-O-S."[16]

But the SS high command quickly came back and canceled Pister's plans to turn Buchenwald over to the Allies; he was to do as previously ordered and evacuate the camp, leaving behind as little evidence of crimes as possible. Of two minds—whether to remain or flee—Pister, on April 3, had 1,500 prisoners marched out, probably to Theresienstadt. This outflow was immediately offset the next day when several thousand inmates from the sub-camp at Ohrdruf arrived at Buchenwald. As stated earlier, the forced march had been one of terror; hundreds of Ohrdruf prisoners had been marched to the point of exhaustion, with many of them executed along the roadside when they could not keep up.[17]

IN A DELICIOUSLY ironic moment, Buchenwald received another prisoner—its first commandant, Karl Otto Koch. After being tried on corruption charges by the SS the previous August, found guilty, and sentenced to death, on April 3 he was taken from his Weimar jail cell and driven up the Ettersberg to the camp he once commanded. He spent a night in a cell in the Bunker and then, the next morning, was secretly removed to the SS shooting range and executed by a firing squad commanded by Pister's adjutant, Hans H.T. Schmidt. Koch's body was then burned in the same crematorium that had consumed so many of his victims. Had the prisoners known that their ex-commandant had been killed by the SS, their shouts of joy would undoubtedly have been heard in Weimar.

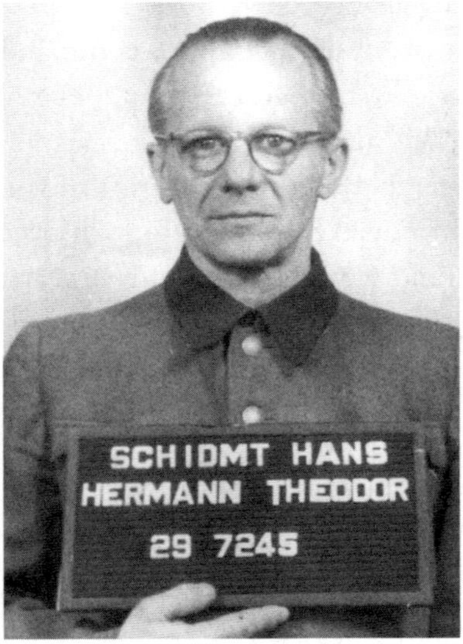

Hans Schmidt, camp adjutant under Pister and the officer in charge of the SS firing squad that executed former commandant Karl Otto Koch on April 5, 1945. (U.S. National Archives)

It remains a bizarre twist of fate that Koch, a man who was responsible for the torture and cruel deaths of tens of thousands of innocent civilians, was executed—not for those crimes, but for corruption. But such was the way of SS "justice."[18]

AT HUNDREDS OF death camps, concentration camps, work camps, and sub-camps, the gates were swung open by the guards upon Himmler's orders, and suddenly the roads and backroads of Germany, Poland, and Austria were clogged with a gray tide of unwashed humanity, marching on a journey to nowhere, a journey to extinction.

One might be tempted to think that the suddenly mobile prisoners would have felt grateful and relieved that they were no longer confined to a stinking barracks, that the fresh air and bucolic countryside would have been a bracing tonic for their spirits, that thoughts of being rescued while on the march or being able to escape into the forests would have filled their heads. For some, to be sure, that was true; a handful of prisoners managed to slip away during the evacuation march. Some were shot, some were recaptured, but a few were able to hide in the woods and make it to safety. For the vast majority, however, the evacuations were an ordeal, a nightmare, the painful prelude to their anonymous, ignominious deaths.

Take, for example, the evacuation from Berga-an-der-Elster—a sub-camp of Buchenwald located thirty-eight miles east-southeast of Weimar. For months, the inmates here were literally worked to death digging and blasting an underground facility inside a mountain for a planned synthetic-fuel plant—the project code-named *Schwalbe V*.

Joining their co-workers from Buchenwald was a detachment of 350 American soldiers—about half of them Jewish—captured during the Battle of the Bulge in Belgium and Operation *Nordwind* in Alsace-Lorraine. The GIs had been transported from their POW camp at Bad Orb, near Frankfurt, and hauled east in cramped boxcars, survived strafings and bombings by Allied aircraft, and found themselves in the same type of wretched conditions in which the concentration camp internees were living.

At Berga, the Americans and the Buchenwalders worked from mid-February until early April, breaking rock during twelve-hour shifts, being exposed to the hazards of mine work without masks or respirators or even the slightest bit of protective clothing, while being beaten by the clubs and truncheons of their overseers and barely surviving on starvation rations.

One of the Yanks, Gerald Daub, a young soldier from New York, was put to work with a big drill breaking off chunks of the tunnel's rock face. "I remember walking through the worksite and seeing these gangs of political prisoners," he said, "working and looking like they were starving and dying, which they were. They were falling and being beaten by their own foremen to get up to work again. It was my impression of Dante's *Inferno*, like my vision of hell—a totally hellish place."

Another GI, Norman Fellman, remembered that his work crew's job was to drill holes in the rock and stuff the holes with gunpowder. "We would all get out of the tunnel and they would blast," he said. "Before the dust had settled, before the noise had stopped echoing, we were forced back into the tunnels. Nobody had any protective gear of any kind. You'd breathe that air, you'd breathe that shit."

Daub added, "The air was just totally filled with stone dust. Everything was coated with it, including your lungs filled with it. And we had no bathing facilities, so you can picture that, after a day or two, we just looked like cement statues walking around."

Besides the unending, back-breaking work in the tunnels, the prisoners at Berga were faced with the usual Nazi brutality, insufficient rations, dysentery, a cold, wet climate, and lice-filled barracks. Even though they had been strong, healthy soldiers when captured, they quickly were reduced to weak, sick, starved, scared, and skeletal slaves, slowly dying.

The order to evacuate Berga came on April 2, 1945, and, the next day, the gates of the American compound were opened and the GIs rousted out to begin their long trek into the hinterlands. The Buchenwald prisoners, too, were released from their vermin-infested encampment beside the Elster River and the two groups hit the road, heading south, but hardly able to put one foot in front of the other.

Theoretically, escape during the march seemed possible, but few had the strength or will to try. Morton Brooks, another of the American captives, said, "The Germans had about four or five [guards] who watched us—not a large number. They really didn't need a large number."

Their evacuation march was typical of the scores of other marches that were then taking place. Medic William Shapiro, one of the 280 Americans on the march from Berga (the other seventy had either escaped from the camp, died of various causes, or had been shot while escaping), recalled, "None of us...had any idea how destructive this march would be to our group. All debilitated, exhausted, emaciated, sick, maimed and cowered soldiers.... This was a walk at a slow pace, interrupted by a break every hour-and-one-half in order to defecate, urinate, or just sit down along the gutters of the road. We were totally unprepared for the horrors that we would encounter—the profound despair, the inability to continue to take another step forward, the discovery of dead buddies each morning, and the wanton, gross murder along the roads."

The marchers trod southward, along the Czech border toward Austria, wandering through rural countryside and the cities and villages of Greiz, Plaun, Hof, Rehau, Selb, Thierstein, and countless more. Ahead of the marching Americans was a long parade of evacuees from other camps, and the GIs continually encountered horrifying scenes of violent death.

The awful human detritus lined the road for hundreds of kilometers. The Americans could see a large body of marchers ahead of them—political prisoners from another camp. The road climbed a rise and, as the Yanks struggled uphill, they noticed up ahead what looked like odd bundles littering the ground. As they got closer, the bundles became clumps of gaunt corpses carpeting the road, sprawled in ditches, and hanging limply from barbed-wire fences. Each one had a bullethole in his head.

During this uphill stretch of highway, prisoner Gerald Daub recalled, "As we approached this hill, we saw a few prisoners lying by the side of the road in these atrocious pleading and praying and frightened positions—all shot. I didn't hear any shooting or see the incidents. We just saw them lying there and it was very grotesque.... All of them were shot in the head. It seemed as though we marched all that day, and practically all we saw were these bodies along the side of the road."

Another American POW, Tony Acevedo, recalled, "Up ahead, the Germans were slaughtering the Jews from another camp. They were slaughtering old people, young people, women, children, everyone. We saw people hanging from the barbed wire fences on both sides of the highway, hanging down, slaughtered by the machine guns of the Germans."

ONE OF THOSE remaining at Ohrdruf was Leo Laufer, a young Polish Jew arrested in 1940 in Łódź, Poland, that country's second largest city, with a population then of 750,000—one third of them Jews who weren't confined to a ghetto. Laufer had already survived five camps: Eichendorf, Auschwitz, Dachau, Sachsenhausen, and Buchenwald; in February 1945 he was transferred from Buchenwald to Ohrdruf.

At the time, according to Laufer, Ohrdruf was "a new camp with new barracks and barbed wire. It wasn't a big camp—just a few thousand people. It was orderly, with nice new barracks, but very regimented, with guards in sentry booths all around. They said that Ohrdruf was created for the hardcore, the ones

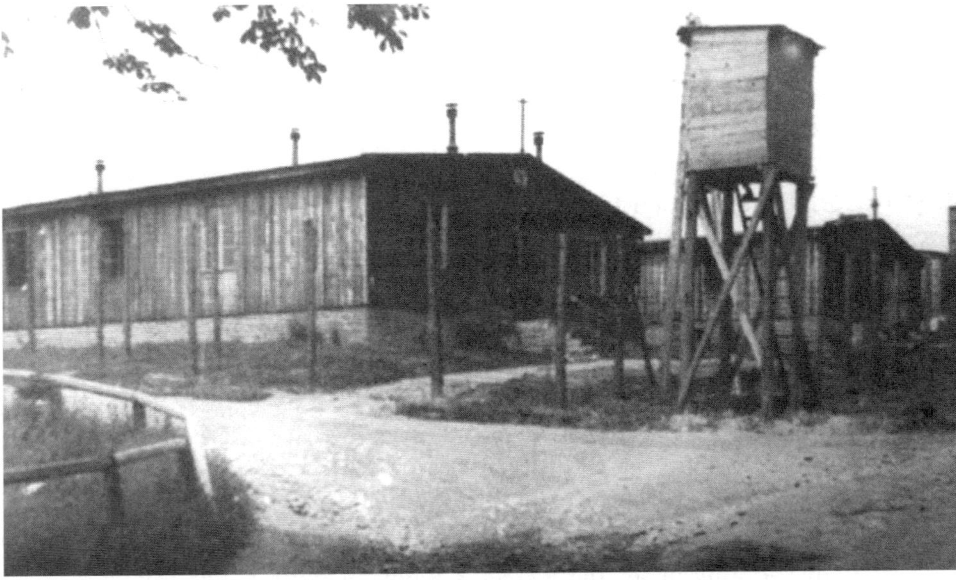

Guard tower and barracks at Ohrdruf camp (U.S. National Archives)

who were not suited for concentration camps like Buchenwald—the most horrible camp I had been in—but I felt fortunate to be alive."

Laufer had already endured an incredible, five-year ordeal. In Łódź his large family of eight children was desperately poor. Although the father, David, had a wealthy cousin who owned a large textile factory in Łódź, the family was virtually destitute; the only source of income came from the finishing of headscarves. Leo said, "I used to go with my father to the factory to bring home unfinished headscarves. My father was the middleman; he would give the headscarves out to very poor peasants in the city who would sew fringe on them. Sometimes my sisters and my mother would do the fringing in the evening in order to save money." When the fringing was completed, Leo and his father would return the scarves to the factory, where they would be paid a few *zloty* for each piece, a portion of which was given to anyone else who had helped in the process. "This is how we made a living, which was very little. I would say that we were not *at* the poverty level, but *below* it."

Even as a youngster, Leo was aware of how hard his mother worked at home. "We had a wooden floor that she scrubbed down every week on her hands and knees," he said. "I don't remember anything that she enjoyed because it was a chore for her to bathe so many children every night. We didn't have a bathroom, and she didn't have any facilities for bathing. We had to bring the water up from downstairs, and she had to put it in a metal tub on the stove to warm it with the wood she chopped. Then she would wash the kids one after the other, cook for them, and put them to bed. We did not have anything. We lived without running water, without toilet facilities, and without gas. We had to chop wood for the stove…and go to the toilet in the backyard of the house."

Leo recalled that the bedroom was so small, "There was no room to walk *through* the room; we had to jump from bed to bed because we had so many beds and no space between them." There were no real mattresses, either; the "mattresses" consisted of burlap bags stuffed with straw and covered with linen.

"When one of the children got sick, they had to stay home and not go to *cheder* [school], and my mother had to take care of them. I loved my father, but I admired my mother. I couldn't understand what a slave she was. My parents had so much love for me and my brothers and sisters, and we would have gone to the end of the world for our parents."

Yet, somehow, even with nothing, the family found the means to be generous. Leo said that every Friday night and Saturday the family would walk a long distance for religious services at a *shtibl*—a single-room synagogue with benches that could accommodate up to twenty-five worshipers. He recalled that a homeless man named Moishe always waited outside of the *shtibl*, hoping that someone would take him home for a Sabbath meal. Invariably, David Laufer invited the man to come home and eat with them. Said Leo, "This was my father's wish, and I respected him for it. My mother used to say, 'Don't worry, children, if there is enough for ten, there will be enough for eleven.' My father always believed that the good things would come after we were gone, not in this life."[19]

Shortly before the German invasion of Poland on September 1, 1939, Leo joined the youth wing of a Zionist group in Łódź known as the "Jabotinsky Group," named for an early Zionist—the Russian Jew Ze'ev Jabotinsky who, during World War I, fought in the Jewish Legion in an attempt to free Palestine from Ottoman Turkish rule. In 1925, Jabotinsky established the Union of Zionist Revisionists, which called for the immediate creation of a Jewish state in Palestine.[20] Leo said, "Our group in Łódź was not very active because we were so far away from Palestine. It was more like a club, just an organization where we got together."

After the German invasion, the anti-Semitic tone in Łódź was definitely turned up. "Poland was ninety-seven or ninety-eight percent Catholic," Leo recalled. "Anti-Semitism was rampant. You could feel it, you could see it, you could hear it. Fortunately, Łódź was not bombed; the city was taken without any shelling at all. As soon as the war in Poland was over, many people suddenly 'became' Germans. We knew that the owner of the apartment house was German—a *Volksdeutsch* [a Pole of German descent with allegiance to Germany]—but we never realized that a lot of the neighbors were also of German descent. Everybody put on a swastika armband; they just came out of the blue."

Leo recalled that the area in which he lived before the Łódz ghetto was established was predominately Jewish, with a sprinkling of Christian families. "We got along with the Christians. In fact, there were Christians in the house we lived in. The house belonged to a *Volksdeutsch*. Of course, they all moved out when the order came that this part of Łódz would be the ghetto."

As a child, Leo had little understanding of the differences between religions and was unaware that, as a Jew, he belonged to a small sect that was hated by a large segment of the population. Even growing up he had quite a few Christian friends. "But I remember as a small child," he said, "my mother used to warn us about two holidays—Christmas and Easter: '*Kinderlach, geh nicht arois.*' ['Children, don't go outside.'] When we asked why, she told us that when the church let out, they were going to kill the Jews. And it did happen sometimes. This is why a mother had to be so protective of her children."

Leo said that his father was a very religious Orthodox Jew and dressed in the traditional long coat, wide-brimmed hat, and had a full beard. "Because he wore his Jewish garb, he became scared to death to go out of the house, because he was afraid that somebody was going to cut his beard off. When they eventually did, he felt terrible because it was so undignified for him. He almost cried, as old a man as he was. He took a handkerchief to put around the part of the beard that was still left, across his face, tied in a knot at the top. He wore it like when you have a toothache. It was degrading, and this kept on for a long time."[21]

To help keep his family alive, Leo got into black market activities that brought in food and money, but another ghetto lad somehow learned about the schemes and wanted in on it, threatening to go to the Gestapo if Leo didn't take him on as a partner; Leo refused. Sure enough, late one night in September 1940, the Gestapo showed up at the Laufers' door. "There was knocking and my father opened the door. The Gestapo man hit my father so hard that he fell down. I got up from bed and went out in my underwear. They said, 'Put your pants on and your jacket,' and they took me and started beating me up even before I got to the Gestapo office. "When I got there, they started beating me so unmercifully that I didn't even know what to say. They wanted to know who gave me my black-market business; I wasn't going to tell them. Even if I did, I had already been beaten up. This ordeal lasted for quite a while. They took me to an isolation cell in the basement and beat me some more. I think I was there almost two weeks. Finally I wound up in the hospital not far away from home."

When at last he was released, Leo learned that the Gestapo had also beaten his parents and siblings. He should have stopped his black-market dealings but didn't. Eventually he was arrested again and put on a train—the first transport to leave Łódz —a long train made up of boxcars. He did not learn until much later that the entire Łódz ghetto would be liquidated. The train stopped at Poznan, and the people were ordered out. They were deloused and had their head and body hair shorn. Then two hundred of them—young men from seventeen to twenty-five—mounted trucks and were transported to a little village named Wolszyn. Outside the village was a farm guarded by armed *Volksdeutsch* militiamen. The Jews from Łódz dismounted from the trucks and were put to work mucking out a large cattle barn; the barn would become their unheated, lice-filled living quarters from October 1940 until March 1941. Lice carry the typhus bacillus, and soon many of the boys contracted the disease; several died each day.

The sub-freezing weather also took its toll; with no winter clothing or proper bedding, many of the young men came down with colds and pneumonia, others with frostbite. By March 1941, the number of boys at the farm had been cut in half by disease and death; no doctor ever came to treat the ill.

"We slept and worked in the same clothes for almost six months," recalled Leo. "We hadn't had a bath or shower in six months. There were no such facilities. There wasn't even a toilet; you just went behind the shed in the open air. The only water we got was from a tin can that we used to bring up from the Dojka River every morning and put in front of the gate. When everybody left for work, we used to take a handful and wash our faces. This was the extent of our hygiene. It was horrible."

No one attempted escape. Laufer said, "It was such a remote area that I don't think any of us knew where it was. And we were guarded night and day." Leo couldn't understand how their guards could be so cruel. "We could never figure out how a Pole, even of German descent, could torture us. They could have given us lodgings; they could have arranged something for us, even though we were slave laborers."

Instead of killing him, the six-month ordeal at Ruchocki Mlyn made Leo

Laufer tougher and more resilient—and more determined than ever to survive whatever the Nazis or his fellow countrymen could throw at him.

He would need every ounce of that determination in the coming years, for the camps at Eichendorf, Dachau, Auschwitz, Buchenwald, and Ohrdruf were still in his future.[22]

EVENTUALLY LAUFER WOUND up at Ohrdruf. Although he didn't know it then, he later learned that the area in which they worked, the Jonastal, "was the most strategic point in Germany at that time. We were dynamiting mountainous areas for the purpose of building caves from which the Nazis could shoot rockets into England. They were also building [an underground] center which, if Hitler had been able to get out of Berlin, would have been his telecommunications center."[23]

Murray Kohn, who was then a sixteen-year-old prisoner with Laufer at Ohrdruf, explained that "the Nazis were preparing the *Führerbunker* in nearby Crawinkel—the final headquarters of Hitler from where he planned to strike a deal with the Americans to join in fighting the Red Army. We worked around the clock—the project was known as the 'Olga' project. We were excavating inside the hills an eighteen-tunnel bunker. Ten thousand people died there."[24]

Like Kohn, Laufer was put to work in the underground construction project at the Jonastal. "We were divided into different *Kommandos*," Leo said. "Everything was military and unbelievably guarded. Of course, they needed labor, and we were there to do the work. They put most of us to work dynamiting mountains, although most of us didn't know how to do it. We put the dynamite in, there was a warning, we got out of the way, and all the rocks would come flying out, chopping off heads, arms, legs—it didn't mean a thing [to the Germans]. We would bring home dead bodies every day."

It did not take long for the hard, dangerous work to wear on Laufer. Fortunately, he had made friends with a Russian POW named Sasha, who worked on a rations detail—the *Kartoffel Kommando*—whose job it was to deliver potatoes to the other camps within a twenty- to thirty-mile radius of Ohrdruf. Laufer said the duty "was nice because the old German [supervisor] really didn't hit us, and he gave us potatoes. I was the happiest person until something happened.

"It was around the first week of March, and you could see the tension. We were unloading a truck of potatoes at one of the [sub] camps. I guess I was too diligent; everybody was already done and I was still trying to get the last potato off the truck with a shovel. This guard, a Ukranian who hated Jews, knew I was Jewish. He said that I took too long and kicked me in the leg." The leg injury soon became infected, requiring Laufer to be taken to the Ohrdruf infirmary. "The wound became so abscessed that pus accumulated and I couldn't walk. I didn't know what to do."

One of the inmate doctors in the infirmary took a knife or a razor and, without anesthesia, opened the festering wound. Despite the excruciating pain, Laufer said, "I felt so relieved. I felt like a new man." Knowing that most people did not survive a stay in the infirmary, Laufer wanted to get out as quickly as possible. After a few days he returned to his old job but found that someone else had taken his place, and so he was reassigned to the dynamite *Kommando* working in the tunnel.

"It was horrible," Laufer said. "If I would have kept on another three weeks, I think I would have been dead, but I guess God was with me. Believe it or not, I was saved by a German." Returning one day from his job in the tunnels, the old German who headed up the potato *Kommando* saw Laufer and asked him why he was no longer in the unit. Laufer told the story of his hospitalization and the German pulled rank to get him reassigned to the potato detail. "The next morning I was back to this *Kartoffel Kommando*, where I worked until the end."

Just before its liberation, the Ohrdruf slave-labor camp had a population of some 12,000 prisoners. As news of the Americans approaching from the west began to circulate among the inmates, everyone felt the end was near. One day an Allied fighter flew low over the camp, strafing the guard towers. A lucky shot by the SS downed the plane and the pilot was captured and thrown into the prison camp, where he was killed. Leo Laufer said, "He was a blond young fellow, but we didn't feel a thing for him because we didn't know who was fighting whom."[25]

FOR THE LEADERS of the Third Reich, the handwriting on the wall spoke very clearly about a bad end looming for them. SS chief Heinrich Himmler was especially consumed with worry about his fate if the Allies should capture him. The trail of blood and ashes from millions of victims of the SS led directly to his doorstep, and he began to think of ways he might be able to escape the hangman's noose. One thing he *could* do, he believed, was to try and cover up the magnitude of his and the SS's crimes. To accomplish that, he had but two choices: either murder all of the remaining inmates of the concentration and death camps and dispose of their bodies, or open the gates of the camps, march the inmates out, and allow the Allies to find only empty barracks.

The problem with the first option was simply that Nazi Germany was running out of time. No matter how efficient the Nazis' mass murder system had become, it would still take weeks, and possibly even months, to kill the hundreds of thousands of people still in the camps and working at slave-labor jobs, and burn or bury the corpses. Himmler feared, and rightly so, that Nazi Germany no longer had weeks or months left to take care of such an enormous task. Added to this problem was the fact that the extermination facilities were no longer in existence, all of them having either been abandoned or captured by the advancing enemy.

The second option seemed much more workable. The camps could be evacuated and the inmates marched under armed guard into the countryside where, devoid of food and medical care, they would begin to die in droves. If Allied armies came across the bodies, Himmler's excuse could be that the inmates had escaped from the camps and, without the care offered by their SS warders, died on their own. If liberating units came close to a group of inmates on the march, the prisoners could be killed en masse by their guards, who would then shed their uniforms and disappear into the woods. No witnesses, no prosecution. Perhaps a case could even be made that the Allied troops had gunned down the inmates, either on purpose or by accident.

Yes, this was the only way Himmler believed he could save himself. And one of the first camps he ordered emptied was Ohrdruf. Eugen Kogon wrote that during a phone conversation on April 2, Himmler left it up to the discretion of Ohrdruf's commandant, SS Captain Oldeburhuis, to liquidate all inmates, such as political prisoners and convicts, deemed to be "dangerous" to the leaders of the Third Reich.[26]

IN EARLY APRIL, probably about the second or third, as the front lines moved closer to his camp, *SS-Hauptmann* Edmund Bräuning,* Ohrdruf-Nord Stalag

* Although Kogon reported that an SS captain named Oldeburhuis was the commandant, former SS master sergeant named Werner Fricke said during his war-crimes trial that Bräuning was the commandant. Records indicating who was actually in charge at Ohrdruf have not been located. (Fricke testimony, U.S. vs. Waldeck, April 16, 1947, NARA, RG-549-000-50-0, Box 435)

III commandant (who previously had been stationed at Ravensbrück),[27] received orders from SS headquarters to evacuate the facility. The inmates were gathered on the *Appellplatz*, the gate was swung open, and most of the prisoners were removed under armed guard. Those who appeared to be too ill or weak were dispatched with a bullet to the brain, while others were inexplicably left alive in their bunks.

In *The Death Marches*, Daniel Blatman posits that the number of prisoners had grown from 1,000 when Ohrdruf opened in November 1944 to more than 13,700 by March 1945. "Ohrdruf became a vast subcamp with subcamps of its own. When it was decided to transfer the Ohrdruf inmates to Buchenwald, the camp commandant received orders from the SD in Weimar to liquidate all dangerous criminal and political elements who might cause problems, but not to harm the Jewish prisoners. Before the Ohrdruf inmates set out on their death march to Buchenwald, more than 1,500 prisoners were mercilessly liquidated. Approximately 12,000 prisoners left and of these only 9,000 survived to enter the gates of Buchenwald three days later. The other 4,000 were shot along the way by the guards, by units of the *Hitlerjugend* [Hitler Youth], and by civilians who took part in exterminating these dangerous enemies of the Reich."[28]

Shortly after the last evacuees left Ohrdruf and with the Americans rapidly approaching, inmate Murray Kohn, who had been a prisoner at Auschwitz and Buchenwald before Ohrdruf, recalled, "Hours before the first Americans appeared at the gates of Ohrdruf, the last remaining Nazi guards managed to execute [inmates] with hand pistols, literally emptying their last bullets on whomever they encountered, leaving them bleeding to death."[29]

Andrew Rosner, an Ohrdruf prisoner, recalled that he was barely alive while he was on the march. "All around me," he said, "I heard the sound of thunder, really the sound of heavy artillery and machinery. I looked for any opportunity to drop out of the march, but any man who fell behind or to the side was shot instantly by the Nazis."

Rosner walked until delirium set in and, as night fell, threw himself off the road and into a clump of bushes. "I lay there, waiting for the inevitable bullet to end my misery. I waited—and waited—and suddenly, *nothing!* No more Nazis shouting orders. No more marching feet. No more people. Alone. All alone and alive, although barely."

He crawled deeper into the woods and fell fast asleep—for how long he did not know. His sleep was violently interrupted as a battle erupted in close proximity to him. "I heard shooting all around me," Rosner said. "I played dead as men ran over me, stumbling over me as they went. I lay there as bullets passed by me and then Nazis fell all around me. Then all was quiet. The battle was over. I waited for hours before I dared move. I got up and saw dead German soldiers laying everywhere."

Famished, Rosner made his way back to the road and began walking toward a small village he could see in the distance where he hoped to find food. Suddenly two German soldiers appeared, one with a rifle that he pointed menacingly at Rosner. "I told him I was lost from the evacuation march," said Rosner, "but he told me that I must have escaped and I knew he was about to shoot me when the other German told him to let me be. It would not serve them well to harm me now. They allowed me to walk away and, as I did, I said a final prayer, knowing that a bullet in the back would now find me for sure. It never did. In the small village I was told to go farther back down the road to Ohrdruf, from where I had come three days before. There I would find the Americans. And so I did."[30]

Not all would be as lucky as Andrew Rosner, however. For many of the inmates, surviving the camps was hard enough; surviving the death marches would be even more difficult.

20
EVACUATING BUCHENWALD

*"The SS ordered the Jews to return to the barracks.
We had obtained a day's delay in our struggle for survival."*

Johannen Goldkrantz
Buchenwald prisoner

IN APRIL, WINTER usually gives up its grip, the air warms, the snows melt, trees begin to show fresh new leaves, and flowers push up from the earth. But early April 1945 atop the Ettersberg remained cold, harsh, wet, and gray, with the omnipresent sense of impending death hanging in the air.

Adding to the general gloom was the fact that KL Buchenwald's commandant, *SS-Oberführer* Hermann Pister, and the rest of the camp administration realized that they were caught in a vise with the Soviets pressing in on them from the east and the Americans pressuring from the west. It was only a matter of time before either American, British, or Russian tanks smashed down the gate, discovered the deplorable conditions of the camp and its inmates, and went on a hunt for the perpetrators. While such a scenario brought a flicker of hope to the inmates, the prisoners were also acutely aware that the Germans likely would slaughter them all before they could be liberated.

It was obvious: the Third Reich was dying, and Himmler's panicky memos to the concentration camp commandants in the first week of April were abundantly clear: Do whatever necessary to conceal the extent of my, your, and our crimes. Above all, get those prisoners with first-hand knowledge out of there.

Following the receipt of Himmler's evacuation order, Pister wondered how he could possibly comply; Buchenwald was bulging with new arrivals. With Allied armies closing in, he must have wondered: *How can I dispose of so many inmates?* He would need over twenty trains to evacuate all the prisoners, but the *Reichsbahn* rail system was being systematically destroyed by swarms of Allied warplanes that had complete and unchallenged mastery of the air. However, like the dutiful bureaucrat he was, Pister began making frantic phone calls, trying to line up trains to carry as many inmates as possible to camps that weren't yet as threatened as his own—Flossenbürg, Dachau, Theresienstadt. What happened to the prisoners once they left Buchenwald would no longer be his concern.[1]

AT 8:00 A.M. on April 6, 1945, with the Americans less than thirty miles away at Ohrdruf and Gotha, the Buchenwald loudspeakers, under Pister's order, crackled out the names of forty-six inmates—inmates believed by the Gestapo to be the ring-leaders of the camp's secret resistance committee. "These inmates will immediately report to the main gate," said the anonymous metallic voice.

As such announcements never portended well for those whose names were announced, the camp underground sprang into action, hiding the forty-six wanted men in non-Jewish barracks, in the Little Camp, or in crawl spaces beneath various buildings. When the wanted men did not immediately report to the main gate, the SS, *Kapos*, and *Blockälteste* began combing the compound, shouting "*Raus! Raus!*" ("Out! Out!") and herding groups of men into the open spaces between barracks for an impromptu roll call. "We haven't seen them," was the common response to the angry, frustrated men searching for the forty-six.[2]

In addition to the forty-six, the SS also wanted all of the Jews rounded up, but the underground had decided that the Jews, like the children, should stay hidden in the camp; some resorted to hiding in the sewers.[3] Johannen Goldkrantz recalled, "When only a small number of Jews reported—a few hundred instead of six or seven thousand—the SS officials were shocked and angry. This was probably the first time such an insubordination had occurred in the camp. The SS ordered the Jews to return to the barracks. We had obtained a day's delay in our struggle for survival.... Personally, I knew well what another evacuation would mean. I decided to hide rather than appear at the roll call. I felt that I had little chance to survive another march into southern Germany."[4]

On that same day, April 6, while Pister waited impatiently for the forty-six prisoners to be apprehended and brought to him, he was handed a message by a courier from the Buchenwald communications center—this message from Heinrich Himmler—telling him that he was to assemble another large group of prisoners immediately and transport them to Flossenbürg; no other details were forthcoming.

That evening, like a man trying to bail a sinking rowboat with a spoon, Pister received a return transport of thousands of inmates from the sub-camps, swelling the total number of prisoners atop the Ettersberg to approximately 48,000.*[5]

Goldkrantz performed another act of insubordination that likely would have gotten him shot had anyone reported him: He removed the yellow six-pointed star from his jacket and sewed on a red triangle with a "D" (denoting he was a German) in its place. He then found a hiding place—a tool cabinet within the now-disused DAW machine hall—where he stayed during the day, returning to Block 49 at night to sleep. He noted, "During the next few days the SS was able to ferret out about two thousand Jews. They simply surrounded [a block], told the prisoners to line up in front, and picked out the Jews. They did this with the help of the green triangles and, sometimes, the senior block elders. On April 8 there were still a few thousand Jews left hiding in the camp."

One evening, after hiding all day, Goldkrantz returned to his barrack just as two SS men, their pistols drawn, entered and ordered everyone outside to form ranks for a roll call. Goldkrantz feared that one of the other prisoners would point him out as a Jew, and that would be that. He said, "The guards then ordered Walter, the senior block elder, to walk with them down the line, look into the prisoners' faces, and identify any Jews. It was the most critical moment of my life, which I will never forget.... Standing at attention in the second row, I stared forward with a frozen expression. Would Walter point me out?

"I was sweating as Walter slowly walked by with the SS guards and looked into the faces of the prisoners. His eyes met mine for a split second as he proceeded to the end of the line. 'No Jews here,' he reported to the Nazis. After the search was over and the SS had left, Walter told me to disappear because too many prisoners in the block knew that I was Jewish."

Goldkrantz made the tool cabinet his full-time residence, venturing out only at night to stretch his legs and find some scraps of food.[6]

To members of the underground, these repeated roll calls and evacuations meant only one thing: The end was near, and soon the SS would begin to liquidate the camp. The moment, therefore, had come to retrieve the carefully hidden weapons and issue them to the squads of men selected for the job. No matter what the Nazis had in store for the prisoners of Buchenwald, the inmates vowed not to go down without a fight.[7]

---

* Beginning on April 7, approximately 28,000 inmates of Buchenwald were evacuated in a series of eight or ten rail transports over a period of several days. (U.S. vs. Waldeck, "Review & Recommendations," p. 23) Harry Stein noted, "On altogether sixty marching routes, some by rail, most on foot, insufficiently dressed and almost without food provisions, in April 1945 approximately 28,000 inmates of the parent camp and at least 10,000 inmates of the sub-camps were en route on marches justifiably referred to as death marches. Probably about one in three inmates either died along the way, of exhaustion immediately after their arrival, or were shot to death by the SS escort units." (Stein, pp. 230-231)

SOMEHOW, DURING ALL the confusion, Buchenwald inmate Eugen Kogon was smuggled out of the camp. Slipping into a safehouse in Weimar, he engaged in some psychological warfare and concocted a bogus letter that was delivered to Pister. It read:

> *Commander!*
>
> *Transports are leaving Buchenwald. They are death transports—like the one from Ohrdruf! The terrible tragedy of Ohrdruf must not be repeated.*
>
> *Dispatched by air to carry out special missions, we have seen with our own eyes the victims of the escort guard units and agitated members of the population along wide stretches.*
>
> *Woe to Thuringia, and woe to the commanders in Buchenwald, if that is repeated. The era of Koch, the Commander of Atrocities, by whose virtue the name of this camp has come to be abhorred by the entire civilized world, would thus be restored.*
>
> *Much has improved under your rule. We know that. Like the rest of the country, you may be in difficulties today—difficulties from which you see no other escape than to send thousands on their way. Stop! Stop immediately!*
>
> *Our tank commanders are on their way this very minute to settle accounts. You still have a chance.*

Kogon, evidently in a fanciful mood, signed the letter "James McLeod, Major, War Office, London." He knew it was a fraud but hoped the Germans did not.[8] He also hoped that the Allies reached Buchenwald before it became another Ohrdruf.

ON APRIL 6, over 3,100 inmates left Buchenwald for Flossenbürg. The following day, two more groups—one of 1,500, the other of 4,500—marched down from the Ettersberg to the Weimar train station. The group of 1,500 was shipped to Leitmeritz, Flossenbürg's largest sub-camp, located thirty-five miles north of Prague; the second group started for Flossenbürg but wound up at Dachau. On April 9, as additional trains became available, two more transports, each loaded with 4,800 prisoners, set out for Dachau; one made it while the other was liberated en route. The next day, 4,500 additional prisoners headed for Dachau; they were intercepted and freed by Soviet forces when the train reached Gera, some thirty-three miles east of Weimar. Two other transports left on April 10—one with 2,000 prisoners on board and the other with 2,780; the first made it to Theresienstadt, but the fate of the second is unknown.*[9]

Over 20,000 inmates were left behind, and they were in a quandary. What should they do if the liberators came near? Should they stay put and trust Pister to keep his earlier word about turning the camp over, intact, to the Allies? Or should they stage a last-minute uprising for which they had been planning and caching weapons? Jacob Werber said, "We realized that we couldn't win since we were in the middle of Germany, but we didn't want to die without resisting and without defending the children. Under no circumstances would we give up the children."[10]

But the march to oblivion had begun. Sixteen-year-old Moniek Goldberg, from Kozenice, Poland, was taken from Buchenwald to Theresienstadt via a jam-packed train. The trip was a nightmare; during the journey the train was strafed by an Allied plane and one of Goldberg's friends was killed. Then, during another air raid, the train's doors were opened and the prisoners were allowed to seek shelter in a farm field. The brief minutes of freedom enabled Goldberg and a few friends to break into a storehouse full of wheat. Scooping the grain into the blankets they carried, Goldberg and the others brought it back to the train, where they shared the raw kernels with their fellow captives.

Chaim Wajchendler, sixteen, was also sent by rail into the hinterlands along with a group of Russian POWs. For four weeks the train rumbled through the countryside, dodging strafing aircraft, stopping only long enough to take on fuel and water for the engine. The prisoners, locked in their boxcars, had been given two days' worth of rations before departing Weimar, but that food was long gone. Wajchendler felt that this was his worst experience as a prisoner. During the journey, he also witnessed cannibalism. When the train finally reached Theresienstadt at the end of April or beginning of May, only 500 or 600 out of the 3,000 prisoners who had departed Buchenwald were still alive.

Another teen from Buchenwald, Salek Orenstein, had been evacuated by rail and had reached the bombed-out city of Chemnitz. At the station Orenstein noticed a crowd of German civilians; a German officer in uniform announced to the crowd that anyone who wished to do so could give the prisoners a drink of water. Orenstein said, "Not one of the Germans lifted a finger to give us a

* After a week-long trip, the April 6th train carrying the 4,500 prisoners ended up, outside the gates of Dachau on April 28 with 2,310 corpses on board; the prisoners had died from starvation and strafing. See Chapter 28 for more details. (Whitlock, *The Rock of Anzio*, p. 357)

drop of water. This I shall never forget.... I thought, 'Have a little bit of compassion. Put yourself in our place. Who knows what the future holds for you?' No one stepped forward, no one showed compassion."

Not everyone left by train; others were forced to walk. One of those leaving Buchenwald was a teenager, Krulik Wilder. Finding his emaciated father in the camp, he attempted to take him along on the forced march into the countryside, but the SS stopped the Wilders at the gate and refused to allow the older man to go because he was sick and very weak. Krulik stated, "I had no choice but leave him on the *Appellplatz*. I was very distressed that I could not save him, but I was so very helpless and utterly lost. I learned later that my father died in Buchenwald. To this day I still cannot get over it. He came so near to freedom, but it was not his fate to survive."

There were flickering moments of hope. During an air raid on the rail yard at Chemnitz, Perec Zylberberg said that the prisoners on his train were let out and allowed to take cover under the cars. "The Allied bombers must have seen our train. At times we could see the pilots of the diving planes. They did not shoot at us. At long last we could almost feel that we were not alone and abandoned."[11]

ARMIN WALTHER, THE Buchenwald inmate and communications expert who repaired the SS radio equipment, recalled, "Access to all offices put me in a position to find out about many important things. As the situation became increasingly tense because of military developments, the camp administration revealed its intention to annihilate the camp by procuring grenades and flamethrowers for use against the prisoners. Thus the prisoners decided to organize for defense, for which the creation of a means of communications with the outside world was needed."[12]

It is believed that as many as seven secret wireless sets had been built over the years by the inmates of Buchenwald, and two are known to have been in operation in April 1945.[13] The possession of such equipment, however, was highly dangerous. A secret radio transmitter had earlier been discovered by the guards at the Mittelbau-Dora camp and, according to Walther, "Twenty-nine prisoners were thrown into the cellblock there; eight were shot, and two hanged themselves."

Nevertheless, a new telegraph transmitter, with a range of twenty miles, had been constructed on April 8 by three Polish inmates and used in an attempt to alert the advancing Allies as to the situation at Buchenwald. Receivers were also built from which the prisoners could learn of developments in the outside world, such as the advance of the Allies on two fronts.

The following message was supposedly transmitted a dozen times on April 8: "To the Allies! To the army of General Patton! We request help. They want to evacuate us. The SS wants to destroy us." There is no reliable indication that, if this or any other S.O.S. messages were sent by the inmates, they were ever received by the Allies.[14]

It has even been reported in some sources that on the afternoon of April 8, a reply was received: "KL Bu. Hold on. We are coming to your aid. Headquarters, Third Army." "Red Triangle," a former Buchenwald prisoner, who has spent many years exhaustively researching matters involving the camp, debunked this message, pointing out, "Even though these [radio transmitters] existed, it is extremely doubtful that the above S.O.S. message was indeed sent and it is even more doubtful that it was received and answered. First of all, if that wireless set had a range of only 20 miles, that message could not have reached any of the units of the U.S. Army which were in the area.... The 4th Armored Division was located in and near Gotha (23 1/2 miles from Buchenwald) or the 6th Armored Division which was in and around Bad Langensalza (32 1/4 miles from Buchenwald). That S.O.S. message could most certainly not have reached the headquarters of the Third Army considering that, on April 8, 1945, they were located in Frankfurt-am-Main (209 miles from Buchenwald)."

The former prisoner also noted, "Considering that, for many weeks, the inmates of Buchenwald had been monitoring radio broadcasts originating from France, Belgium and Luxembourg, it is of course possible that they knew that there was a U.S. Third Army and that George S. Patton, Jr. was its Commanding General; however, how could they possibly have figured out in advance that the area of Weimar and Buchenwald would have been overrun by the Third Army?

"Then, as far as the reply by the Headquarters of the Third Army is concerned, it would most definitely not have been addressed to "KL Bu"—an abbreviation which was strictly used by the SS administration of the concentrations camps."

Red Triangle further stated that if the message had been brought to Patton's attention, he obviously would have been informed that Buchenwald existed and likely would have issued instructions regarding what to do when his units reached the camp. Yet, General Patton—as well as the rest of the U.S. Army—was still in the dark when it came to being aware of the existence of Buchenwald.

"Last but not least," said the former prisoner, "if that S.O.S. message would indeed have been received and answered, entries to that effect would have been made in the official records of the Headquarters of the Third Army as well as in those of the units which may have intercepted it, yet that message and its reply are not mentioned in any journal or report issued by any unit of the U.S. Army which operated in the area west of Buchenwald on April 8, 1945, and remained there until April 11, 1945."[15]

But the question remained: Could Patton's Third Army reach Buchenwald in time to prevent a complete slaughter?

21
OVERRUNNING OHRDRUF

"I could hardly believe what I was seeing. The stench was terrible. Many of us cried like babies."

William F. Charboneau, Jr.
American liberator of Ohrdruf

GENERAL PATTON HAD, on April 3, 1945, ordered the 4th Armored Division to head immediately for Gotha, a town over twenty miles west of Weimar, and an important rear-area supply base for the German army. William M. Hoge, the 4th Armored's commanding officer, decided to split his command and send Combat Command B to Gotha and Combat Command A to Ohrdruf. Patton also requested that a 3,000-man regimental combat team from the 89th Infantry Division be attached to the 4th Armored.[1]

Colonel Jesse Harris, commander of the 355th Infantry Regimental Combat Team (CT5) of the 89th Division, recalled that he was directed to proceed to the 4th Armored's command post at Bad Homberg: "There I was briefed by the Assistant Division Commander as to the nature of the operation. He provided me with a map and indicated a point on the outskirts of Gotha where I was to have at least a battalion of infantry prepared to carry out mop-up operations in Gotha. The battalion was to be in position by 7:00 A.M. the following morning, April 4th. As the Combat Team had been alerted for the move, we were able to get underway about 4:00 P.M. During the move from Rudesheim to Gotha, approximately 150 miles, we were forced, because of blown bridges, to detour from the Autobahn down muddy, unimproved roads. In crossing one of the streams it became necessary to call upon the tank destroyers to use their towing cables to tow our trucks across the muddy stream. Fortunately, we met little enemy resistance so the entire Combat Team was in position at the appointed time.

"The 3rd Battalion, 355th, joined with the tanks of the 4th Armored Division in the assault on Gotha. The mopping-up operation moved rapidly against light opposition and was completed by noon. General Hoge, C.G. 4th Armored Division, called a meeting of the three Combat Team commanders and myself as commander of CT5. The meeting was brief and General Hoge indicated that the operation had gone well. No mention was made of the concentration camp, which has led me to believe that General Hoge and members of the 4th Armored Division were unaware of Stalag Ohrdruf-Nord."[2]

Harris was correct; no one knew about Ohrdruf-Nord Stalag III. It would the first Nazi concentration camp to be liberated by U.S. forces.

Early on the morning of April 4, the 8th Tank Battalion ran into a group of Hitler Youth armed with panzerfausts near Ohrdruf, but "this opposition was quickly reduced and [the town of] Ohrdruf taken with little difficulty."[3] Had the armored column been dispatched a day earlier, they might have captured Field Marshal Albert Kesselring* and the headquarters of *OB West,* who were at the Ohrdruf command center before fleeing.[4] The April 1945 After-Action Report of Combat Command A, 4th Armored Division, indicates that higher headquarters learned from a prisoner-of-war two weeks earlier that the German High Command was establishing a headquarters and communications center in the area of Gotha, Ohrdruf, Erfurt, and Arnstadt, and that "the mission of the division had been changed from seizing the high ground to the north of Eisenach to that of seizing the communications centers at Gotha and Ohrdruf, the objective of Combat Command 'A' being Ohrdruf." The report noted that enemy defenses were strong and "considerable opposition" was encountered.

Meanwhile, a small group of American soldiers—the 355th Infantry Regiment's Intelligence and Reconnaissance Platoon** of the 89th Infantry Division (which was under the operational control of the 4th Armored Division)—came across a row of empty SS barracks on the outskirts of Ohrdruf while, on a nearby hill, was clustered a group of low, dirty, and weather-beaten wooden buildings behind a double barbed-wire enclosure beneath now-vacant guard towers. This was the slave-labor camp.

Meanwhile, the inmate Andrew Rosner, who had escaped from the death march and was hiding in the woods outside of Ohrdruf, ran into some GIs who stopped and questioned him, then escorted him into town. "I was immediately surrounded by Americans and, as their officers questioned where I had been

* Kesselring was one of the few officers Hitler could still trust. Previously commander of German forces in North Africa, then Italy, and finally in Western Europe, Kesselring was supposedly Hitler's "master of defense," despite the fact that defeat was imminent and inevitable. (Liddell Hart, p. 671)

** The 355th Infantry was part of Colonel Harris' Combat Team 5 of the 89th Infantry Division. Other units in CT5 were the 914th Field Artillery Battalion, Company C of the 602nd Tank Destroyer Battalion, and Company C of the 707th Tank Battalion, plus additional supporting units. It is often claimed that the 4th Armored Division liberated the Ohrdruf camp, but it was elements of the 4th Armored that captured the *town* of Ohrdruf at 3:20 P.M. on April 4; elements of the 4th Armored did not enter the Ohrdruf concentration camp until April 6, 1945. ("Red Triangle," "Inside the Vicious Heart" monograph)

and what had happened to me, GIs were showering me with food and chocolate and other treats that I had not known for almost five years [of captivity]." Rosner was sent to an army field hospital to begin recovering from his ordeal.[5]

Leo Laufer, too, had been sent on the forced march a couple of days before the Americans arrived. "We were marched out," he recalled. "In the background you could hear the artillery. We knew that this was the end. Guarded heavily by men with machine guns, we marched for about five or six hours."

As the thousands of Ohrdruf inmates trudged along the road through a dense forest, Laufer and three others decided on an escape plan. The quartet was comprised of Laufer, a lad from Warsaw, another from Holland, and the Russian POW Sasha; in spite of their various languages, they somehow managed to communicate. Because of his military training and experience, Sasha was elected the group's leader. As they marched, Sasha told them to slip off their wooden shoes because they were too noisy and would slow them down once they decided to make a break for freedom. Their blankets and metal food containers were also discarded along the route in anticipation of making a fast getaway.

The four men worked their way to the front of the long column of marchers and then, as darkness fell and the nearest guard appeared to relax and look the other way, bolted into the forest. The guards fired in their general direction, but missed. Deeper into the woods the men ran and hid; no one followed them.

"We wondered where we should go," Laufer said. "Nobody knew the terrain or where we were. But we knew that somebody—the Americans or British or Russians—were coming toward us, so we felt the best way to go was back toward the sound of the fighting instead of the direction the Germans had been taking us."

The group eventually decided that they would go back to Ohrdruf; if the camp was going to be liberated, then that's where they wanted to be. "The next morning we reached the camp," Laufer said. "We ran across the highway [and] into the woods. There was a lot of shooting going on. It was unbelievable. It was like firecrackers. We didn't know what was going on. We were scared to death to go into the camp, but we remembered that when we used to go to work we could see an air-raid shelter on top of the mountain, so Sasha said that's where we should go. So we went up the mountain."

The four men, armed only with rocks, entered the darkened concrete structure. It was empty. Sasha told the other three, "If anybody walks in, I don't care if he is a guard or one of ours, kill him." Laufer thought the group would be in the bunker for just a few hours and then could emerge. But there was shooting, artillery fire, and bombing going on all around their position. They remained hidden.[6]

AFTER THE CAMP was reached, a recon party from the 24th Armored Engineer Battalion, Combat Command B, 4th Armored Division, headed out to find S-III, the rumored underground communications center south of Ohrdruf. Leading the recon party was Lieutenant J. Leavitt Anderson. "I suppose they should have sent the signal company, but they sent us instead," he said.

After much searching, Anderson and his men finally spotted the entrance to a tunnel dug into the side of a mountain in the Jonastal. "You could drive right into the entrance with a halftrack," Anderson said. "There were no German troops there at all. We went in and went down some stairs—the place was huge; it went ten stories down. This was the central telephone exchange for the entire German army. The lights were on in the tunnels and everywhere there was electronic equipment of all sorts."

When Anderson's group reached the lowest level, they saw large electrical cables spreading out in several different directions. "Somebody had cut these cables with an ax," Anderson recalled. "I went to the end of the tunnel following one of the cables. It ended outside about a mile away in what looked like a little shed."[7]

After the underground facility was discovered by Anderson and his men, the Intelligence officer of the 4th Armored Division notified VIII Corps: "Ohrdruf area reports three large partially completed telephone centrals located.... Contained huge signal stocks mainly telephone, some radio equipment and great quantities carrier equipment valued at five million dollars. Request guards and EELS* men immediately."[8] VIII Corps then sent a message to Third Army noting, "In Ohrdruf a huge communications center of the entire German Army has been installed in preparation for a retreat from Berlin.... Immense underground radio stations, cable, and telephone switchboards large enough to serve a city were set deep in concrete tunnels."[9]

* The author was unable to find a reference for this acronym. However, Dr. Richard J. Sommers of the U.S. Army Military History Institute suggested the possibility that the acronym was misspelled and that "EELS" was intended to be "EEIS," which stands for "Enemy Equipment Intelligence Service." He said, "The 4th Armored Division had just captured all this special enemy equipment related to communications and now some experts were needed to identify it." (R.J. Sommers e-mail to author, December 11, 2007)

WITHOUT FOOD OR water, time passed with excruciating slowness for Leo Laufer, Sasha the Russian, and the other two escapees hiding in the mountaintop bunker. Early one morning, from their elevated position, the four famished ex-prisoners saw activity in the valley below them. "We saw tanks and artillery down there," Laufer said. "I'm talking about an army settling down below. We didn't know what to do. We were so hungry we could have eaten sand. We had no water, no food. We were almost dead. Finally, we decided to go down."

Using rags as a flag of peace, they slowly walked toward the military encampment. "We looked horrible and downtrodden," Laufer said. "We had striped uniforms and Mohawk haircuts so the [German] civilians could recognize us as prisoners if we ran away." The quartet cautiously approached a group of soldiers. "We didn't even know if they were Americans. All we saw on a truck was white stars; we didn't know if it was Russian or British or what. Sasha said, 'It's not the Russian army.'

"When we came down, they talked to us in English but we didn't understand. We started talking in German. Nobody understood us; we couldn't converse with them. Finally one of their guys called somebody. I knew later on that he was an officer because he had two bars. He was very nice. He was a doctor. Fortunately, he was of Czech descent, so we spoke a little Polish, which is similar to Czech. We told him who we were and I showed him the tattooed numbers on my arm."

The captain told the GIs who were pointing rifles at the quartet to relax. Then the four were given food and water—a terrible mistake, for their ravaged digestive systems couldn't hold the sudden inrush of rich food. "All four of us collapsed as though we were dead," said Laufer. "They took us to a little makeshift hospital and pumped our stomachs and revived us. It was the most horrible experience we went through after liberation."

But they were alive. And they were free.[10]

IN ADDITION TO finding the communications center, the Americans began pouring into Ohrdruf-Nord Stalag III, which was still littered with corpses. An 89th Recon Troop officer reported that his men entered the camp and "saw first-hand the horror of life in a Nazi concentration camp. We radioed our troop headquarters for instructions and were told to remain there, keeping the inmates contained (this was hardly necessary, as most were in their bunks, hardly able to walk) while Headquarters contacted the infantry to relieve us." It took nearly three more hours before the 3rd Battalion of the 355th Infantry arrived and took control of the situation.[11]

Among the first GIs to enter the camp was Sol R. Brandell, a scout with the Intelligence and Recon Platoon, 2nd Battalion, 355th Infantry Regiment. He saw a small building with a sign, *Krankenhaus—Achtung: Typhus* ("Hospital—Warning: Typhus") and went inside, only to be greeted by the sight and smell of "about twelve or thirteen bodies lying in two-high wooden bunks and emitting the worst stench of rotten flesh, blood, and feces that I had ever before encountered, so intense that it stopped my breath and I had to escape to the outdoors, which didn't smell as bad."

After he regained his composure, Brandell went on a cursory inspection of the camp, coming across an immense pit that contained what he estimated to be the bodies of 6,000 to 7,000 naked corpses [a former inmate said there were 9,000 bodies], covered with a thin dusting of quick-lime.[12] He recalled that one of the soldiers in his group, a devout Roman Catholic, caught sight of the death pit, "let out a loud wail, dropped to his knees, clasped his hands and prayed to God amidst loud sobs, with tears running down his cheeks. Although we had both been in 2nd Battalion for at least the last eight months, including stateside training at Camp Butner, North Carolina, I had never before realized he could be such a compassionate person."[13]

Stanley N. Hodson, a private in the 355th Infantry, wandered over to another large pit, this one obviously used for mass cremation as it was crisscrossed with a makeshift grid of warped steel rails and blackened logs on which burned bodies were still visible. A liberated inmate told him that the enormous grate "was made of steel rails and brush and logs by the prisoners, who were then forced to lie on top and be shot there, then more logs were brought, and more prisoners, until the pile was high enough. Then tar was poured over them and the pyre lit. There were long poles with steel hooks on them used for turning the bodies over. Even so, they didn't do a good job. The bodies were still there, some only charred, some half burnt. Off to one side some graves were dug about two feet deep. They were filled with rainwater. The rain had washed some of the dirt away and a man's leg was showing." Disgusted, Hodson said, "These people [German civilians] could not help but see those living zombies."[14]

Another member of the 89th, Bruce Nickols, recalled, "As we stepped into the compound, one was greeted by an overpowering odor of quick-lime, dirty clothing, feces, and urine. Lying in the center of the square were sixty-seventy dead prisoners clad in striped clothing and in disarray." Nichols said someone told him that the prisoners had been executed the day before "because they were too weak to march to another camp. The idea was for the SS and the prisoners to avoid the approaching U.S. Army and the Russians."[15]

Ralph G. Cole, another 89th Division GI, said that inside the camp entrance was the body of "a young American aviator, still dressed in his flight gear.* The crematorium was filled with the partially consumed bodies of many people, some still smoldering and smoking.... Nearby in a warehouse were piles of bodies covered with lye, awaiting cremation. In one locale, a body was still on a roasting-type campfire, treated as you might roast a pig. There were almost no survivors, as the Nazis had killed as many prisoners as possible to prevent anyone from telling what had happened."[16]

Staff Sergeant Wencie Higuera, with Headquarters, 2nd Battalion, 355th Infantry Regiment, also remembered seeing the dead American pilot. The corpse had a bullet hole in the back of the neck. Higuera knelt down and inspected a tag attached to the aviator's uniform. "It said he was Mitiek Wagner of Gardner, Massachusetts," recalled Higuera.[17]

Technician fifth grade William F. Charboneau, Jr., with the 89th Division's 1st Battalion, 355th Regiment, said, "I could hardly believe what I was seeing. The stench was terrible. Many of us cried like babies. Even today, my eyes fill up when I think of it. I was only nineteen years old at the time, but I think I became a man that day."[18]

A filthy, emaciated Polish inmate suddenly approached another 355th soldier, Ralph G. Rush. In broken English, he told Rush that some of the guards were still in the camp, disguised in the prisoners' striped uniforms until they could escape. "He asked me for my gun," Rush said; the inmate wanted to take revenge on some of his tormentors. Rush initially told him no, but then relented, giving him a captured German Luger pistol he had picked up after a previous battle. The prisoner went off in search of retribution.

Under the orders of his sergeant, Rush and others of the squad then made

* Probably the same aviator that Leo Laufer recalled being shot down.

a sweep of the headquarters building and the commandant's office. Everything was neat and orderly, and Rush, looking for some sort of souvenir or keepsake, swiped a slide rule from off the commandant's mahogany desk—a slide rule he kept and later used in college.

After a short while, the young Pole returned to Rush and handed back the Luger. "He had tears in his eyes," Rush recalled, "as he returned the empty gun and empty ammo clips, and cried as he thanked me over and over for helping him and his people. He said, 'Some of the guards would not harm anyone again.'"[19]

Bruce Nichols noted that he was very upset by the flagrant disregard for human life he saw at Ohrdruf. "The whole experience was far beyond my understanding. I wrote a letter to my parents describing the experience, which was read at a local gathering of businessmen. It was widely disbelieved."[20]

Michael Hirsh, author of *The Liberators*, wrote that Stanley Friedenberg, a member of a Counter Intelligence Corps unit that was prowling the countryside in search of evidence of possible war crimes, reached Ohrdruf where he encountered a swimming-pool-size pit filled with decomposing, lime-dusted bodies. "I took one picture," he said, "that's all I could take because it was such a horrible sight. How can one human being do this to another, no matter how much you hated them…? How could it be? Is there a god?"

Hirsh noted, "Even as a member of CIC, Friedenberg had had no idea about the concentration camps. At that point in the war, news of them had not made it down the chain of command. Some officers in the line units knew the Russians had run into them, and [Lieutenant Colonel Albin F.] Irzyk says there were 'undercurrents about concentration camps, but I don't think the impact—it never came until Ohrdruf. To see it, to see it'—he pauses, searching for the right word—'it's staggering, staggering.'"[21]

Private first class Eric Leiserofef was a German-American Jew serving with the 89th Division's Company E, 353rd Regiment. Although Company E was located several miles from the Ohrdruf camp, Leiserofef obtained permission from his commanding officer to visit it and search for any relatives who might be there. He found no family members but later learned that some of his relatives died at Buchenwald and at other death camps. He also recalled getting a certain amount of satisfaction in talking with some of the locals in the town of Ohrdruf. While no one admitted having anything to do with the camp—or even having any knowledge of it—Leiserofef pointed to himself and said, "I used to get a great kick out of telling them I am Jewish—'*Ich bin ein Jude*.'"[22]

The After-Action Report of Combat Command A, 4th Armored Division, described the camp: "This was Ohrdruf-Nord, work camp for the Buchenwald concentration camp. When the troops entered, they found twenty-nine bodies on the ground in front of the administration building. A short distance away was a gallows and not far beyond it a shed in which fifty-two naked bodies were stacked in tiers of four, covered with what appeared to be powdered lime. They apparently had been awaiting transportation to pits in the forest where between two and three thousand others had been buried during the six months the camp had existed. Most had died of disease, but most also had marks on their faces and heads and bruises on their bodies. A third group of nine charred torsos lay among ashes under a rough incinerator made of railroad ties and rails. Those in front of the administration building were the most recently dead—all shot in the back of the neck.

"Ohrdruf-Nord had no gas chamber or high-performance crematorium. The deaths there were caused by disease and neglect, helped along by overwork and brutality. The inmates had been employed at digging a tunnel, probably as a site for an underground factory. A thousand had been there a week before the

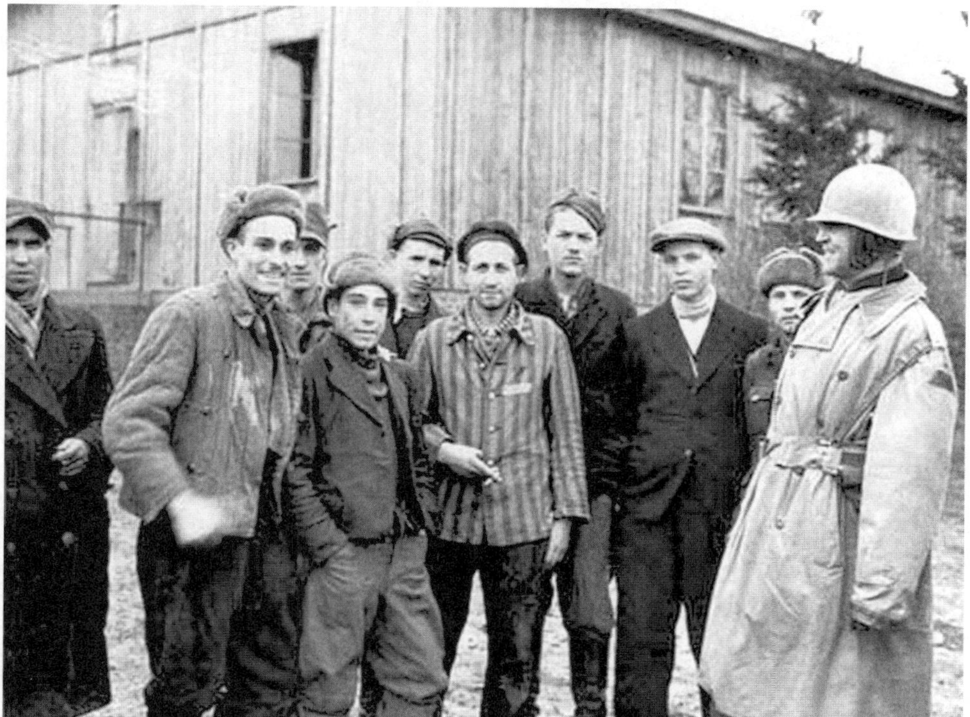

Colonel Hayden Sears (right) meets with a group of Ohrdruf prisoners who were freed when his CCA, 4th Armored Division, liberated the Buchenwald sub-camp on April 4, 1945. (U.S. National Archives)

Americans came. In the succeeding days the guards had marched those who could walk away to the east. Two buses had come to take out the bedridden sick. By then American artillery fire could be heard coming close, and the commandant lost his nerve, sent the buses away empty, and shot the prisoners with his pistol. A dozen men had hidden in the camp buildings and survived to tell about the last days at Ohrdruf-Nord and to identify the dead, among whom was an American pilot who had been imprisoned there after being shot down nearby."[23]

"Colonel [Hayden A.] Sears, commander of CC 'A,' ordered the people of Ohrdruf to the concentration camp to view the ghastly scene left by their army. 46 [SS] prisoners were captured by CC 'A' in patrol activities around Ohrdruf. The mayor and his wife, while professing no knowledge of the affairs of the camp, later committed suicide."[24]

It was true. Sears had ordered a group of Ohrdruf citizens to tour the camp so they could see what their government and countrymen had been up to. Lieutenant Colonel James H. Van Wagenen, the 4th Armored's military government officer, told the town's mayor, Albert Schneider, to be one of the first to

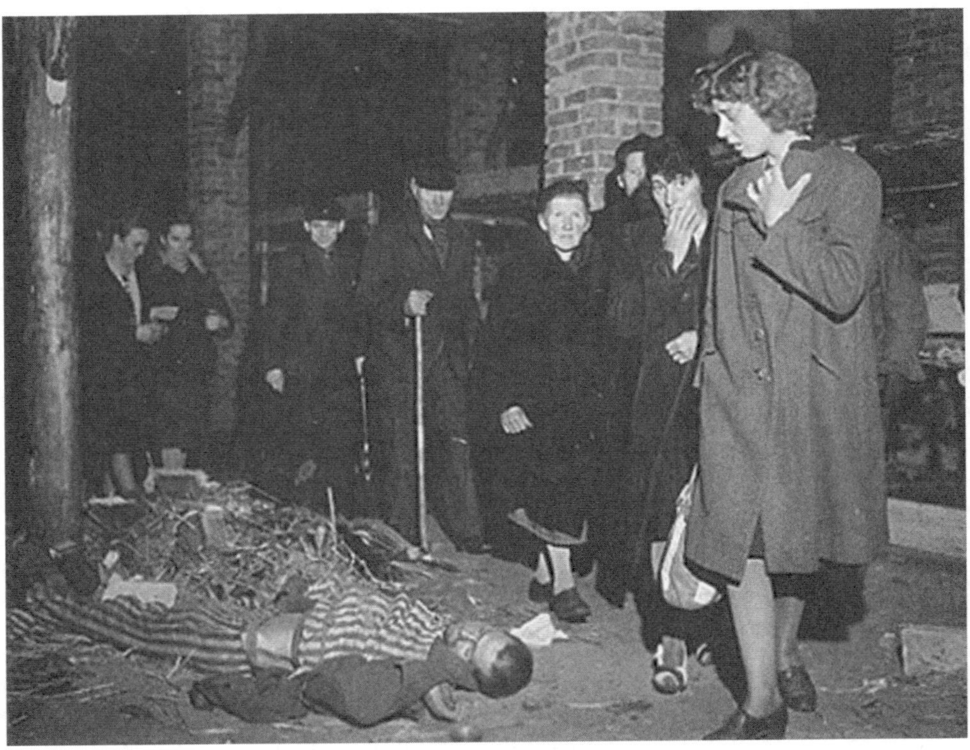

Civilians from Ohrdruf display various reactions during the forced tour of the camp near their city, April 4, 1945. (U.S. National Archives)

visit the camp, as the Army's official history noted:

"Schneider had been a [Nazi] party member since 1933, but he had also been an honest and conscientious mayor, and he had not skipped town ahead of the Americans as other Nazi officials were doing. He was shocked by what he saw. Admitting there had been rumors in the town, he claimed simply not to have believed Germans capable of such atrocities. On Van Wagenen's orders, he agreed to summon twenty-five prominent men and women who were to be taken to view the camp the next morning.

"In the morning, a soldier who had been sent to fetch him after he failed to appear at the stated time found him and his wife dead in their bedroom, their wrists slashed. G-2 investigators concluded the Schneiders' suicides were motivated by sincere shock and regret over what had happened in their town. One of the most frustrating psychological problems of the early occupation was going to be how to make the German people realize the horror of the concentration camps. In Ohrdruf, however, after the Schneiders' suicides and after others had been taken to see the camp, the citizens seemed to be convinced."[25]

THE LIBERATORS OF Ohrdruf were genuinely shocked and outraged at what they saw, but it should be remembered that the citizens of the United States had known for over a decade, thanks to frequent and regular newspaper reports, of the incarceration, persecution, and systematic slaughter of Europe's undesirables. The fact is that the U.S.—both at the personal and governmental levels—was well aware of the atrocities taking place and failed to tell American troops about them and did little or nothing to stop them.

While the GIs who stumbled onto Ohrdruf were stunned, sickened, and revolted by what they found, there were even greater horrors waiting down the road at Buchenwald.

22
THE LIBERATION OF BUCHENWALD

"The decisive moment had come."

Thomas Geve
Buchenwald prisoner

SS-OBERGRUPPENFÜHRER UND General der Waffen-SS Prince Josias zu Waldeck und Pyrmont was now Hermann Pister's official pain-in-the-neck.

As the American Army approached his palatial home and headquarters in Kassel, Waldeck kept one step ahead of the advancing enemy, first going to Weimar and then, on March 31, up the hill to Buchenwald. Seeing thousands of prisoners still behind the electrified barbed wire, Waldeck stormed into Pister's office and demanded to know why the commandant had not followed Himmler's orders to finish evacuating the camp. Flustered, Pister began immediately to do so, but a furious Waldeck told Pister that the camp commandant was now his subordinate, and that he—Waldeck—was now in charge of the evacuation.[1]

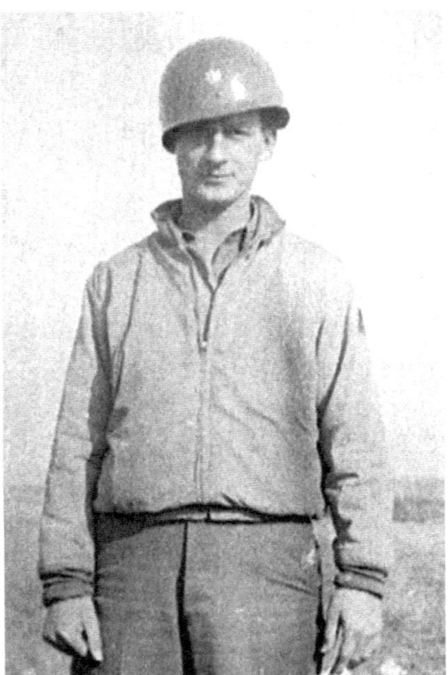

Captain Robert J. Bennett (shown in July 1945 as a major), commander of the Southern Column of Combat Team 9 and Keffer's superior (Courtesy Bernd Schmidt)

But no sooner had Waldeck assumed command of Buchenwald than the situation deteriorated irretrievably. On April 11, 1945, the Southern Column of Combat Team 9 (commanded by Captain Robert J. Bennett) of the 9th Armored Infantry Battalion (Major Gilman E. Morse), Combat Command A (Colonel Albert E. Harris), 6th Armored Division (Major General Robert W. Grow), was charging eastward, having made a lightning advance of sixty-three miles since morning.

Even on that late date, and despite the fact that the sub-camp at Ohrdruf had been overrun by Combat Team 5 of the 89th Infantry Division on April 4, the existence of Buchenwald was still largely unknown to the GIs of the 6th Armored

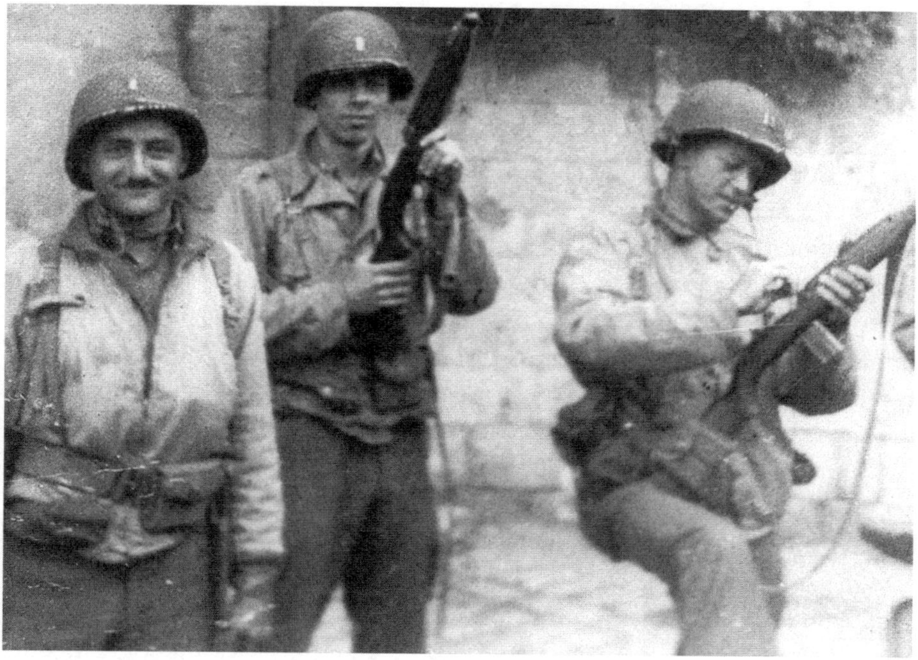

Lieutenant (later Captain) Frederic Keffer (center) "somewhere in France," summer 1944 (Courtesy Leslie Keffer Rego)

Division; they were operating with military maps on which neither the name Buchenwald, nor the names of any of the other concentration camps, appeared.[2]

AT DAWN ON April 11, inmate Johannen Goldkrantz was still asleep in his tool-cabinet hiding place in the disused DAW machine hall. "A camp policeman entered the hall," he said, "and must have heard a noise coming from the tool cabinet where I hid. Perhaps I had moved while asleep, because I hadn't heard him come into the hall. He opened the cabinet, saw me, and warned me to leave or the SS would kill me. He told me the entire camp was being evacuated."

"I was half frozen, hadn't eaten anything for two days, and could hardly move. I roamed the camp, watching for SS guards. Many barracks were now standing empty. The fresh morning air revived me a little. I noticed other shadows moving around between the blocks. At about 9 A.M., I saw a group of

German political prisoners standing near a block and quietly discussing the situation. They were looking toward the camp gate and keenly watching any action coming from there. From their conversation I understood that there were still thousands of inmates in the camp, although daily ten to twelve thousand prisoners were being evacuated on foot. These middle-aged Germans were analyzing the situation, and my impression was that they were part of the underground. I kept hanging around to hear more. They ignored my presence and didn't chase me away."[3]

At about the same time, Pister was meeting with Franz Eichorn and Senior Inmate Hans Eiden to give them a stunning piece of news: Allied forces were approaching, and he and the rest of the SS were preparing to leave the camp; the camp would be the prisoners' responsibility once the departure took place. An hour later the loudspeakers blared, "All members of the SS are to leave the camp immediately!" It would take some time, however, before all the guards and staff members could comply with the order.[4]

One of the inmates, a German named Thomas Geve, recalled, "We heard a wailing like we had never heard before. The Germans called it the 'Tank-Alarm Siren.' The decisive moment had come. On the periphery of the forest we saw a party of greycoats with steel helmets running, SS guards who had retreated with cases of ammunition and machine guns. Later on we saw more of them; they were running faster but only a few of them were armed with rifles. Then the surrounding area was quiet again and the uncertainty dragged on."[5]

As the morning wore on, the popping sounds of small-arms fire and the boom of artillery rolling from the direction of Erfurt to the west made the camp guards very nervous and gave the remaining prisoners hope that liberation was close at hand. Twenty-three-year-old inmate Robert Max Widerman said that at about 10:15 A.M., the sound of aircraft engines was heard. He and the others around him looked up to see two planes circling low overhead, the white American stars on their olive-drab wings plainly visible. The outpouring of emotion was spontaneous. "A huge roar, the cumulative sound of all our voices, rose up as we screamed at the planes," Widerman recalled. "We tore off our shirts and waved them.... Inmates hugged each other, jumping up and down, dancing, laughing with tears running down their cheeks, and shouting with incredible joy. Those too ill and weak could only smile; they understood what was happening. It was almost impossible to fathom that this day had actually arrived, that our miseries had come to an end, that we had survived."

Widerman then glanced around and was astonished at the sight: "As we looked at the guard towers, we saw that they were empty. There was an unusual silence hanging over Buchenwald. We knew in our hearts that this was the day."[6]

AT SOME POINT—accounts vary as to exactly when—the International Committee, the camp's underground resistance group—moved into action. The detonating of a grenade by the inmates was the signal for the "self-liberation" of Buchenwald to begin—a liberation that had been planned for years. Men whose spirits, whose hope of survival, had been crushed into the mud by an army of sadistic brutes suddenly knew that the hour of their redemption was at hand, redemption that they themselves would help bring about—or die in the attempt.

From numerous hiding places under the hospital and barracks, the inmates' arsenal—ninety-six rifles and carbines, 100 pistols, and one machine gun—magically appeared, along with boxes of ammunition and 123 grenades. The resistance leadership authorized the distribution of weapons to several hundred men who had volunteered to strike back at their oppressors.[7]

Nine hundred members of the camp' underground militia had been pre-organized into 189 combat sections and seven intelligence sections of three to six men each and assigned specific tasks; some were to assault and take over the main gate, while others were to overpower any guards that remained. Still others were to set up a protective ring around the barracks that held the children and adolescents. One of the sections—all Russians—took off in the direction of the hamlet of Hottelstedt. Many of the others headed east, toward Weimar, in hopes that the city had been captured by the Allies—as well as in hopes of finding food. One of the inmates, Max Feuer, recalled, "We expected to defend ourselves. We counted now that they—the guards—will try to exterminate the camp. For this moment we were prepared to fight the guards."[8] Quickly the armed inmates ran to their pre-assigned positions, expecting at any moment to encounter the SS moving in to slaughter them. But the majority of the guards were either gone or in the process of fleeing.[9]

The political prisoner Otto Roth rushed to the main gate, where he found several inmates milling around, wondering what to do. He instructed inmate Fritz Freudenberg to reach inside the window of the guard station and press a button that unlocked the gate. Freudenberg did so, recalling, "This triggered the electric lock and the camp gate opened.... Now that the camp gate stood open, the inmates came running towards it, first singly, then in larger masses. Several of them had rifles! The stream of inmates poured onto the barrack grounds and took possession of the rifles and ammunition that were to be found there."

Another inmate found the main control box for the electrified fence and shut it down. A ladder was produced from somewhere by Freudenberg, and inmates climbed up and occupied the unmanned watchtower above the main gate. Otto Roth noted, "Immediately following the occupation of the main gate, the camp senior Hans Eiden followed and raised the white flag on the tower. The central loudspeaker system was put back into operation and in a short address the entire camp was informed that the control of the camp had been taken over by the International Committee."[10]

Robert Max Widerman recalled seeing "inmates from the Big Camp who had organized underground groups, hundreds of them, carrying arms they had smuggled and hidden for such a day, running toward the barbed-wire fences. They cut huge holes in them, went into the woods to search for fleeing SS."[11]

In addition to their smuggled weapons, the now-free inmates broke into the guards' armory and grabbed 1,500 rifles, eighteen light machine guns, four heavy machine guns, and 180 *Panzerfaust* anti-tank weapons.[12]

Firing broke out throughout the compound; the inmates were in revolt and shooting their weapons at the guards, who were in a panic and trying to flee. Elie Wiesel recounted in his autobiographical novel *Night*, "Armed men appeared everywhere. Burst of gunshots. Grenades exploding. We, the children, remained flat on the floor.... The battle did not last long and around noon, everything was calm again."[13]

A group of inmates at the southwestern corner of the camp forced open the gate between Towers Two and Three and captured an SS man trying to escape from the detention-cell building—the first German prisoner taken that day by the inmates. Another German soldier, also near the main gate, was stripped of his rifle and ammunition; he then took off running in the direction of Weimar.* Within fifteen to twenty minutes, the "Battle of Buchenwald" was over. Casualty figures differ; "Red Triangle" told the author that only one SS guard and one prisoner were killed in the brief shoot-out while Louis Gros recalled that no guards were killed; a handful of inmates were wounded before the remaining guards ran for their lives.[14]

---

* Eventually the inmates would capture 120 SS men and place them in custody under heavy guard in Block 17, then turn them over to the Americans. ("Red Triangle," letter to author, June 10, 1997)

IN THE EARLY afternoon of April 11, Combat Team 9's operations officer noted in his report that, after witnessing an airstrike on the village of Grossmölsen, evidently requested by the 4th Armored Division operating to the 6th Armored Division's south, Captain Bennett's patrol from CT9 ran into enemy resistance at the village of Hottelstedt, about two miles northwest of Buchenwald, where it engaged an unknown number of defenders in a brief firefight. There is some confusion as to exactly what happened next.

According to the division's newspaper, the *Armored Attacker*, Captain Frederic Keffer, the battalion's S-2 (Intelligence) officer on the scene, told a reporter that CT9 captured fifteen German soldiers at Hottelstedt. Keffer said, "We no sooner had lined them against a wall preparing to send them to the rear when fifty Russians came up the road, recognized some of the SS men as former guards at the prison and started to attack them. We had to hold them off at the point of guns."[15]

Another version, provided many years later by Captain Robert J. Bennett, commanding the Southern Column of CT9, indicated that the inmates had armed themselves before leaving the concentration camp and had chased a group of guards down the road and into Hottelstedt. They were in the process of "roughing them up" when the GIs showed up and intervened.[16]

However it happened, the Russian POWs managed to convey to the Americans the fact that they were inmates of a horrible concentration camp located just up the road behind a heavy screen of trees. Despite the fact that he had no knowledge of a concentration camp in the area, Bennett nevertheless disregarded his orders not to stop or slow down, and made the decision to send a small reconnaissance party along the narrow country lane to scout the situation up ahead. Although he had with him a platoon of five Sherman tanks from Company C of the 15th Tank Battalion, Bennett did not want to risk them in case the Germans were planning an ambush along the heavily wooded road. Instead, he sent forward a four-man scouting party, headed by Captain Keffer, in a six-wheeled M-8 armored car. Accompanying Keffer were Berlin-born Technical Sergeant Herbert Gottschalk, radio operator Private First Class James Hoyt, and driver Sergeant Harry Ward. At about 4:30 P.M., two of the Russians climbed onto the armored car to guide Keffer to camp.

Moving cautiously up the tree-lined road toward Buchenwald, Keffer arrived at the camp approximately fifteen minutes after leaving Hottelstedt. When they cleared the trees they saw the barbed-wire perimeter and, beyond, a sea of barracks. They could see thousands of scrawny men, dressed in shabby rags, milling about, singly and in groups. Some of them carried weapons; a few caught sight of the approaching Americans and began cheering and waving. The Yanks saw no German guards.

A number of different stories have emerged over the years, with some GIs claiming to be liberators when, in fact, official records show that their units were nowhere near Buchenwald or Weimar on April 11, 1945. Even some contemporary reports are confused or in error. For example, inmates noted in Camp Report No. 1, "On the evening of April 11, 1945, the first two American tanks approached the quarry from the north at 1 p.m. An hour later, twelve tanks reached the stalls in the northern section of the camp and engaged the SS in heavy combat. At about 2:30 p.m. they overran the SS [barracks] area. A short time later—at 2:45—the inmates began an operation to disarm the remaining SS men and take control of the camp."⋆ [17]

Another document ("Buchenwald: A Preliminary Report") written by Lieutenant Edward A. Tenenbaum and a civilian named Egon W. Fleck says that they also arrived at the camp on April 11, but their unit or team is unknown. Red Triangle commented that the seventeen-page document "does not show when Tenenbaum and Fleck arrived at Buchenwald and when they left it and from where they came and to where they went on the days they drove to and from Buchenwald. The omission of these very important details is so exceptional in connection with the preparation of official military reports that it makes [their report] a worthless document in spite of the fact that it contains a considerable amount of valuable information." Red Triangle noted that other, more reliable, information indicated that the two men first arrived at the camp on April 13—two days after its liberation.

Further, as Red Triangle pointed out, Tenenbaum later told a reporter that he was a lieutenant with the 4th Armored Division, while other documents show him being with the Psychological Warfare Branch of Patton's Third Army. As Red Triangle wryly noted, "Tenenbaum must have had an unusual capacity for telling tall tales," and that his claim that he arrived at Buchenwald on April 11 "is nothing other than a ludicrous fabrication."[18]

⋆ This report contradicts Keffer's reports. It is possible that inmates mistook his M-8 armored car for a tank. Also, U.S. Army records do not indicate that "two tanks" approached from the north, nor that "twelve tanks" engaged the SS in heavy combat in the barracks area; Bennett had five tanks, and they remained in Hottelstedt for most of the day. The Buchenwald inmates' Camp Report No. 1 also indicates, albeit incorrectly, that two French soldiers (Lieutenant Emmanuel Desard and Sergeant Paul Bodot), acting as scouts for the U.S. 4th Armored Division reached and entered the camp at around 5:00 P.M. and that Keffer and his patrol did not arrive until 5:10—contradicting Keffer's recollection that he arrived somewhere between 4:30 and 5:00 P.M. (www. Buchenwald.de/en/473)

Keffer told Ward and Hoyt to stay with the M-8 outside the enclosure while he and Gottschalk entered the camp through a gaping hole in the wire that had been made by the inmates when they took over the camp. What Keffer and his men found would stay with them for the rest of their lives.[19]

Keffer and Gottschalk were immediately swarmed upon by a crowd of foul-smelling, deliriously happy inmates, all of them excitedly cheering and babbling in incomprehensible tongues. Keffer was told the name of the camp, but the name "Buchenwald" had little meaning for him at that time. Suddenly, Keffer found himself lifted off the ground by a score of hands and carried around "on the shoulders of the crowd like a conquering hero."[20]

Keffer later wrote, "What an incredible greeting that was. I was picked up by arms and legs, thrown in the air, caught, thrown again, caught, thrown, etc., until I had to stop it, I was getting so dizzy. How the men found such a surge of strength in their emaciated condition was one of those bodily wonders in which the spirit sometimes overcomes all weaknesses of the flesh. My, but it was a great day!"[21]

Inmate Louis Gros said that he caught a glimpse of Keffer entering the camp: "He enters at a walking pace. We don't have the time to discern whether he smiles or not. And why should he smile? In half a tick, we discover that his uniform…his officer's insignia, shoes, and behavior can belong only to an American. And that one is our liberator, the first to enter the camp, to confirm our state as free men—free and rescued from the Nazi tyranny, definitely! Then twelve arms, maybe more, apprehend him, raise and throw him into the air, once, twice, ten times! He literally flies, such as a disjointed puppet until, tired of that exhausting sport, he shouts a forcible 'Stop!', which is promptly obeyed. Sensing that scene, I suddenly feel taken by an intense emotion. My tears release irresistibly because they have been repressed for too long a time. I have no shame; never have I felt so alive, so existing, than at that supreme instant!"[22]

Keffer said, "I was slowly pulled and pushed through the crowd towards a headquarters building. There I met some of the leaders of the prison underground who were now in control. I told them I would radio for medical help and for food, and I requested them not to let the former prisoners, if they could help it, wander far outside the camp and possibly unwittingly interfere with our military progress. Then I managed somehow to return to the scout car, give all the food we had to the camp, and drive back to our main column [at Hottelstedt]."[23]

Keffer also radioed Captain Bennett to apprise him of what he had found and to request that food, water, and medical help be dispatched to the camp as soon as possible.* At 5:35 P.M., Keffer and his advance party left Buchenwald; the camp was now under the complete and sole control of the inmates.[24]

After the Americans left, Johannen Goldkranz, the prisoner from Bendzin who had survived so much and was barely alive at the moment of liberation, made his way to the roll-call area. "I saw armed inmates bringing in a few SS guards," he recalled. "These were the guards who had manned the watchtowers and been unable to get far enough away." Weak and exhausted but happy, he went back to Block 49 and fell asleep.[25]

At around 7:30 P.M., some two hours after Keffer's patrol departed Buchenwald, two more officers from the 6th Armored Division—Captain Edmund Coates (Assistant G-1, Personnel) and Captain Charles Davidson (Assistant G-5, Military Government)—reached the camp, made a more thorough inspection than Keffer had been able to do, interviewed a number of inmates (which probably also included a meeting with the leaders of the camp's underground resistance force), then departed for the division command post approximately two hours later. Coates and Davidson took with them the news that 900 political prisoners had been executed by the Nazis just a week before the 6th Armored Division had arrived.[26]

ROBERT MAX WIDERMAN noted that, after the arrival of the Americans, the heavy mantle of fear and death had been lifted off the camp as if by magic, transfiguring the grim, monochromatic landscape into a bright and hopeful vision. "Flags from all European nations had appeared, flying from the tops of the barracks," he said. "The whole camp took on a different tone. There was constant laughter, mixed with the eerie feeling we had of believing without believing what had just happened to us. The GIs [later] distributed food—things we hadn't seen for years, and in large quantity. The tragedy is that many survivors died from overeating food too rich for them after such a long time of starvation."

As though in a dream, Widerman and two friends walked out of the camp's gate and into the fresh air of the vacant SS barracks area of the camp, all the while reciting a mantra: "We are free! We are free!" as if only by repetition could

* It took several days for the supplies to reach the camp, however, because combat units did not carry additional provisions with them. Without prior knowledge of Buchenwald's existence, neither the 6th Armored Division, nor any other supporting units, could have anticipated the extraordinary situation they would encounter. The relief of Buchenwald became the responsibility of Third Army's military government (G-5) sections, mobile field hospitals, and other service units. As other units subsequently reached the camp, the GIs, stunned by the overwhelming need, generously gave away their rations to the starving inmates—an act of kindness that was, in many cases, literally more than the inmates could stomach.

they finally get themselves to believe it. "I was bursting with excitement," he said, "realizing that I was a human being again and not a set of numbers." He also realized that he was not going to die at the hands of the SS.[27]

Singly and in small groups, SS guards began reappearing at the camp under the watch of former prisoners with their fingers on the triggers of Mauser rifles and Schmeisser machine pistols. Some of the guards sported black eyes, bruised cheeks, and fattened lips, evidence that some of the prisoners had taken a little revenge on their former keepers.

Food was also on the minds of the newly freed. Johannen Goldkranz recalled, "I woke late the next morning. I heard people speaking of soup being given out in the kitchen. I rushed there and received a bowl of hot, thick, fatty soup with meat and other solid food in it—the first good meal I had eaten for a very long time. It was delicious. I finished it and immediately had to rush to the toilet. My stomach had not digested fat for so long that it reacted violently." For the next several days, Goldkranz teetered between life and death. Injections of glucose by an American doctor saved his life.[28]

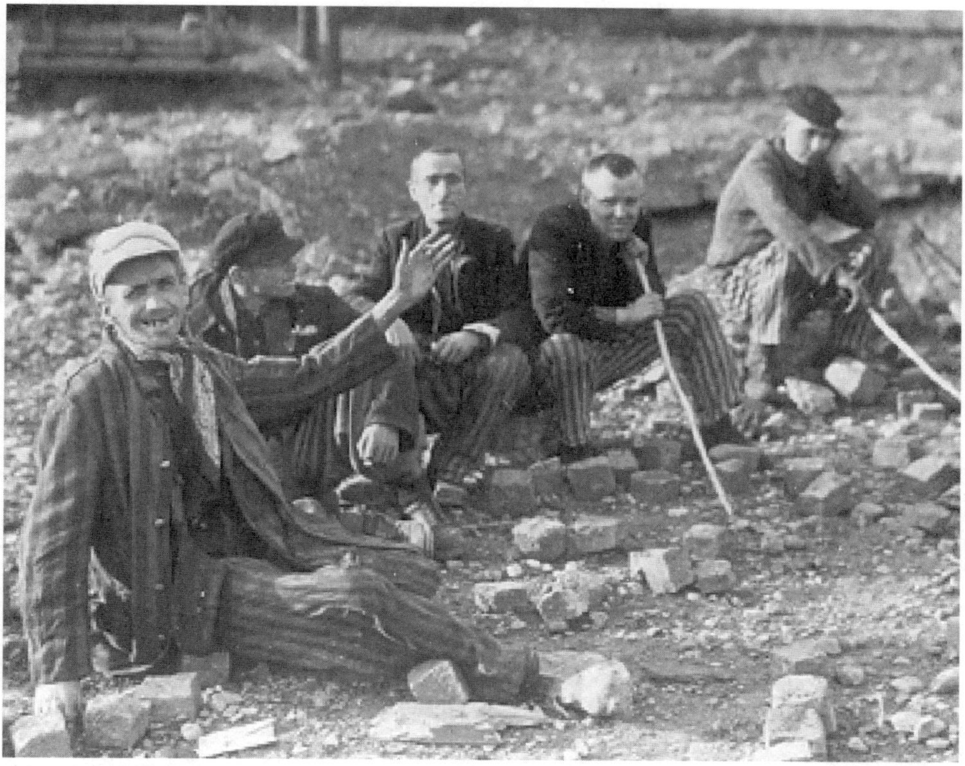

Newly liberated prisoners at Nordhausen/Mittelbau-Dora pose for the photographer. Some are happy while others seem apathetic to their changed circumstances.
(U.S. Army Military History Institute, Paul T. Hiser Collection)

SIXTY MILES TO the northwest, at the rocket factory at Nordhausen and Buchenwald's slave-labor sub-camp known as Mittelbau-Dora, a similar scene was being played on that historic day of April 11. At those two facilities, units from Brigadier General Doyle O. Hickey's 3rd Armored and Major General Terry Allen's 104th Infantry Divisions marched through unguarded gates and found 2,700 unburied bodies and 3,000 "living skeletons."[29]

"Only a handful could stand on rickety, pipestem legs," noted Al Newman, a reporter for *Newsweek* magazine. "Their eyes were sunk deeply into their skulls and their skins under thick dirt were a ghastly yellow. Some sobbed great dry sobs to see the Americans. Others merely wailed pitifully, and one poor, semiconscious Jew…who kept crying '*Ey yaah*' will haunt my dreams for many years."[30]

WITH BUCHENWALD NOW liberated, it was time for the U.S. Army to take care of the next order of business—the capture of Weimar.

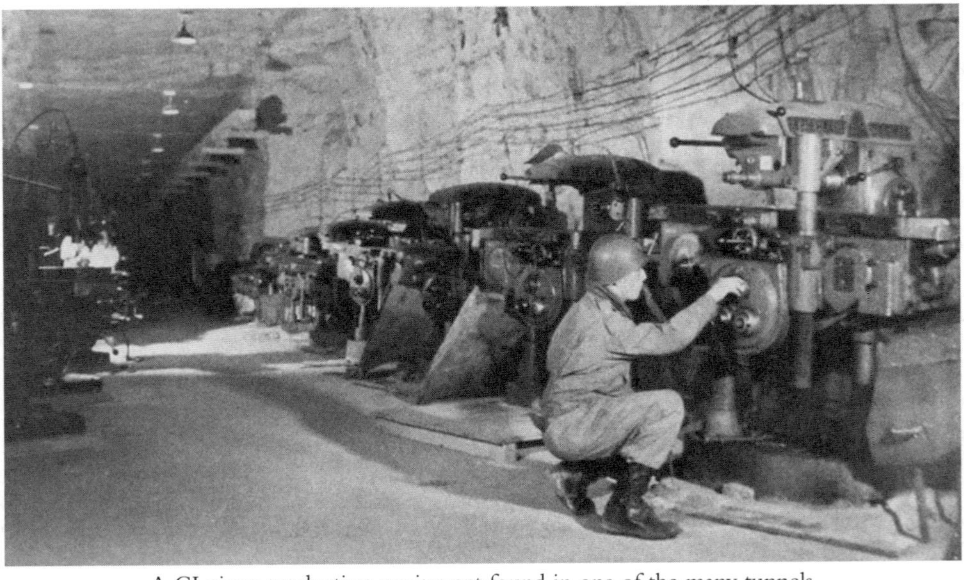

A GI views production equipment found in one of the many tunnels at Nordhausen, May 1945. (U.S. Army Military History Institute, Paul T. Hiser Collection)

23
THE SURRENDER OF WEIMAR

"Your city is surrounded and untenable. Surrender and you will be treated according to the rules of the Geneva Convention."

Colonel Normand O. Costello
80th U.S. Infantry Division

AS THE SUN set on the glorious day of April 11, 1945, negotiations for the surrender of Weimar took place in the village of Troistedt, three miles south of Weimar. With the nervous mayor of Troistedt standing by, the surrender ultimatum was drawn up by Colonel Normand O. Costello, commander of the 80th Infantry Division's Combat Team 319, and Lieutenant Colonel Paul Bandy. It read: "To the Commander of Troops, District Weimar, German Army: The Third American Army advances once more triumphantly. We propose to pass through this district and through historic Weimar. In as much as our superiority is now overwhelming, as your leaders are requiring you to fight needlessly, the honorable but unconditional surrender of Weimar and of the troops in its vicinity is demanded forthwith.

"Therefore, in order to save your city Weimar from unnecessary destruction and to prevent further shedding of blood, you will accept this offer at once. Send an emissary at once to the place directed by the bearer. The rules of the Geneva Convention will be strictly adhered to in all matters. An affirmative answer must be received at the time and the place directed by the bearer or the city of Weimar will be shelled. The American army once again is marching triumphantly forward. Your city is surrounded and untenable. Surrender and you will be treated according to the rules of the Geneva Convention."

Bandy handed Costello's ultimatum to the mayor of Troistedt, who then pedaled his bicycle into Weimar and delivered the surrender demand to his counterpart, Lord Mayor Otto Koch (no relation to Karl Otto Koch). In a hurriedly called executive session with the Weimar police chief, Burgermeister Koch prudently decided that the wisest course of action was to surrender; the police chief concurred. The burgermeister of Troistedt was sent back to Colonel Costello the next morning with the acceptance of the surrender terms.[1]

Before he arrived, however, Howard E. Congdon, with Battery B, 905th Field Artillery Battalion, 80th Infantry Division, recalled, "On the morning of

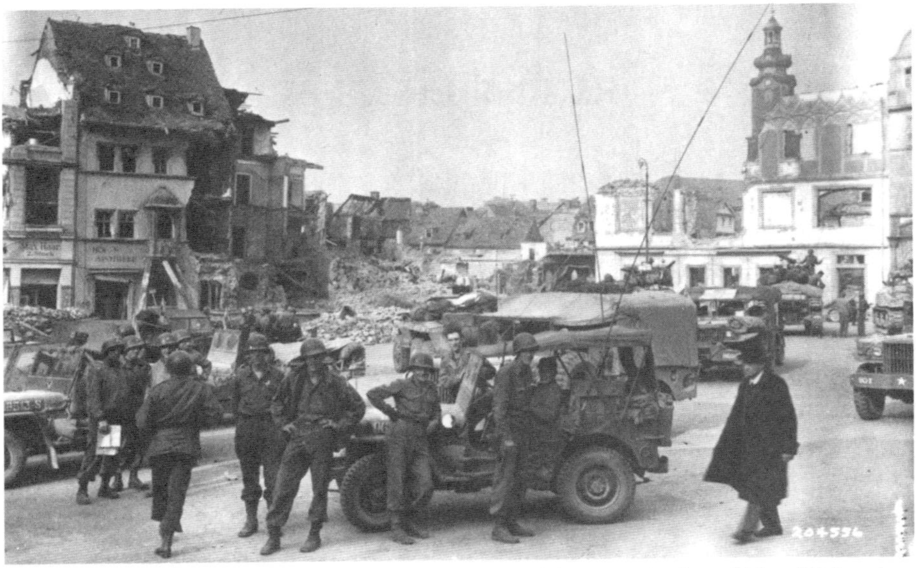

GIs from the U.S. 80th Infantry Division strike a confident pose in the rubble of Weimar's Marktplatz, April 1945. (U.S. National Archives)

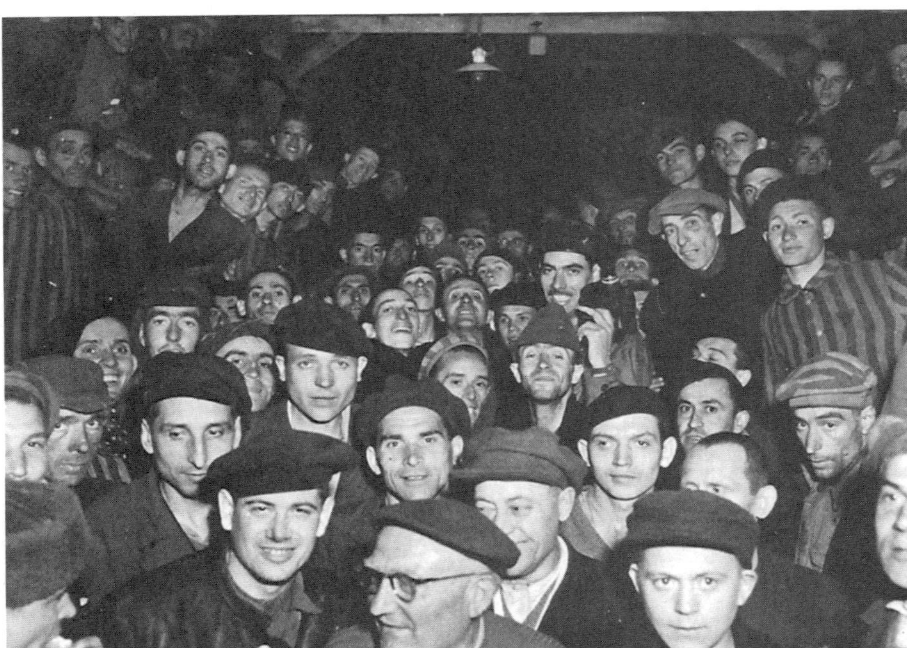

Free at last! While some of these liberated prisoners are smiling, many appear to be unsure about what the future has in store for them. Photo taken April 14, 1945. (U.S. National Archives)

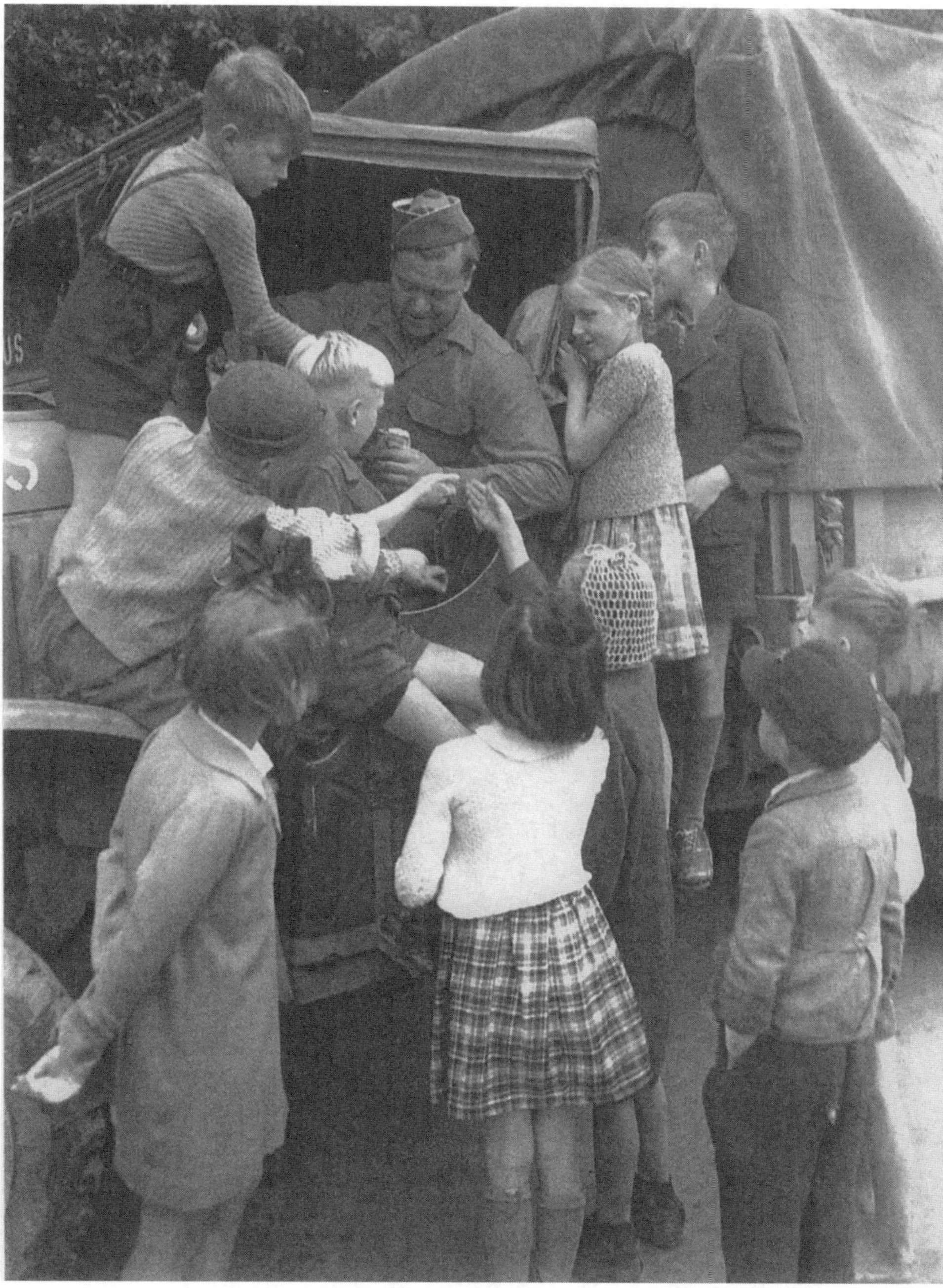

An American soldier is swarmed on by Weimar children as he hands out treats.
(U.S. National Archives)

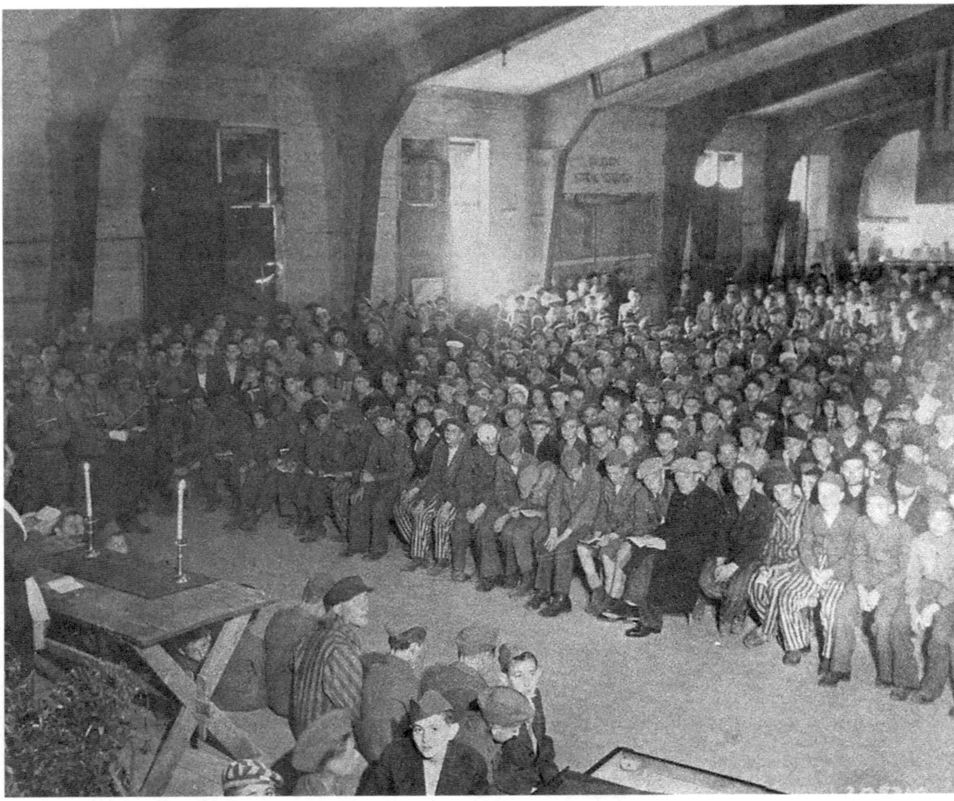

The Buchenwald theater is turned into a synagogue for a worship service shortly after American units took control of the camp. (Buchenwald Memorial)

April 12, our company was in Troistedt.... I was in on the preparations for the attack [on Weimar] which seemed like a perfect textbook plan. Weimar had been offered the chance to surrender by 9 A.M., and American fighter planes were even circling over the city as a threat. Just before the deadline, about 8:30 A.M., we noted a man on a bicycle riding toward us from Weimar. He wore a long black frock coat and a tall black hat (like Abe Lincoln) and he turned out to be the [Troistedt] mayor."[2]

Accompanying the Troistedt mayor was an interpreter, Dr. Erica Fischer, who spoke fluent English; her mother, Henrietta Hansen Schirmer, had been born in New York City, and she and her mother were living in a bomb shelter in Weimar. The surrender document was finalized and Mayor Koch was informed.

Shortly thereafter, Mayor Koch arrived in Troistedt in his limousine and agreed to the terms of surrender. Captain Lawrence A. Degner, the 80th Infantry

Division's military government officer, rode in the limo with the mayor, followed by Costello and four jeeps, plus a contingent of well-armed ground troops led by Captain William H. Chamberlain of the 2nd Battalion of the 80th's 319th Infantry Regiment.

When they marched into Weimar's destroyed main square at mid-morning, 2,000 citizens were there, many waving and cheering as if they were being liberated, while a few hard-liners turned their backs on their conquerors. The Weimar police force also lined up in the streets and turned over their weapons to the Yanks.[3] From the windows and balconies of Weimar's shattered buildings, where once Nazi flags were proudly draped, now fluttered only the white flags of surrender.[4]

THE THIRD REICH was in its death throes. On April 12, the U.S. 2nd Armored Division, part of a three-million-man Allied force on the Continent, was reported to be sixty-three miles from Berlin, while the Soviet Third and Fifth Shock Armies—the vanguard of several million troops—were closing in on Berlin from the east. Aware that Berlin would be part of the Soviet zone of occupation when Germany was defeated, Eisenhower had no intention of allowing Americans to become involved in a bloody street-by-street, building-by-building fight for the German capital; he was content to let the Soviets do that. Despite the protestations of Churchill, Ike felt the prestige of taking Berlin was not worth the lives of thousands of American soldiers. He and Omar Bradley had discussed the situation; "They both agreed that heavy casualties were an unacceptable price to pay for a prestige objective," wrote Antony Beevor.*[5]

On April 12, the *New York Times* also noted rumors that Adolf Hitler was dying and that Heinrich Himmler was preparing to take control of Germany. (In reality, Hitler was very much alive, but would not be so for long.) Another article in the *Times* said that five million European Jews were estimated to have been killed by the Nazis, giving Americans the first real hint of the scope of the Third Reich's crimes. But the end of the Hitler regime could not come soon enough for those still clinging to life.[6]

* Ike's judgment proved to be correct; some 352,425 Soviet soldiers (of whom almost a third were killed) became casualties during the desperate, two-week battle to capture the city. (Beevor, p. 756)

THREE MORE VISITORS arrived at Buchenwald on April 12. At approximately 2:30 P.M., an 80th Infantry Division jeep with three men inside pulled into the compound. The men were Major E. Coe Kerr, Jr., Assistant G-3 (Operations officer) of the division; Capitaine Pierre Chatenay, a French liaison officer; and the driver, a Private Mitchell.

While there, Kerr encountered Count Raoul de Lubersac, a French nobleman who spoke fluent English because his mother was an American and lived in Jericho, New York—only a short distance from Kerr's home town of Glen Cove—and knew the Kerr family. Seeing the desperate conditions within the camp, Kerr had de Lubersac climb into the jeep and, at about 4:00 P.M., they left Buchenwald to find a unit that might have a field radio with which they could request more assistance. At about 6:45 P.M., a detachment of about fifty or sixty men from Company A, 317th Infantry Regiment, 80th Infantry Division, arrived at Buchenwald. The company commander, Captain J. P. "Woody" Woodside, had orders to disarm the prisoners but decided to disobey the order. "The fellows [prisoners] had more machine guns that I had men," Woodside said.[7]

As the Americans probed deeper into the camp, they encountered hundreds of children—dirty, ragged, emaciated children—but *alive* children. Somehow they had been hidden by the adult inmates for months in anticipation of just this day. The authors of *The Children of Buchenwald* said of this discovery, "The soldiers went from barracks to barracks until they reached number 66. What they saw there magnified their horror. Hundreds of children, all boys, silently gazed at them with huge, deep-set eyes from faces resembling those of elderly men. They were Jewish children from Poland and Hungary aged eight to twenty."

The American commander sent out a message to higher headquarters: "Have found a thousand Jewish children in Buchenwald. Take immediate measures to evacuate them."[8]

One of the children at Buchenwald, a fourteen-year-old by the name of Meyer, had narrow but vivid memories of the liberation: "I was very small and did not really understand what was happening. For me, liberation meant that there was suddenly bread to eat. I went to Weimar and stole a bicycle. It was the first bicycle in Buchenwald and I watched it constantly." The tires needed air and Meyer asked a Ukranian, who, for some unknown reason, had a tire pump, if he could borrow it. The Ukranian said yes, but on the condition that he be allowed to take a ride on the bike. "He never came back," said Meyer sadly.[9]

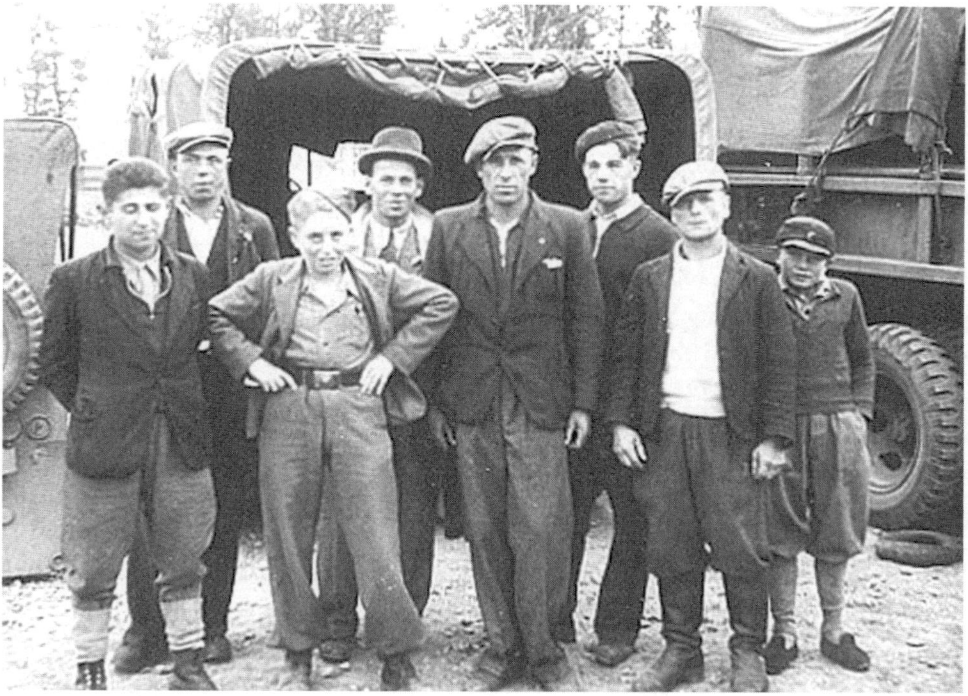

Polish men and boys, all former prisoners, prepare to leave Buchenwald for refugee camps and then repatriation to unknown destinations.
(Photo by Edwin Bonde, June 28, 1945, Courtesy Alan Bonde)

Another boy, named Alex, recalled that, when the Americans arrived, they gave him a whole loaf of bread. "Afraid that I wouldn't get any more," said Alex, "I saved part of it, an act that may have saved my life. Many others died of overeating."[10]

Another of the children, eight-year-old Yisrael Meir Lau of Piotrkow, Poland, recalled the moment when an Army chaplain laughed with joy, then broke down in tears and embraced him. The chaplain asked how old Lau was.

"What does it matter? I'm older than you," said the solemn Lau.

Taken aback, the chaplain asked why Lau made that statement.

"Because you laugh and cry like a child. I don't cry, and I haven't laughed for a long time. Tell me, who is older, me or you?"

Yisrael Meir Lau would live to become the Chief Rabbi of Israel.[11]

ACCORDING TO THE 80th Infantry Division's G-1 Journal, on April 13 heavy fighting was still taking place at the Nohra airfield and at Erfurt, thirteen miles west of Weimar, where Field Marshal Albert Kesselring, in charge of the defense of the West, had been headquartered until April 11.

The 80th Division supply officer was directed to procure as many blankets as possible for the freed inmates of Buchenwald. G-4 (Supply) noted that they had also found innumerable numbers of bolts of cloth of heavy cloth material of approximately blanket width. G-4 was directed to truck the bolts to the camp, where the tailor shop would convert the cloth into blankets.[12] Plenty of food was also found in the Buchenwald camp larder. GIs going through the storehouse discovered 3,000 loaves of bread, 150 tons of potatoes, thirty to forty tons of rye grits, and thirty tons of margarine. Additionally, the clothing depot contained a large supply of shoes and clothing. The soldiers looked at the abundance stored at Buchenwald and then at the emaciated prisoners in their filthy, worn-out rags and wooden shoes, and just shook their heads in anger at the incomprehensible unfairness of it all; someone would have to pay for this, they vowed.[13]

24
IKE AT OHRDRUF

"We are told that the American soldier does not know what he is fighting for. *Now, at least, he will know what he is fighting* against.*"*
General Dwight D. Eisenhower at Ohrdruf

UNTIL APRIL 13, 1945, when the *New York Times* published the first news about the liberation of the camp, the name and even the existence of Buchenwald was, arguably, unknown to most Americans. But the electrifying news of the camp's liberation—and, in fact, the entire Third Army's dramatic eastward push—was overshadowed by the news of the death of sixty-three-year-old President Franklin Delano Roosevelt of a massive cerebral hemorrhage at his vacation home in Warm Springs, Georgia. On that day, the *New York Times* devoted ten full pages to FDR's death but only three sentences—sixty-nine words—to the story of the liberation of Buchenwald—and not until page eleven.[1]

Vice-president Harry S. Truman had assumed the reins of power, but few people knew anything about him and no one had any idea what would happen to the American war effort now that their commander-in-chief was gone.*

The unexpected news of Roosevelt's passing hit many American soldiers overseas with unusual force. Captain Mel Rappaport, with Combat Command B, 6th Armored Division, was at division headquarters when the news came in over the radio. "It was a real shock," Rappaport said, remembering that he had cast his very first vote in a presidential election in September, 1944, while occupying a very wet foxhole east of Nancy, France, with German artillery fire playing in the background. "It was President FDR all the way against Governor Tom Dewey of New York. I was always a huge FDR fan and I really admired him. I cannot recall how FDR's death hit the other men; the war was going on all around us, so we went back to work."[2]

ON THAT SAME day of April 13, 1945, Generals Eisenhower, Bradley, and Patton arrived at the town of Merkers, some fifty miles west of Weimar, to inspect

* Hitler, as might be expected, was ecstatic at the news. Josef Goebbels, the Nazi propaganda minister, crowed, "My Führer, I congratulate you! Roosevelt is dead! It is written in the stars that the second half of April will be the turning point for us." (Shirer, pp. 1440-1441)

a recently discovered salt mine that, according to XII Corps Commanding General Manton S. Eddy, contained the Third Reich's entire gold reserve. At the bottom of the deep shaft, the generals stepped from the elevator into an immense, dimly lit vault. According to Patton's aide, Colonel Charles R. Codman, everywhere were "boxes, crates, stacks of paper currency, gold coin and bullion, jewels, paintings, dental bridgework and fillings. More than one hundred million dollars' worth, Colonel Bernstein [from the Finance Section of SHAEF] estimated. In a corner by itself [were] a dozen sizable bales of Reichsmarks."*[3]

But the excitement of finding the enormous treasure was overshadowed later that day by news of something far less enjoyable: Ohrdruf. "At Walker's suggestion," wrote Patton, "we drove to Ohrdruf and visited the first horror camp any of us had ever seen. It was the most appalling sight imaginable. A man who said he was one of the former inmates acted as impresario and showed us first the gallows, where men were hanged for attempting to escape.... Our guide then took us to the whipping table.... The feet were placed in stocks on the ground and the man was pulled over the table, which was slightly hollowed, and held by two guards, while he was beaten across the back and loins. The stick which they said had been used, and which had some blood on it, was bigger than the handle of a pick. Our guide claimed that he himself had received twenty-five blows with this tool. It later developed that he was not a prisoner at all, but one of the executioners. General Eisenhower must have suspected it, because he asked the man very pointedly how he could be so fat. He was found dead the next morning, killed by some of the inmates...."

---

* The salt mines at Merkers were used by the Reichsbank to store the bulk of its gold reserves in order to prevent it from being destroyed by the increasing Allied air raids on Berlin. Elements of the U.S. 90th Infantry Division, acting on tips from French displaced persons who worked in the mines, came upon the underground treasury on April 6, 1945, which also contained scores of crates filled with priceless paintings from Berlin art museums. Gold and silver bars, along with a considerable amount of currency, coins, jewelry, and even gold teeth and fillings from the mouths of death camp and concentration camp victims, filled the mines. It was later estimated that the value of the treasury was approximately $520 million in 1945 dollars.

One of the more interesting items found was the 3,300-year-old carved and painted limestone head of the ancient Queen Nefertiti, which had been removed from Egypt by German archaeologists in 1913 and has been displayed at the Berlin Museum ever since. Despite repeated Egyptian requests for its return, it is, at this writing, still there.

The treasure was later handed over to an international organization for safekeeping. In 1998, the Tripartite Gold Commission, which had been established to handle various claims to the treasure, received permission from fifteen claimant nations to distribute and donate it to a Nazi Persecution Relief Fund to help survivors of the Holocaust as compensation for victims of Nazi persecution. (www. archives.gov/publications/prologue/1999/spring/nazi-gold-merkers-mine-treasure; Patton, *War As I Knew It*, pp. 291-292; *New York Times*, April 12, 1945)

A former Buchenwald inmate informed the author of his own experiences regarding compensation: "These German 'reparations' were a joke, considering that, for thirty-nine months of captivity and sixty years after my liberation, I received exactly $8,636.35, which means that my monthly compensation [for my incarceration] was $221.14, or $7.38 per day.' ("Red Triangle," letter to author, June 4, 2007)

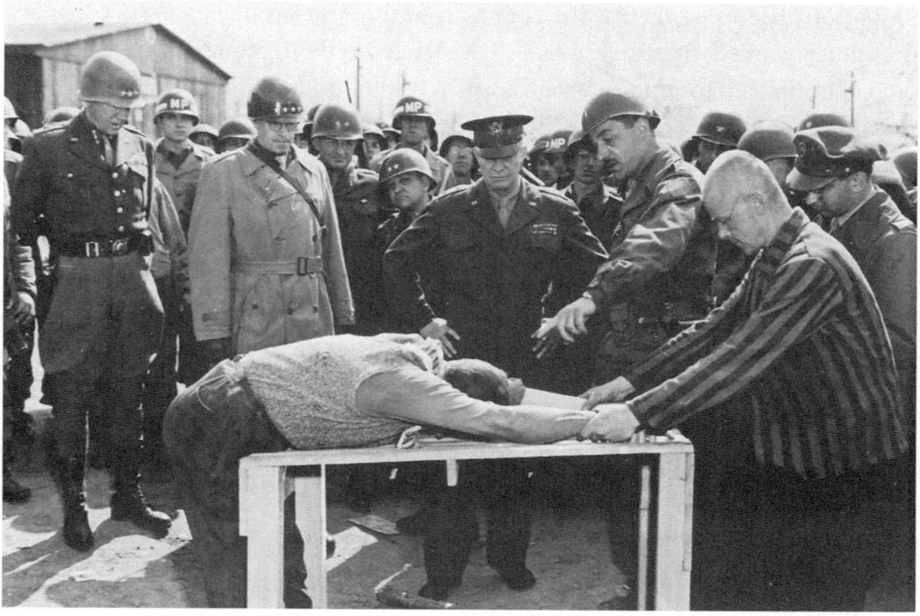

Generals Eisenhower, Patton (left), and Bradley are shown how prisoners were stretched over a special table and whipped at the Ohrdruf slave-labor camp, April 13, 1945. Between Bradley and Eisenhower are Generals Middleton and Gay. (U.S. National Archives)

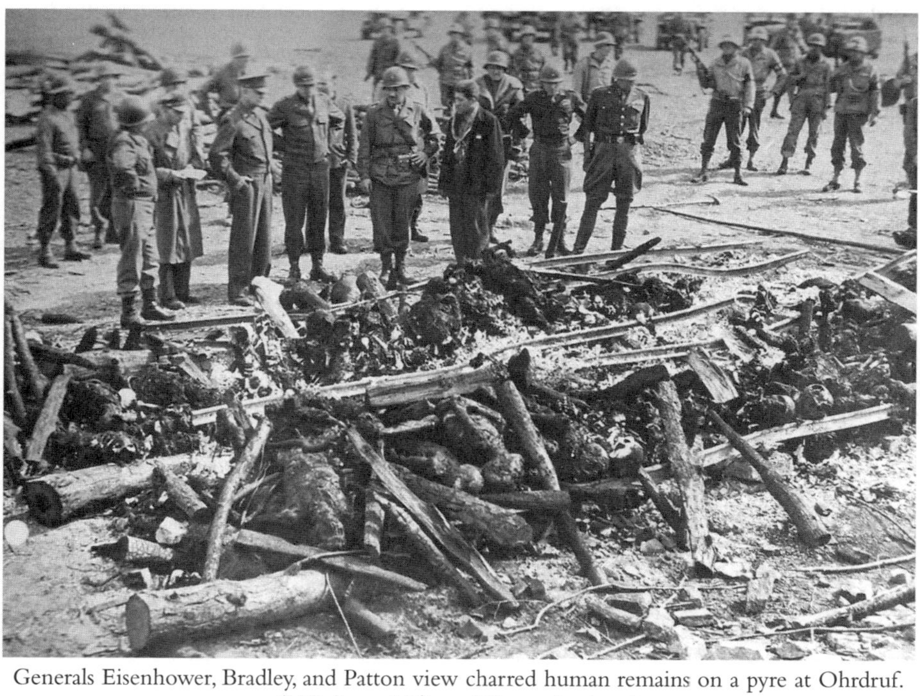

Generals Eisenhower, Bradley, and Patton view charred human remains on a pyre at Ohrdruf. (U.S. Army Military History Institute)

Patton also noted that, at the approach of the American army, "the Germans thought it expedient to remove the evidence of their crimes. They therefore used the inmates to exhume the recently buried bodies and to build a sort of mammoth griddle of 60 cm. railway tracks laid on a brick foundation. The bodies were piled on this and they attempted to burn them. The attempt was a bad failure. Actually, one could not help but think of some gigantic cannibalistic barbeque. In the pit itself were arms and legs and portions of bodies sticking out of the green water which partially filled it."[4]

Through the camp the generals and their entourage walked, dumbfounded, outraged, one horrific scene followed by another that was even worse. "We were spared nothing," said Codman. "The gallows...the whipping racks, the butcher's block for the cleaving of jaws and smashing out of gold fillings. The half-filled and still-smoking ovens of the crematories. The general officers present all are men who have seen much of life in the raw, yet never on any human faces have I witnessed such horror and disgust. At one point General Patton frankly disappeared behind the corner of a building and was violently sick to his stomach."[5]

Patton, the controversial firebrand commander of the U.S. Third Army, known as "Old Blood and Guts"—an officer who once inspired his troops in battle by telling them to grease the treads of their tanks with the intestines of German soldiers—could not stomach what he saw at Ohrdruf. "He went off to a corner thoroughly sick," wrote Robert D. Murphy, diplomat and senior political advisor to Eisenhower, who accompanied the group. "The inmates liberated by our forces were skeletons...many of the captives [had been] professional soldiers and they pulled their wasted bodies in gallant salutes as Eisenhower, Patton, and their staffs passed them. It was enough to make strong men weep—and some American officers did so unabashedly."[6]

In his 1948 best-selling memoir, *Crusade in Europe*, Eisenhower wrote, "...I saw my first horror camp. It was near the town of Gotha. I have never felt able to describe my emotional reactions when I first came face to face with indisputable evidence of Nazi brutality and ruthless disregard of every shred of decency. Up to that time I had known about it only generally or through secondary sources. I am certain, however, that I have never at any other time experienced an equal sense of shock."[7]

Eisenhower wasn't the only top American leader horrified by the discovery of Ohrdruf. Omar Bradley wrote in his memoirs, *A Soldier's Story*, "Third Army had overrun Ohrdruf...and George [Patton] insisted we view it. 'You'll never believe how bastardly these Krauts can be,' he said, 'until you've seen this pest-hole yourself.' "

Bradley went on, "The smell of death overwhelmed us even before we passed through the stockade. More than 3,200 naked, emaciated bodies had been flung into shallow graves. Others lay in the streets where they had fallen. Lice crawled over the yellowed skin of their sharp, bony frames. A guard showed us how the blood had congealed in coarse black scabs where the starving prisoners had torn out the entrails of the dead for food. Eisenhower's face whitened into a mask. Patton walked over to a corner and sickened. I was too revolted to speak. For here death had been so fouled by degradation that it both stunned and numbed us. Within a week we were to overrun others and soon the depravity of Buchenwald, Erla, Belsen, and Dachau would shock a world that thought itself inured to the horrors of war."* [8]

Lieutenant General Hobart R. "Hap" Gay, Third Army Chief of Staff, noted in his diary, "The evidence of inhuman treatment, starvation, beating and killing of these prisoners of war by the Germans was beyond the American mind to comprehend. Hundreds and hundreds of bodies were left around the area. Some 200 or more had been dug up, apparently with the idea of burning them so that there would not be evidence of their inhuman treatment, but the [American] advance had been so rapid that they had to leave them on the burning pyre.

"The commanding general of XX Corps [Major General Walton H. Walker] had brought as many soldiers as he could possibly spare to see this, using it as evidence of what they might expect should they be captured by the Germans, and also as an inkling, perhaps, of what treatment should be afforded to people of such sadistic temperament."[9]

Colonel Codman wrote home to his wife: "After lunching at [Eddy's] XII Corps we flew to [Walton's] XX Corps at Gotha, and from there proceeded to the overrun German concentration camp at Ohrdruf. In the midst of this lovely spring countryside, a festering wound. Rows of hideous wooden barracks surrounded by a double enclosure of barbed wire. Even before reaching the entrance, the smell of death and corruption was almost overpowering. An officer from XX Corps, still pale and shaken, received us. 'They tried to eliminate the evidence before we arrived,' he said, 'but as you see, they were not very successful.' "

Noting that one of the young American enlisted men accidentally bumped into a former Ohrdruf guard and laughed nervously, Codman wrote, "General

---

* "Erla" was the name of a company—Erla-Werke—that utilized slave labor at its facilities at the Buchenwald sub-camp of Thekla, near Leipzig; 464 half-dead inmates were freed there on April 11, 1945. "Belsen" refers to KL Bergen-Belsen. ("Red Triangle" ex-Buchenwald inmate, letter to author, June 4, 2007)

Eisenhower fixed [the GI] with a cold eye and when he spoke, each word was like the drop off an icicle. 'Still having trouble hating them?' " Ike asked.

When the revolting, stomach-churning tour of the abattoir was concluded, Ike turned grimly to the others and said, "I want every American unit not actually in the front lines to see this place. We are told that the American soldier does not know what he is fighting for. Now, at least, he will know what he is fighting *against*."[10]

War correspondent Meyer Levin, accompanying the high-ranking officers, wrote, "We had known this. The world had vaguely heard. But until now, no one of us had looked on this. This morning we had not imagined we would look on this. It was as though we had penetrated at last to the center of the black heart, to the very crawling inside of the vicious heart."[11]

The average GI who saw the horrors of Ohrdruf also had something to say about them. Sergeant Peter A. Belpulsi, Battery B, 66th Armored Field Artillery Battalion, 4th Armored Division, said, "It made me vomit." Private First Class Richard C. Lukehart, Company B, 10th Armored Infantry Battalion, 4th Armored Division, noted, "It was horror beyond belief." After the war, Technician Third Grade Norman Sue, Company C, 53rd Armored Infantry Battalion, 4th Armored Division, said that so few people believed the scenes of degradation he described that he stopped trying to describe them.[12]

Captain Harry C. Butcher, Eisenhower's naval aide, noted that Ike interviewed several surviving prisoners through an interpreter "and said that their stories of starvation, cruelty, and bestiality [sic] were so overpowering that he felt sick. In one room he had seen twenty to thirty naked men killed by starvation. Patton refused to enter. Said he would upchuck if he did, but Ike said he had forced himself to see the bodies, as he wanted to be able to have firsthand evidence to combat anyone in the future who would say that stories of the atrocities were 'propaganda.' I told him I thought we should give responsible people at home an opportunity to see the ghastly scenes for themselves. He is planning to ask the War Department to select a group of editors and publishers to visit the camps."[13]

Two days later, Eisenhower, perhaps acting on Butcher's suggestion, wrote to General George C. Marshall, the Army Chief of Staff in Washington, D.C.: "The things I saw [at Ohrdruf] beggar description.... I made the visit deliberately, in order to be in a position to give first-hand [Ike's emphasis] evidence of these things if ever, in the future, there develops a tendency to charge these allegations merely to propaganda."[14]

Ike also sent communiqués to both Washington and London, "urging the two governments to send instantly to Germany a random group of newspaper editors and representative groups from the national legislatures. I felt that the evidence should be immediately placed before the American and British publics in a fashion that would leave no room for cynical doubt."[15]

LEO LAUFER AND his three fellow Ohrdruf survivors had meanwhile been well taken care of by the GIs—deloused, clothed, shod, fed, and given medical treatment. Laufer recalled the April 13 visit to Ohrdruf by the Army's top brass: "While we were staying at the camp, we saw a big entourage coming. Of course, we campmates, not knowing a word of English, didn't understand what it was all about. Little did we realize who these people were. It was General Eisenhower, General Bradley, and General Patton."

After the tour, Laufer said the U.S. Army "brought a lot of people from the city, including the mayor of the town, to show them what had transpired in this camp. They looked at the dead bodies and at the camp and they just shook their heads like they didn't know this had happened. Being an inmate, I cannot conceive that they didn't see. We marched from the camp to the town square every day, day in and day out, on our way to work in the tunnels. If a mayor of a town didn't see thousands of people walking through the square with striped uniforms, he must have been blind. Or maybe he didn't want to know. He claimed he didn't know that a camp existed. I heard that, afterwards, he and his wife went home and they hanged themselves."

With lots of free time and nowhere to spend it, Laufer began exploring the area around the camp. He said he went into Gotha one day and saw an American GI guarding what used to be the main bank in town, but which had been converted into the headquarters of an American anti-aircraft battalion. Trying to strike up a conversation with the guard, Laufer discovered that the guard, from the Bronx, spoke Yiddish, which is similar to German. Laufer asked him if he might be able to work in the headquarters kitchen. "Just a minute," the guard told him and went inside to check with his commanding officer, who was also Jewish. The GI returned shortly with the news that Laufer could have a job.

Laufer was instructed to take off his prison uniform. "They gave me a GI uniform, a little Eisenhower jacket without insignia, and a pair of pants," he said, "and then they gave me a little room where they prepared a GI cot with

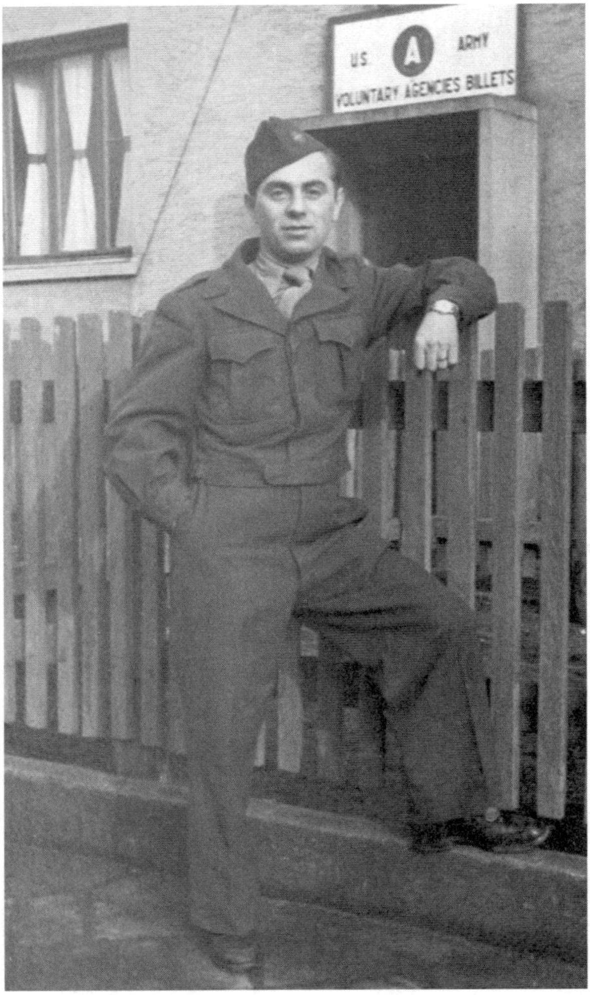

Leo Laufer (formerly Shmuel Lieb), photographed in 1947 in Hanau, Germany. He is wearing an army uniform with UNNRA (United Nations Relief and Rehabilitation Administration) insignia. (Courtesy Leo Laufer)

a green blanket and a pillow and they said, 'This is your place to sleep.' And they took me to the kitchen and told me I would become what they called in their vernacular a 'KP'—Kitchen Personnel, which was very good. This kitchen was good; you could always have food. I was very happy."[16]

Not happy, however, was General Patton, who had just heard about Buchenwald. He steeled himself to visit it.

25
PATTON AT BUCHENWALD

"Ohrdruf was the first, and all of us prayed the last, concentration camp any of us would ever see. No such luck. Within forty-eight hours XX Corps had overrun a far bigger one north of Weimar, the notorious Buchenwald...."

Lt. Gen. George S. Patton, Jr.
Letter to his wife, April 15, 1945

UPON RECEIVING WORD of 6th Armored's discovery atop the Ettersberg, General Patton ordered his aide, Colonel Charles R. Codman, to alert hospital teams to the situation, get food up the hill, and get himself to Buchenwald immediately and come back with a full report. Codman made the calls, arranged for some photographers, and then, accompanied by Third Army's French liaison officer, a Colonel Réthoré, drove there as fast as possible.

The two men passed through the rubble-strewn streets of Weimar, then headed up the "Blood Road" to the camp. Codman saw the main gate to the prisoner enclosure—the punishment "Bunker" and wooden tower from which a black flag flew, erected by the inmates on April 13 when they received the news of Roosevelt's death—describing the gate thusly: "If you didn't know what it was, you might take it for the entrance to a third-rate amusement park."

Once inside the camp, Codman and Réthoré were met by a greeting party of high-ranking French officers—political prisoners who had been incarcerated for "crimes against the Reich." The two visitors were shown the crematorium and, outside it, a wagon stacked with thirty or forty naked corpses around which flies buzzed. Codman noted, "Prisoners who died from 'natural causes' were simply carted into the ground floor of the crematory proper and tossed into six coke ovens, in which are still to be seen the charred remains of the last overhasty and incomplete job that the arrival of our troops interrupted."

Codman then described what he was told about the fate that awaited those who were brought in for execution: "Here, according to eyewitnesses whom I have no reason to disbelieve, were brought prisoners condemned of capital crimes—for example, attempting to escape, insubordination, stealing a potato, smiling in ranks—usually in groups of twenty or so at a time. They were lined up against the walls [in the basement] each one under a hook fixed at a height of about eight feet from the floor.... A short slip-noose was placed about the

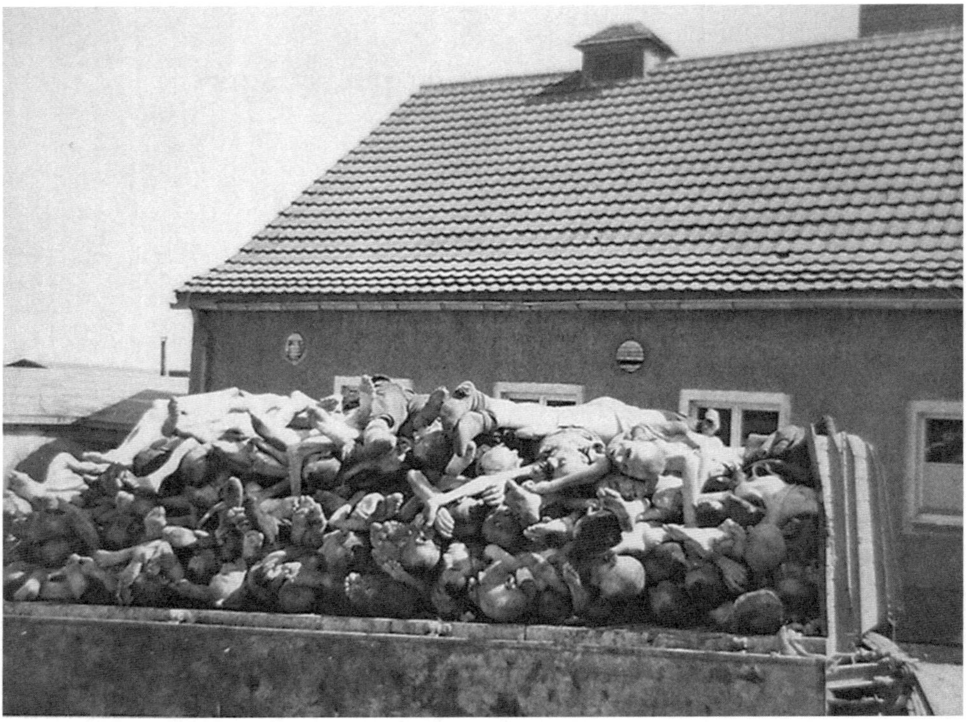

A wagon full of corpses outside the crematorium provides mute testimony to the cheapness of life at Buchenwald. (U.S. National Archives)

neck of the condemned, who was then raised by the guards the distance necessary to affix the end of the noose to the hook.

"If the ensuing strangulation took too long to suit the mood of the guards, they beat out the brains of the condemned with a long-handled club resembling a potato masher.... The remains were then placed on an elevator which lifted them directly to the crematory proper...."

Codman and Réthoré were then guided to the killing chamber of Block 61 to witness the conditions there; some inmates still inhabited it. "An emaciated specter of a man who had managed to get to the latrine and back was attempting to crawl up onto the first shelf [of the bunk bed]," wrote Codman. "It was only three feet from the floor, but he could not make it. As he collapsed, his shirt—he had no other clothing on—fell open.... Two of the inmates who accompanied us picked him up by the shoulders and placed him on the shelf. So much for Barrack 61. Barrack 47 was like it, but frankly, I hadn't the stomach."

Fluent in French, Codman conferred with a number of now-freed French

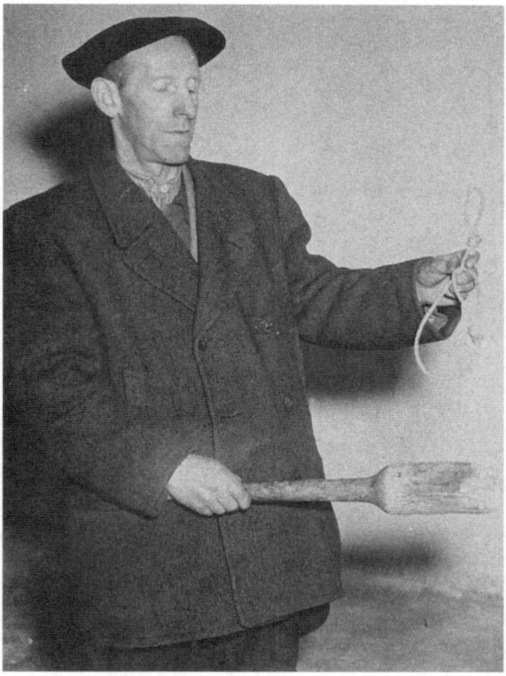

Rene l'Hopital, former aide-de-camp to Marshal Foch, and a prisoner at Buchenwald since February 1945, shows a wooden mallet and a short noose. Patton's aide, Colonel Codman said, "If the ensuing strangulation took too long to suit the mood of the guards, they beat out the brains of the condemned with a long-handled club resembling a potato masher." (U.S. National Archives)

inmates about their experiences and came away sickened at the violence, the sadism, the diabolical methods of torture, the sheer inhumanity that had reigned supreme at the camp. After returning to headquarters, he wrote to his wife, "I have taken a bath, changed my clothes, smoked two packs of cigarettes, but the overpowering moral and physical stench of Barrack 61 remains in my nostrils—the sour-sweet stench of death, dysentery, and despair. Perhaps it is meant to."[1]

NO MATTER HOW revolted he was by Ohrdruf, General Patton, unlike Ike and Bradley, steeled himself to tour Buchenwald—an experience that seared his soul. He noted in his memoirs that the camp, "was apparently much worse than the one at Ohrdruf." He flew to Weimar on April 15 and went through the camp with Major General Walton H. Walker, commander of XX Corps. "This camp was in the vicinity of a factory largely engaged in the construction of parts for the V-1 [sic] bomb and of artillery caisson," Patton wrote, "and is a monument to the accurate bombing of our air force, because they completely eliminated the factory without putting a single bomb in the camp, which was contiguous."*

Like his aide Codman, Patton also visited the barracks, an experience that

* As noted in Chapter 15, this statement is not totally factual; parts of the camp *were* hit.

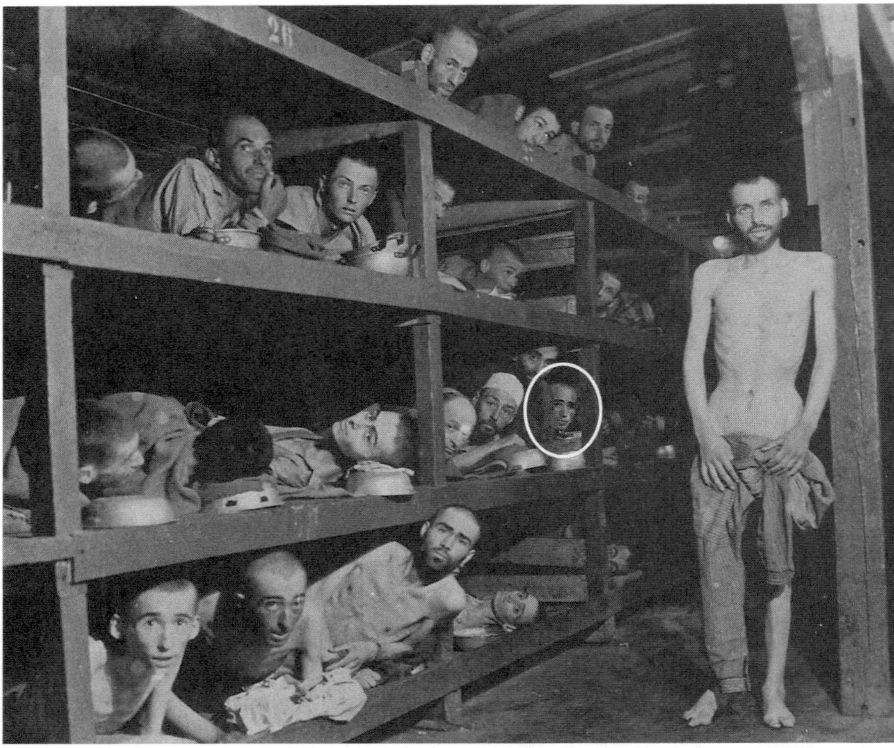

A post-liberation photo (April 16, 1945) of the interior of one of the barracks. The future Nobel Prize winner Elie Wiesel is circled. (U.S. National Archives)

thoroughly repulsed him. "I walked through two buildings," he said, "each with four tiers of bunks on a side. The bunks were at right angles to the gangway and were built so that they sloped slightly toward the front, and so that the fecal matter and other refuse left by the prisoners trickled down under their chins onto the floor, which was at least three inches deep in filth when I went through." He also observed that the inmates "looked like feebly animated mummies and seemed to be of the same level of intelligence." And, like Codman, Patton was escorted to see the crematorium and all its attendant horrors.

Patton said that his guides also pointed out to him that in Buchenwald "there were a number of allegedly eminent physicians whose professional rectitude had been so completely destroyed that they had been persuaded to perform some very abominable experiments on their fellow inmates. One case was reported in which eight hundred slaves had been inoculated with anti-typhus vaccine and then inoculated with the typhus bug. Of the eight hundred, some seven hundred died, and the experiment was considered unsatisfactory. Colonel Odom* asked some of these doctors if there was anything he could do for them. One said yes, that he was making a very interesting experiment on a human brain and needed some carbon black. The human brain, apparently, was still alive."[2]

An anonymous corporal from Tacoma, Washington, assigned to XX Corps headquarters, recalled seeing a very angry Patton leaving the camp: "Our C.O., Captain Mordy, asked me to drive him to just-liberated Buchenwald. As we drove up to the gate, General Patton's jeep drove out. [Patton] sat stony-faced as he passed by. We found ourselves inside the camp. All about us the starved, ragged inmates presented a sad picture. We met an English-speaking inmate who guided us. He took us to a barracks where, in bunks, lay the emaciated moribund, those who were obviously dying. It was a macabre scene I can never forget."[3]

Not only had Patton been shocked by the stacks of corpses scattered around the camp, their dead eyes staring at him, he was also incredibly angry. He was angry that the Germans had done this to other human beings, and even angrier that the townspeople of Weimar, who undoubtedly knew what had been going on atop the Ettersberg hill for eight years, silently condoned it and even profited from it. Reminded by General Walker that the mayor of Ohrdruf and some of the townsfolk had been forced by Colonel Hayden Sears to tour the Ohrdruf camp after its liberation, Patton decided to do the same with the citizens of Weimar. Patton would find the mayor and order a thousand of the good burghers of Weimar to tour the camp.[4]

First, however, he had another task. Upon returning to his headquarters, Patton said, "I immediately called General Eisenhower and suggested he send senior representatives of the press and photographers to get the horrid details. General Eisenhower not only did this but also got Congressmen to come over. This was the camp where we paraded some fifteen hundred citizens of Weimar to give them a first-hand knowledge of the infamy of their own government. In honesty, I believe that most of them were ignorant of much that had gone on there."[5]

He also followed up his phone call with a letter to Ike: "We have found at a place four miles north of Weimar a similar camp, only much worse [than Ohrdruf]. The normal population was 25,000, and they died at the rate of about a hundred a day. The burning arrangements, according to [Lieutenant] General [Hobart R. "Hap"] Gay [Third Army Chief of Staff] and Colonel Codman who

---

* Charles B. Odom was Patton's personal physician throughout World War II, as well as the Third Army's surgical consultant. (Patton, pp. 110-111)

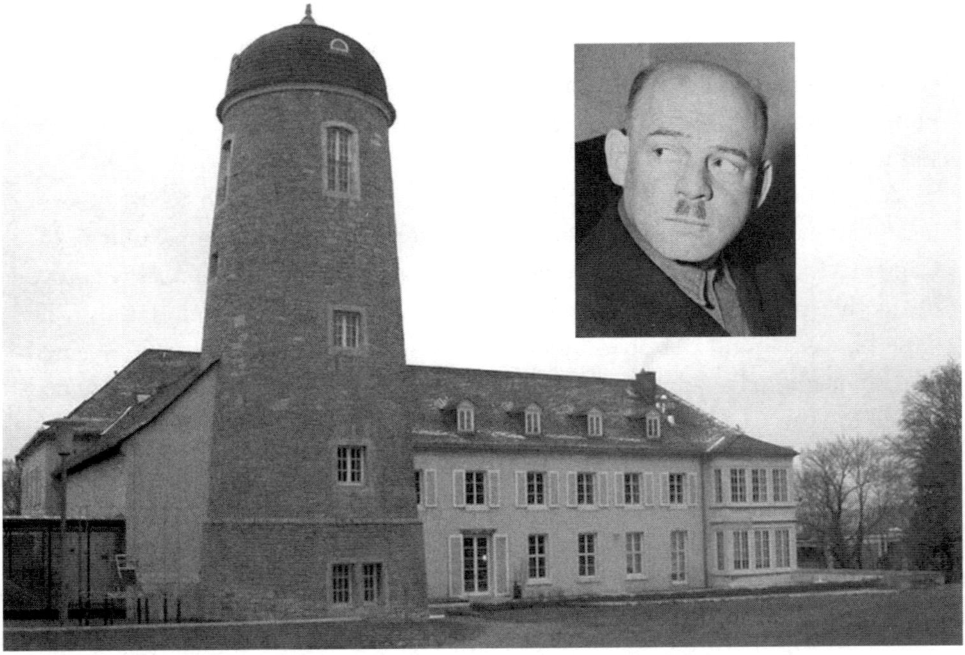

Haus Sauckel, former Weimar offices of Thuringia *Gauleiter* Fritz Sauckel, was used by General Patton as his temporary Third Army headquarters. (Courtesy Bernd Schmidt) Inset: Fritz Sauckel (U.S. National Archives)

visited it yesterday, were far superior to those they had at Ohrdruf. I told the press to go up there and see it, and then write as much about it as they could. I also called General Bradley last night and suggested that you send selected individuals from the upper strata of the press to look at it, so that you can build another page of the necessary evidence as to the brutality of the Germans."[6]

ANDREA KLOSS, THE daughter of Erich Kloss, the acting mayor of Weimar, recalled the events of April 12, 1945, while Weimar was under siege. She said that on that day, while hiding in the basement of her home, she could hear the whistling of artillery shells as they flew over Weimar. The first Americans she recalled seeing were riding in their *kleinen Wagen*—"small cars," i.e., jeeps—followed by tanks and trucks that entered the center of town.

Later on, she received word that Weimar's mayor, Otto Koch, had just been arrested by the Americans. Her father and two others were selected as candidates to take Koch's place and were subjected to an interrogation by the U.S. Army's CIC (Counter Intelligence Corps); Kloss was then appointed mayor. The townspeople began barraging the new mayor with complaints about GIs looting their homes, but Kloss could do little except pass the complaints on to the occupiers.

At 11:00 P.M. on April 15, a U.S. Third Army captain named Calloway knocked on the new mayor's door with an order that he was to immediately report to General Patton at the temporary Third Army headquarters set up in the villa formerly used by *Gauleiter* Fritz Sauckel as his offices. Because Andrea spoke fluent English, she went along as translator; Calloway drove the two to the luxuriously appointed headquarters. There they found Patton at his desk, flanked by members of his staff.

Andrea was struck by Patton's "*eisernem, kalten Gesicht*"—his "iron, cold face." He confirmed Kloss's position as acting mayor and began to dictate the terms of the appointment. The first order was to tell the acting mayor that at noon the following day—Monday, April 16—there would be a thousand-person march from Weimar up to KL Buchenwald, preferably by local members of the Nazi Party. Kloss said that he had no such list of members.

Patton then directed him to order the police to gather more than a thousand residents at random who were to bring with them sufficient food and water to last them from noon until four in the afternoon. Patton said that the composition of the group should be five hundred men and five hundred women, with two-thirds of them being from affluent neighborhoods and the rest made up of as many Nazi Party members as possible. They would march up to KL Buchenwald to see with their own eyes what Hitler had made the Germans do. If Kloss refused, then Patton would have him arrested for failing to obey an order.

Kloss hesitated briefly, trying to decide if he should refuse to carry out the order and allow himself to be arrested. "I initially protested that the people of Weimar had no knowledge of the details of the camp," Kloss said he told Patton. "If evil has been done, it should also be noted that Hitler had also done good things."

Patton cut the mayor off, telling him that he had not been brought there to talk, but only to listen. Kloss noted that, although he felt the general's reasoning was wrong, and the tour would be humiliating for the townspeople, such a visit to the camp might actually do some good. Patton added some details, such as only healthy people from eighteen to forty-five should take part in the march, that an ambulance would accompany the marchers, and that *dass keine Absicht vorlag, zu quälen*—"it was not his intention to torment" the marchers.

Kloss agreed to obey the order, adding that he and his family would accompany the marchers on the visit, for he felt the need to suffer along with his fellow countrymen. But Patton refused the suggestion on the grounds that the mayor, who had a heart condition, was too old to make the climb. The officers offered Kloss a car to take him up the road, but he declined. His worried daughter, Andrea, protested but Patton, unrelenting, said that Captain Calloway, along with doctors and the ambulance, would be by his side in case of any emergency.

For her part, Andrea did not know how it would be possible to force a thousand citizens "*um dort die greulichen dinge anzusehen, von denen wir gehört haben*" ("to see the horrible things at the top of the hill of which we have heard"). Perhaps the police would be able to assist in the undertaking.

With the meeting concluded, Calloway drove Kloss and his daughter to the Weimar police station for a late-night meeting with Police Captain Hentschel. There they discussed the following day's march and decided that each policeman would be responsible for gathering from eight to ten men and women, "*vorzugsweise aus den besseren Stadtvierteln*" ("preferably from the better neighborhoods"). Kloss and his daughter finally returned home, exhausted, at 1:00 A.M., wondering and worrying about what the morrow would bring.[7]

AT AROUND MIDNIGHT on April 15-16, 273 members of the U.S. 120th Medical Evacuation Hospital, Semi-Mobile, reached Buchenwald. Warren Priest, a surgical technician assigned to the 120th, recalled, "We smelled Buchenwald long before we saw it. That whole area was overwhelmingly and intrusively affected by the odor of death in the camp. You couldn't escape it. Reaching near the top [of the Ettersberg hill], I suddenly encountered human forms. We had been trained not to fraternize, so I didn't say anything.... They moved to the side of the pathway and got down on their knees and put their hands together prayerfully and looked up and smiled. It was one of those moments when expression was all nonverbal."[8]

The greatest and most immediate problem facing the Americans was the lack of sanitation in the camp. The water-main system had been destroyed by explosives, and the latrines—pestilential during the best of times—were completely unusable. Trucks hauling water trailers were driven up to the camp, and portable showers and toilets put into operation.

The barracks, of course, were overcrowded with both humans and vermin, and the inmates were in various stages of starvation. Field kitchens were set up and ten ambulances would take two days to transport 600 of the worst cases from the camp hospital to a better facility in Weimar. Two thousand others were admitted to the 120th's facilities over the next five days to be treated for malnutrition, dehydration, and diarrhea. In addition, doctors found 320 cases of tuberculosis and sixty cases of typhus—probably leftovers from the medical experiments.

Each patient was stripped, had his clothes burned, and was dusted with DDT to kill lice. Everything within the blocks—beds, bedding, furniture, etc.—was also burned, then the barracks were given a thorough scrubbing down because most of the liberated prisoners would be required to remain in the camp until their status could be established and some final determination of their future made.

New cots and bedding were trucked in from U.S. Army Quartermaster supplies. When the hospital ran out of beds, patients were placed on cots and even on pads of blankets on the floor. Vast quantities of medications, bandages, and surgical instruments were taken from captured German army medical supply depots

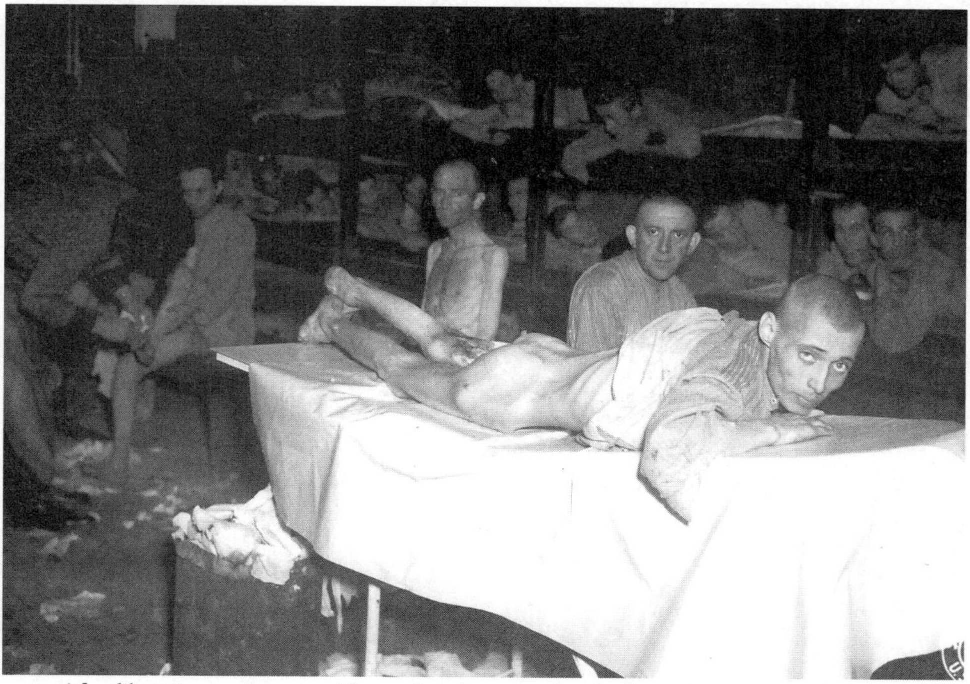

After liberation, an inmate with a serious leg wound waits for an American medic while another former prisoner (left) has his foot injury treated. (U.S. National Archives)

and requested from U.S. Quartermaster stocks. Everything possible was done to save the lives of those whom the Nazis had brutalized. Within three days of the arrival of the 120th, the death rate at Buchenwald had dropped from one hundred a day to less than thirty.[9] Approximately 4,700 sick inmates from the camp infirmary, barracks, and Little Camp were carried to buildings in the former SS barracks area, which had been converted into infirmaries.[10]

The 120th Medical Evacuation Hospital's official report said, "Since conditions were so terrible at Buchenwald Concentration Camp, it was declared unfit for nurses and [the] unit's nurses were detached to 121st Evacuation Hospital operating in the vicinity of Gotha.... An inspection of Buchenwald Concentration Camp was made by Col. [William E.] Williams and his officers on 17 April 1945 to devise a plan of operation and that afternoon work was

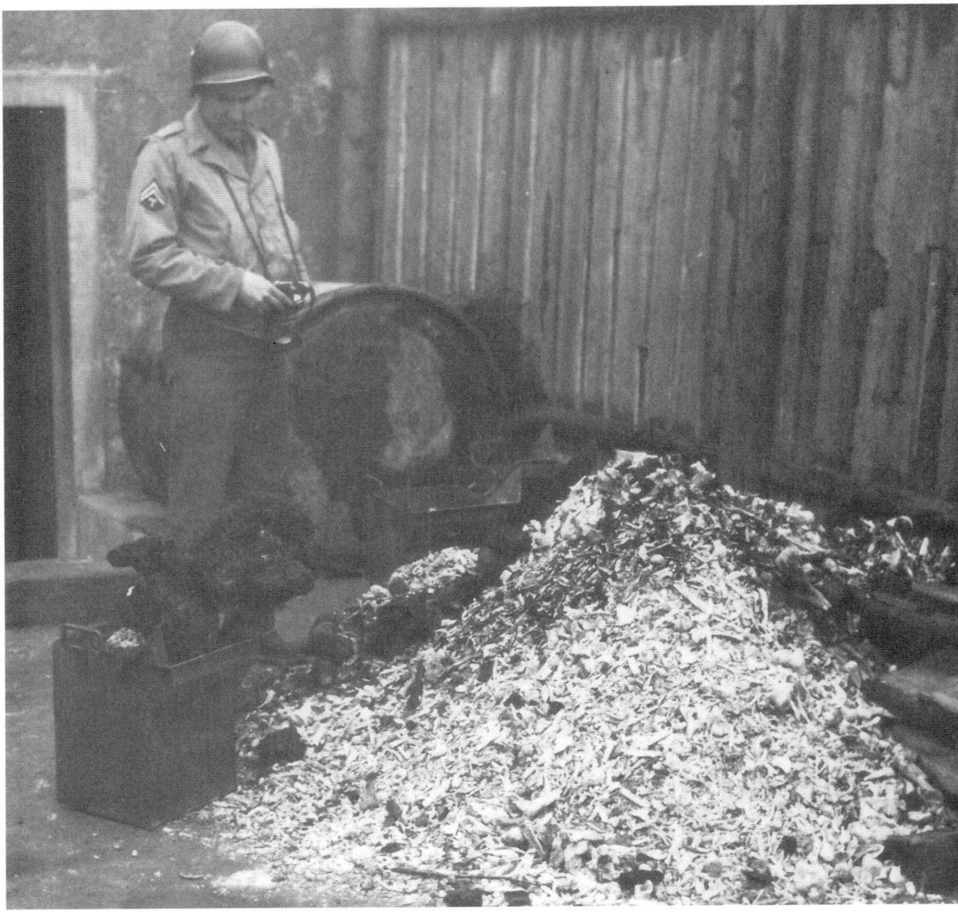

An American soldier prepares to photograph a pile of cremains outside the crematorium. (U.S. National Archives)

started in the camp.... During the first few days...a mess was set up in the Buchenwald camp to help feed the inmates. Food consisted of soft and liquid diet (i.e., soup, milk, oatmeal, and meat stew)."*[11]

Captain Charles Mullinex was an American physician serving with the 76th Medical Battalion of the 6th Armored Division. On April 15, 1945, in a letter to his family, Dr. Mullinex recounted what he was told about how the SS mistreated the prisoners: "Five men in two beds put side by side with one blanket for all of them. No anesthesia was used on the patients and if they died, well, it made very little difference. The entire theme of the camp was as long as a man could work he existed, and if he could not, or if he caused any trouble whatsoever, he was murdered....

"The Germans with their scientific interest had a little exhibit for the advancement of medicine. Some of the inmates were [deliberately] infected with various deadly germs and then when the disease was known to be full blown, the victim [was] killed and that particular part of his body mounted in formaldehyde. One prisoner must have had some interesting tattooed figures on his chest, because I saw the skin with the figures mounted in a glass container. I also saw three or four lungs, a neck and parts of the head.

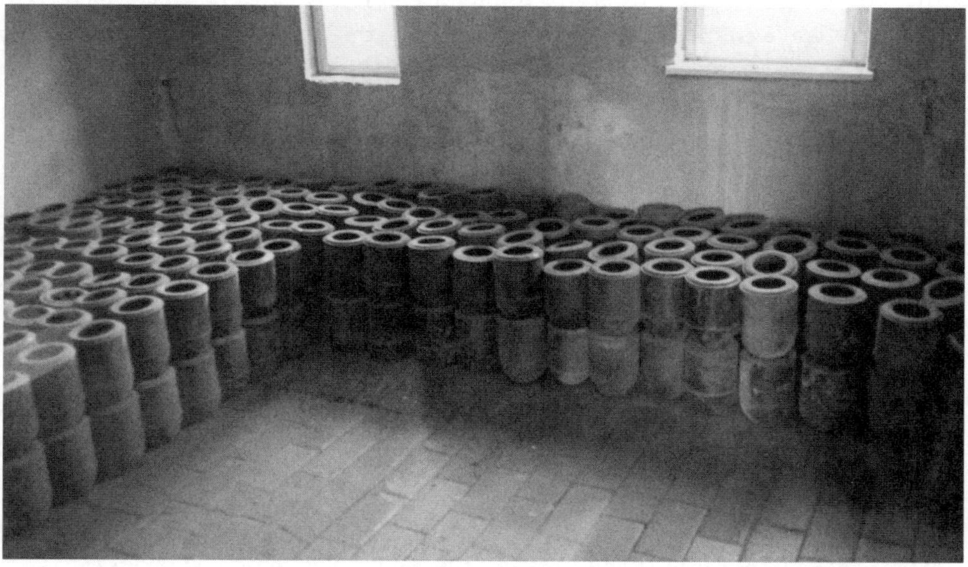

Ceramic urns in which ashes were randomly dumped and returned to family members of victims at Buchenwald—for a fee. (Author photo)

* Medical teams did whatever they could to comfort the dying and keep the desperately ill former prisoners alive, but, despite the great improvement in medical care, hygiene, and food, however, twenty-five percent of the inmate patients were beyond recovery and died in the subsequent weeks. (Stein, p. 240)

"All of this I have seen and now I will tell you a little of what my guide told me concerning some of the other camps. Some had women as well as men, and he had been in one of these co-ed camps. When the women entered they were seen by a doctor. If they were over 40 and if, in his opinion, they could work along with the younger women, he gave the guard a "thumbs up." However if he thought they could not work, he gave the guard a "thumbs down" and within a few hours these women, along with the older women, were killed.

"Some younger women were used in a very ["]noble["] way for the advancement of obstetrics. They were inseminated and then, 8 1/2 months later, a Caesarian section was done with no anesthetic. New methods of technique, procedure, and observations were made and then the women were killed.

"This is a little eye-opening into the 'Greater Germany,' and I really wonder if they are human...."[12]

Army photographer Walter Halloran, a member of the 165th Signal Photo Company, also found himself one of the earliest visitors to Buchenwald. Having gone ashore at Normandy with the first wave and captured some of the most memorable images of the invasion, he was no stranger to scenes of death and destruction, but Buchenwald caught him off guard. "There was a rumor among the advancing American troops of something unbelievable and indescribable," he said. "We were accustomed to brutality by this time in the war, but we weren't hardened enough for all this."

One of his most indelible memories was seeing three inmates, two of whom were holding up the one in the middle who wore no pants. "They tried to come to attention and the most robust of the three tried to salute us, if you can imagine that," Halloran said.

He recalled that he was shooting pictures of the stack of naked corpses on a wagon outside the crematorium when a thought struck him: "Every one of these men was a father, a son, a fiancé. Every one had someone who considered him the most precious thing in their life. But now these men's dignity had been completely stripped from them, and they are just carcasses piled on a cart. And I tried to keep from vomiting."[13]

Halloran also noted that the medical attention the inmates received was "phenomenal. A big problem was trying to get the prisoners in a position where they could eat normal food. All Americans are generous, and all of them wanted to give food to these people. But even one little square of a Hershey bar could be fatal, and the medical people tried to stop the soldiers from sharing their food."[14]

THE WEIMAR POLICE force went through the town on April 16, knocking on doors, selecting people at random and ordering them, without much explanation, to report to the main railroad station before noon with enough food and water for the day.

A crowd of over a thousand dutifully gathered before noon next to the main railroad station along Schopenhauerstraße, on the city's relatively undamaged north side, where Mayor Kloss introduced himself to them, explained that he was the newly appointed acting mayor, and told them the purpose of their gathering and subsequent march up the Ettersberg. Andrea Kloss recorded her impressions of that morning: "To my amazement—instead of the expected gloomy faces, clenched fists, and police officers struggling to control the crowd—I see the biggest line of people whose faces are curious or indifferent, with packages of provisions under their arms, and in lively conversation.... Many have even come voluntarily." Herself depressed with a sense of foreboding about what the tour would reveal, Andrea Kloss decided not to go on the journey; she returned home.

At noon, the line of people began moving west on Schopenhauerstraße for a couple of blocks until it intersected with Ettersburgerstraße, then turned right. Mayor Kloss noted with dismay that Captain Callaway, who had promised to watch over him during the march, was nowhere to be seen, but at least the mayor had a small car in which to ride. A number of American military vehicles along the journey carried what Kloss believed were reporters and photographers.

On they walked for over five miles beneath trees shading the flat road, then turned left at Blutstraße—the "Blood Street," constructed by the inmates in 1938. Here the road, on which they had been forbidden to travel for years, began its upward tilt. The climbing became harder now, and the breathing was labored. Jackets and coats came off as the heat of the day began wearing on the marchers. Some halted briefly to rest or take a drink but were quickly hurried along by the armed American military escort.

Up the road the townspeople continued to plod. Who knew the road was so long, so steep? Those who had visited the Bismarckturm for a dinner at the restaurant or a picnic on the lawn or a view of Weimar from the top of the tower before it became off-limits could not remember the trek being so arduous. And still they marched on, the sun and heat unrelenting. At last they passed, on their left, the gray stone tower that served as the local landmark and was visible for miles around. A few hundred yards more and then it came into view—KL Buchenwald—with its three-story SS barracks buildings, the ominous guard towers, the tall square smokestack of the crematorium, and the surrounding barbed-wire fence. Even in its benign state under a brilliant sun and blue sky, the camp appeared somehow sinister, as though it were a living, breathing beast that was about to expose itself to the gentle, refined citizens of Weimar.

As the group approached the main gatehouse, they saw a number of American soldiers in military uniform and gaunt men in gray-and-blue striped prison garb waiting for them. No one was smiling. Kloss said that, at the gatehouse, confusion seemed to reign as the visitors were organized into groups; the women and girls who had come up from Weimar were angry at being herded first from one line to another and then back again. "It was good that the American soldiers accompanying them did not understand German," he commented.[15]

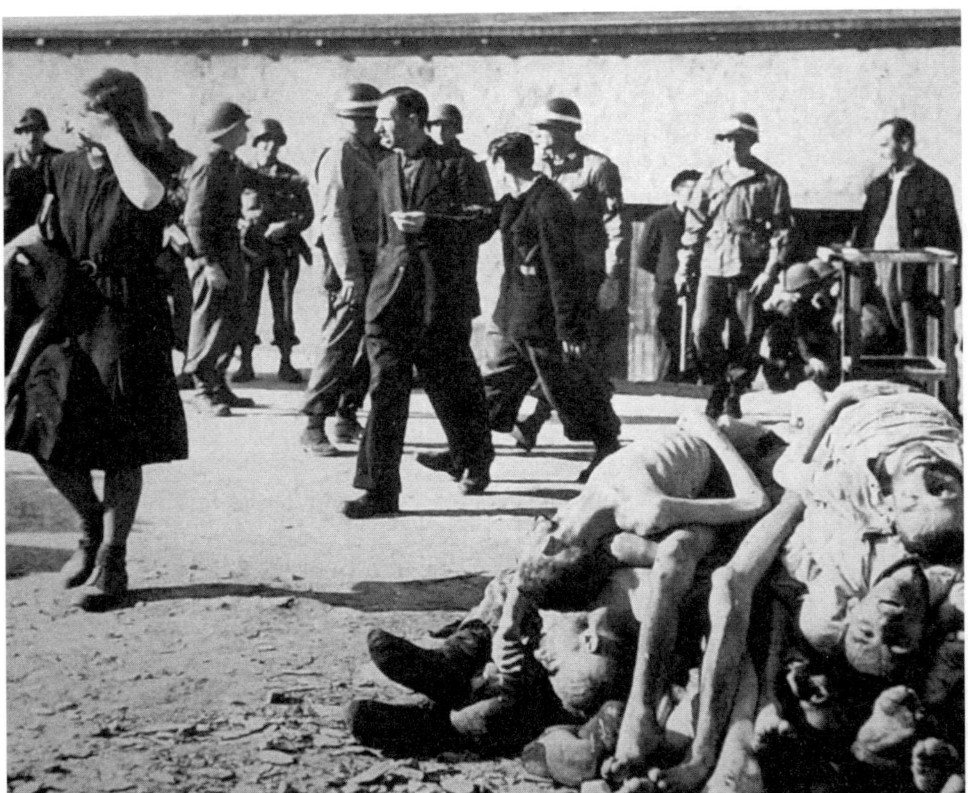

A woman from Weimar covers her eyes while two men behind her avert their gaze from the stack of corpses outside the crematorium. (U.S. National Archives)

After more delays, the irritated civilians began entering the camp in groups of 150, passing through the gatehouse where they were confronted with a table laden with grisly items that looked like props from some horror film: pieces of tattooed human skin, a couple of shrunken heads, and human organs preserved in glass containers of formaldehyde. A German-speaking man explained what the items were, and how they had been obtained. Then it was off to the crematorium.

One GI recalled, "An interpreter met them at the gate, marched them around, and, according to the word I heard later, carefully explained in great detail what had been going on in the camp. In fact, all the interpreter would have needed would have been a few words and a pointed finger. The evidence was all there; the pile of bodies still stacked; the [oven] doors in the crematorium now all open, and more of the trays pulled out with their contents visible."[16]

Army photographer Walter Halloran said, "The first group [to go through] was the men, and of course they were older men because all the young men were in the army. We were so angry we wanted to shoot some of them. They were just rigid and they looked straight forward, not a glance at what was there. Everybody, of course, said they had no idea this was going on."[17]

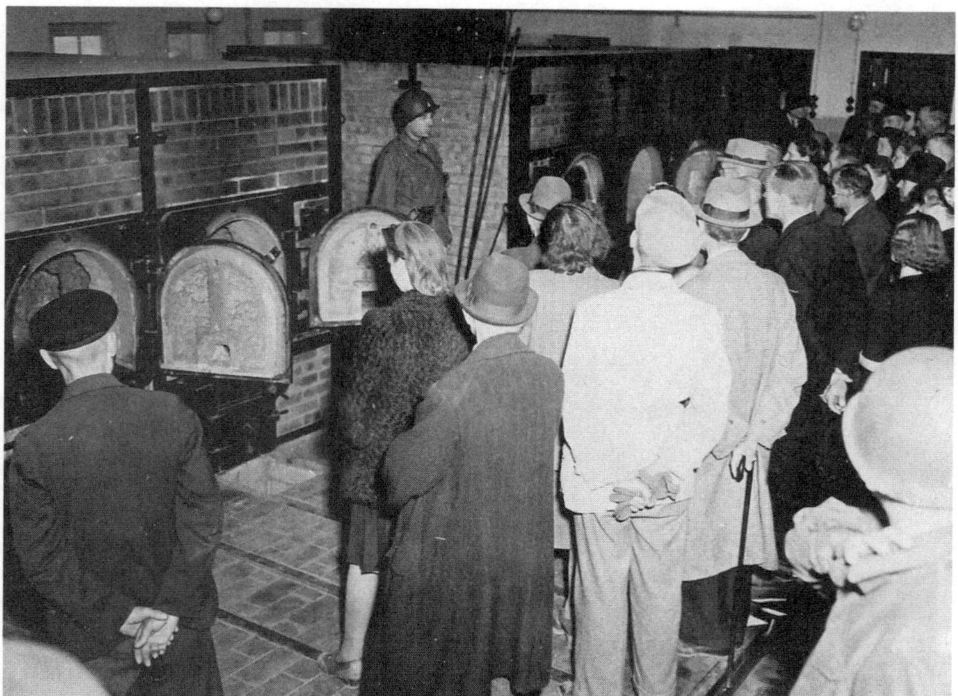

A German-speaking American officer describes the purpose and function of the crematorium ovens to an assembled group of Weimar citizens. (U.S. National Archives)

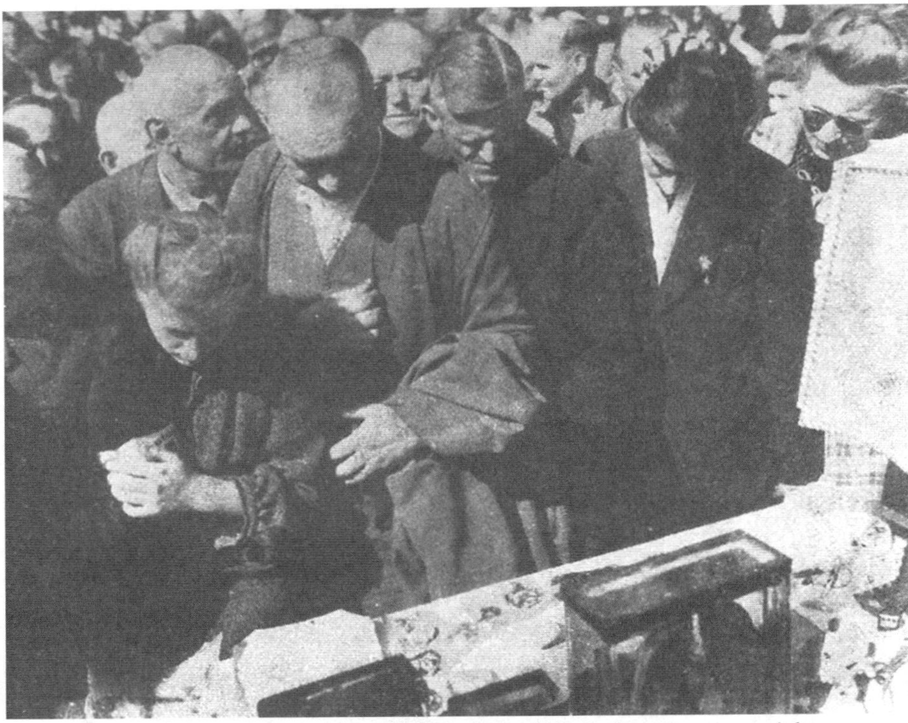

Weimar citizens view examples of the Buchenwald Pathology Department's human experiments. (U.S. Army Military History Institute)

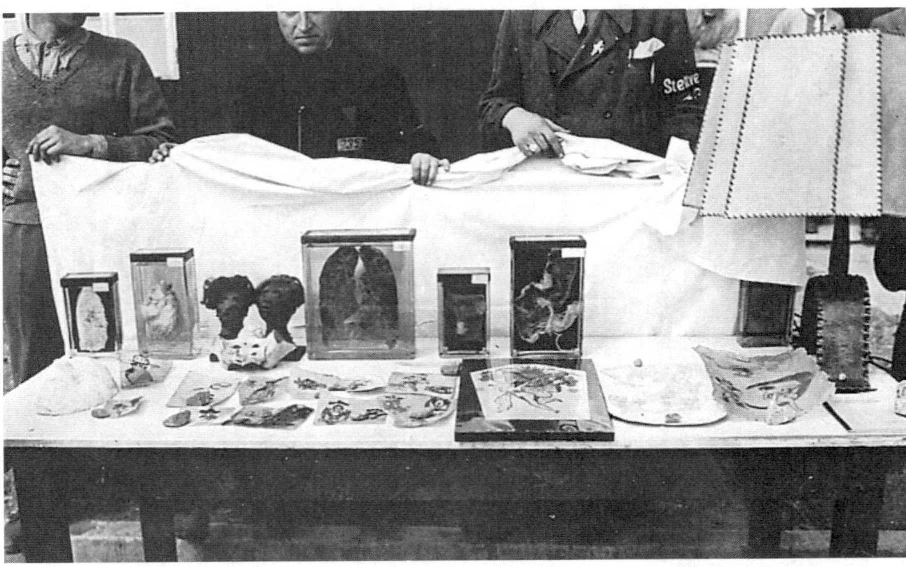

What the people saw: a table full of grisly artifacts, including preserved human tissue and organs, tattooed skin, shrunken heads, and a lampshade made with human skin. (U.S. National Archives)

For his part, Mayor Kloss was skeptical when German-speaking American officers explained what had been going on at the camp, dismissing what he heard as "American propaganda lies."[18]

The tour went on mercilessly, unsparingly. Those Weimar civilians with weak stomachs and tender dispositions wept and vomited. Others remained stone-faced, not wanting to show their conquerors visible signs of remorse, masking their emotions behind impassive glances at the corpses stacked outside the crematorium, the gallows, the ovens, the table with its shocking evidence of torture, abuse, and unspeakable crimes against humanity.[19]

Kloss wasn't buying what he saw and was being told by the former prisoners. He later wrote, "It was obvious that the prisoners would, in some cases, also confirm the false information out of hatred and anger. Of course, it was not likely that all prisoners would distort the truth. Their statements had value for me only if they were eyewitnesses to the processes in question. I know how easily it is to make a mountain out of a molehill." Even after being shown lampshades purportedly made from tattooed human skin, Kloss remained unconvinced. "Only hearing from prisoners who had themselves witnessed the skin being removed and processed would be sufficient proof for me," he noted in his memoirs.

Even after walking through Block 46, the building in which typhus experiments were conducted, the mayor again refused to believe that unwilling subjects were exposed to the disease and used as lab rats to test the vaccines. At another site, the horse stables, a former Russian inmate explained how thousands of his countrymen were killed there with a bullet in the neck. At last conceding that murders were indeed committed, Kloss could only wonder why they were not carried out in a more humane manner.[20]

One GI recalled that, once the tour was over and the group started back down the road to Weimar still under armed guard, someone made a wisecrack and some of the civilians laughed. The officer escorting the group was not amused, however, and marched them back up the road and made them go through the camp again. This time there was no laughter.[21]

Exhausted from the multi-hour tour and barely able to stand, the mayor returned home late in the day, finally grudgingly willing to admit that what Buchenwald represented was "outrageous."[22] But, like many Germans, even the incontrovertible evidence of atrocities was insufficient to totally convince them that what they saw with their own eyes was nothing more than "American propaganda." Disbelief that the Holocaust and its attendant horrors actually occurred, however, would not be a symptom confined solely to some Germans.

MAJOR LORENZ SCHMUHL, an officer on the staff of Third Army's G-5 Section and the first American to be put in charge of Buchenwald after its liberation, wrote in his journal on April 16: "Out to Camp [Buchenwald] bright and early, went through the Camp and saw things that I did not believe was [*sic*] possible. Saw thousands of living skeletons, nothing but bones with skin drawn over them and breathing. Looked over the torture house and the crematory, where thousands of bodies had been burned, parts of skeletons were visible in the ovens. Also saw the room where they hung, shot, and beat people to death. The walls and clubs were blood stained. Saw piles of human ashes. Sights to [*sic*] horrible to mention. Lamp shades, book covers, etc. made from Human skin. When a man came into Camp that was tatooed [*sic*] and the guards or Officers, Officers Wives wanted the skin, the man would be killed that night. One of the Officers' wives* had hand bags, uppers of her slippers and gloves made from human skin. Wonder what kind of people would do these things, surely not human beings."[23]

WITH BUCHENWALD NOW in American hands, more evidence of atrocities began to come to light. Five days after touring the camp on the morning of April 15, 1945, with Commandant Rene l'Hopital (former aide to Marshal Ferdinand Foch, the supreme commander of Allied armies in World War I and a prisoner at Buchenwald since February 1945), Brigadier General Eric F. Wood, Lieutenant Colonel Charles H. Ott, and Chief Warrant Officer S. M. Dye wrote in their report: "The 20 April [1945] Paris edition of the *Stars and Stripes* carried on page 2 a story regarding the use, by the SS officers of the camp, of tattooed human skin for souvenirs. This story is true in every respect. Commandant l'Hopital stated that the wife of one of the SS officers [no doubt Ilse Koch] started the fad; that any prisoner who happened to have extensive tatooing [*sic*] on any part of his body was brought to her; that if she found the tatooing satisfactory the prisoner was killed and skinned; that the skin with the tatooing was then tanned and made into souvenirs such as lampshades, pictures, book ends, etc; that about 40 examples of this artistry were found in SS offices and quarters in the camp. This

* Undoubtedly a reference to Ilse Koch.

statement was confirmed by 1st Lt. Walter F. Emmons. And we ourselves saw 6 examples at Camp HQ, including a lampshade."[24]

Efforts to save those clinging to life in Buchenwald and the other camps shifted into high gear. The U.S. Army's official history noted, "The 12th Army Group had assigned responsibility for the concentration camps to the Displaced Persons Executive (DPX), and on the day after liberation First Lieutenant Walter F. Emmons, commanding DP Detachment 10, took charge in Buchenwald. He had food and clothing brought in from German stocks in Weimar and Jena and set up an emergency hospital in the SS barracks, where inmate physicians gave seventy blood transfusions from the American blood bank the first day. On the fourth and fifth days, to reduce the death rate, which was far less than before but was still about twenty a day, the 66th Medical Battalion and a complete 500-bed evacuation hospital came in with enough medical supplies to treat the 5,000 cases needing immediate attention. By then 700 cases had been treated, and Germans had been put to work improving the sanitation."[25]

WHILE THE THIRD Reich was in its death throes, Heinrich Himmler was planning to escape justice and Berlin, where Russian shells were raining down in unremitting fury. After expressing birthday wishes to his Führer in the Chancellery bunker on April 20, the *Reichsführer-SS* met that evening at Gut Harzwalde, his masseur Felix Kersten's villa outside Berlin, with Norbert Masur of the World Jewish Congress and trying to pass himself off—incredibly—as the savior of the Jews.

Yes, large numbers of Jews had been cremated, Himmler admitted to Masur, but it was only to stop an outbreak of typhus—and typhus was the reason so many Jews had died, he said, not because of any deliberate act by the Nazis. Himmler went on to try and lie his way out of any involvement in the mistreatment of Jews. It was *he*, he explained, who had wanted only the *deportation* of the Jews, but not even countries that were friendly toward Jews would take them. Then, once the war began, Himmler said, "We came into contact with the masses of the Eastern Jewish proletariat, and this created new problems. We could not have such an enemy in our back," he told Masur.[26]

As John Toland wrote in his biography of Hitler, "Himmler protested that he had always intended turning over the camps to the Allies without resistance. Hadn't he done so with Bergen-Belsen and Buchenwald? And look what he got in return: faked atrocity pictures [and fantastic stories of cruelty and murder] being circulated by the Americans! And when he let 2,700 Jews go to Switzerland [in late 1944], the foreign press claimed that he had done so only to get himself an alibi."

Himmler asked Kersten to fly to SHAEF headquarters and meet with Eisenhower to arrange for a truce, with the further aim of convincing Ike to shift hostilities toward Germany's and America's common enemy—the Soviets. Then, to show that he was not a monster, he arranged to have a thousand Jewish women released from Ravensbrück and sent to neutral Sweden.

Meeting later that day with Walter Schellenberg, head of the Nazis' foreign intelligence service, Himmler appeared to be a nervous wreck. According to Toland, "Once Schellenberg began criticizing the unrealistic policy of evacuating all the concentration camps, [Himmler] pouted like a scolded child. 'Schellenberg, don't you start too,' he said. 'Hitler has been raging for days because Buchenwald and Bergen-Belsen were not completely evacuated.'"[27]

Germany's enemies were drawing the noose tighter around the Nazi state's neck. On April 22, elements of the Soviet 47th Army came across KL Sachsenhausen north of Berlin and found 3,000 sick and starving inmates, half of whom were women, still inside. Thirty-three thousand other prisoners had been sent on death marches before the Russians arrived.[28]

ALTHOUGH 1945 WAS less than four months old, 13,969 prisoners had already died that year in Buchenwald, while more than 12,000 had perished on the evacuation marches into the countryside.

American officers tried to determine the exact number of persons who died during Buchenwald's nearly eight years of operation, but it was no easy task. According to SS documents, 33,462 died in Buchenwald and another 23,083 in Buchenwald's satellite camps. Normally fastidious record-keepers, the Nazis were obviously overwhelmed by the task of recording so many deaths and became sloppy in their accounting practices. Among those executed before 1944, thousands were listed as "transferred to the Gestapo," their true number and fate unknown. After 1941, over 8,000 Soviet POWs were executed *en masse* and anonymously; their names were not even recorded. Furthermore, prisoners arriving from other camps and selected for immediate execution were not entered into the camp registers.

Walter Bartel, in his 1960 book, *Buchenwald: Mahnung und Verpflichtung—Dokumente und Berichte*, assembled the following numbers:

- Deaths according to SS records: 33,462★ (all causes, including illness, overwork, exposure, beatings, male deaths at the main camp, and the American air raid of August 24, 1944)
- Executions of Soviet POWs by shooting (estimate): 8,483
- Executions by hanging (estimate): 1,100
- Deaths during evacuation transports and marches (estimate): 13,500
- Total: 56,545

SS documents also show that a total of 238,380 persons were incarcerated at one time or another at Buchenwald; if this count is accurate, Bartel's estimated 56,545 who are believed to have died in the main and sub-camps is a death rate of nearly 24 percent.[29]

Of course, these are just numbers, impersonal statistics, mere digits representing persons without names, persons no one but their immediate families probably remember today. But it is important not to forget that each one was a living, breathing human being, with hopes and dreams and aspirations. Who knows how their lives might have enriched those around them had they lived? Who knows what musical compositions or literary works one or more of them might have written? What works of art they might have created? What medical or scientific breakthroughs they might have achieved? What instruction they might have given in a classroom that would have inspired others and enriched mankind's pool of knowledge? What goodness they might have brought to the world? Or simply what children they might have brought into the world who would have done great things? Unfortunately, we will never know, for they will forever remain the forgotten, anonymous dead...just a set of numbers.

★ According to a document in the U.S. National Archives ("Report on Concentration Camp Buchenwald – Atrocities - Annex A"), 32,705 death certificates were discovered on file at KL Buchenwald.

26
TOURIST DESTINATION

"Before this, you would have said all these stories [of atrocities] were propaganda, but now you know they aren't."

American soldier
quoted in *Newsweek*, April 30, 1945

BECAUSE MANY OF the Buchenwald political prisoners were of the communist or socialist persuasion, they felt that, now that Buchenwald was liberated and fascist Germany was dying, their political point of view should replace the Nazi system and that a new nation built on socialist principles should rise from the ashes of the old.

Consequently, a document known as the "Buchenwald Manifesto" was drafted by Dr. Hermann Brill, a Social Democratic politician and a now-freed Buchenwald prisoner. On April 19, the ten-point manifesto was read over loudspeakers to thousands of ex-inmates at a memorial gathering on the *Appellplatz*, and printed copies were distributed. Brill's document, a sort of German

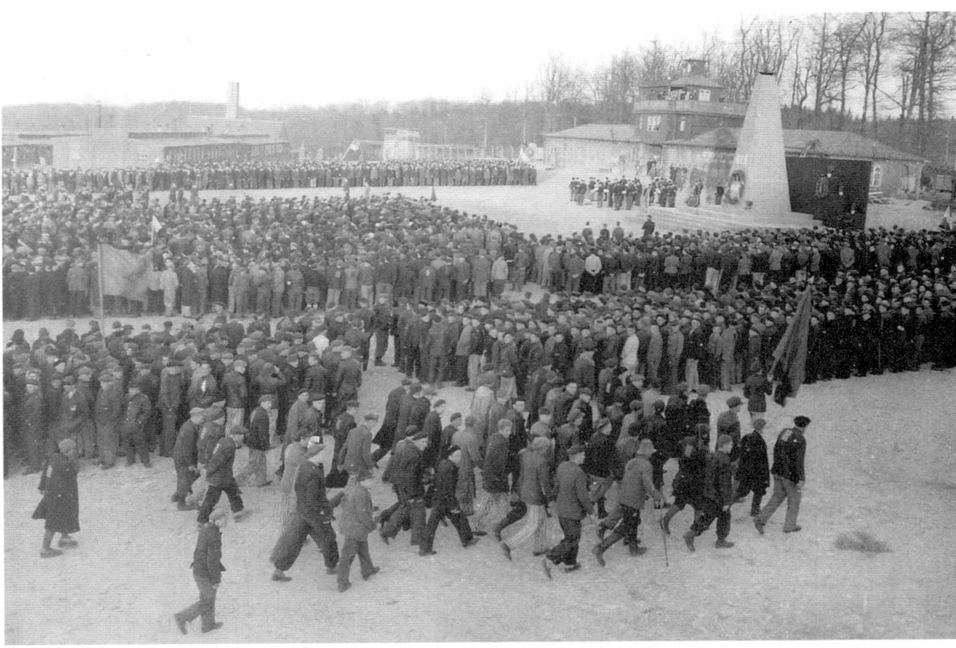

After the camp was liberated, thousands of freed inmates formed up for one last gathering on the *Appellplatz*. (Buchenwald Memorial)

Declaration of Independence that listed grievances against the old order, said that Democratic Socialists had endured unbelievably harsh punishment and suffering because "we believed that under the dictatorship we had to work for the ideas and goals of socialism and for the maintenance of peace" in order to set the agenda for the post-war future of Germany, Europe, and mankind.

Brill pointed out that those who survived the horrors were "therefore authorized and obligated to tell the German people what measures are necessary in order to save Germany" from collapse and to be able to return the country to the ranks of civilized nations. Brill called for the end of fascism and militarism in Germany—a task that could be accomplished only if all anti-fascist forces united "in an unbreakable alliance" and a "new type of democracy" was formed. According to Brill, only an economy rebuilt upon socialist principles could ensure a new direction for the German people.

Richard Bessel, author of *Germany 1945*, said, "The tone of the [Buchenwald] Manifesto was significant. The experience of Nazi rule had reinforced the sense of rectitude and moral authority among Germany's 'democratic socialists' and the conviction that the hour to realize their visions for a post-war Germany had arrived."* [1]

FOR THE NEXT several weeks—even before the final surrender of Germany on May 8, 1945—Buchenwald became a tourist attraction, with the bodies still there, laid out in all their stark nudity for the visitors to see. Based on Ike's request, George Marshall set in motion visits by U.S. congressmen, senators, and newspaper publishers and editors; the British also sent a Parliamentary delegation—eight from the House of Commons and two from the House of Lords.[2]

A report by the U.S. Army 120th Evacuation Hospital noted, "On 19 April 1945 the camp was visited by a body of ten British Members of Parliament to see at first hand the conditions at the camp. They were conducted through the camp and wards and were very favorably impressed by the work being done by this unit. On their inspection they were shown prisoner barracks, children's quarters, the camp crematorium, the notorious 'Block 61' [where inmates were killed by lethal injection] and the SS barracks which had been taken over for use as wards. They spoke with some of the patients through interpreters and found the patients

* Brill's vision of a socialist Germany did not materialize, at least not in the West. After Germany was partitioned into East and West, the eastern half was run under a harsh, Soviet style of communist government and economy while the West followed a more strongly "democratic" and capitalist path.

to be grateful for the care being taken of them by the Americans."[3]

After their tour, the British Parliamentary delegation reported, "We have endeavored to write with restraint and objectivity, and to avoid obtruding personal reactions or emotional comments. We would conclude, however, by stating...that such camps as this mark the lowest point of degradation to which humanity has yet descended. The memory of what we saw and heard at Buchenwald will haunt us ineffaceably for many years."[4]

The next official delegation came from Washington, D.C., as part of a group that had flown to Europe to visit three camps—Buchenwald, Nordhausen, and Dachau. The 120th Evacuation Hospital's report noted, "On 21 April 1945, we were honored by a visit by U.S. Senators sent to investigate the Buchenwald Concentration Camp [Alben W. Barkley (Kentucky), C. Wayland Brooks (Illinois), Walter F. George (Georgia), Leverett W. Saltonstall (Massachusetts), Elbert D. Thomas (Utah), and Kenneth S. Wherry (Nebraska)]. As on the two previous days, a tour of the camp was made and our distinguished visitors left with a clear picture of what they had come to see.

"We were relieved from duty on 23 April 1945 but by this time, food had been procured and transported to the camp to provide the patients with a ration comparable to an 'A' ration [an Army meal using fresh, refrigerated, or frozen ingredients, as opposed to canned or dried]. Since Buchenwald Concentration Camp was our first chance to function since arriving on the continent, both the officers and enlisted men worked hard to prove their capabilities. Each person felt that he was accomplishing something and in addition to efficient and cooperative work from all sections, morale was raised to a higher degree."[5]

On the heels of the senators came a group from the U.S. House of Representatives: Clare Booth Luce (Connecticut), Gordon Canfield (New Jersey), Leonard W. Hall (New York), Ed V. Izac (California), Henry Jackson (Washington), John C. Kunkel (Pennsylvania), Carter Manasco (Alabama), James W. Mott (Oregon), James P. Richards (South Carolina), Dewey Short (Missouri), R. Ewing Thomason (Texas), and John M. Vorys (Ohio).[6]

"They likewise were horrified at living conditions and the treatment of the inmates by the Germans," observed the 120th Evacuation Hospital's report, "and were greatly impressed with the progress made by this unit in correcting these conditions...."[7]

The Congressmen were shaken by what they had seen. Representative Kunkel told the press, "If you tried to tell the actual facts, you'd get into a story of obscenity and filth that would be unprintable." Representative Jackson

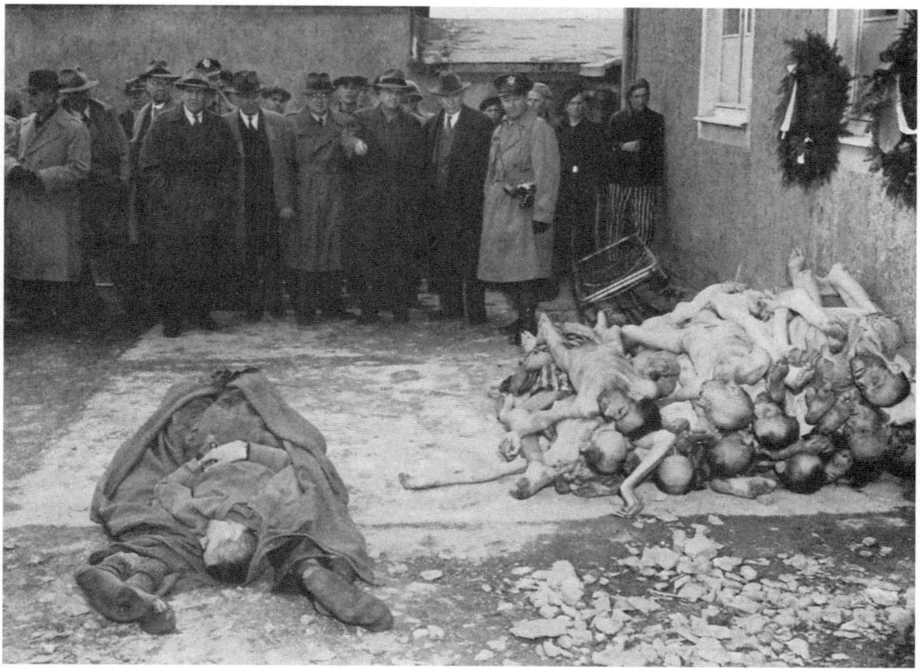

A group of American congressional delegates view corpses outside the Buchenwald crematorium. (U.S. National Archives)

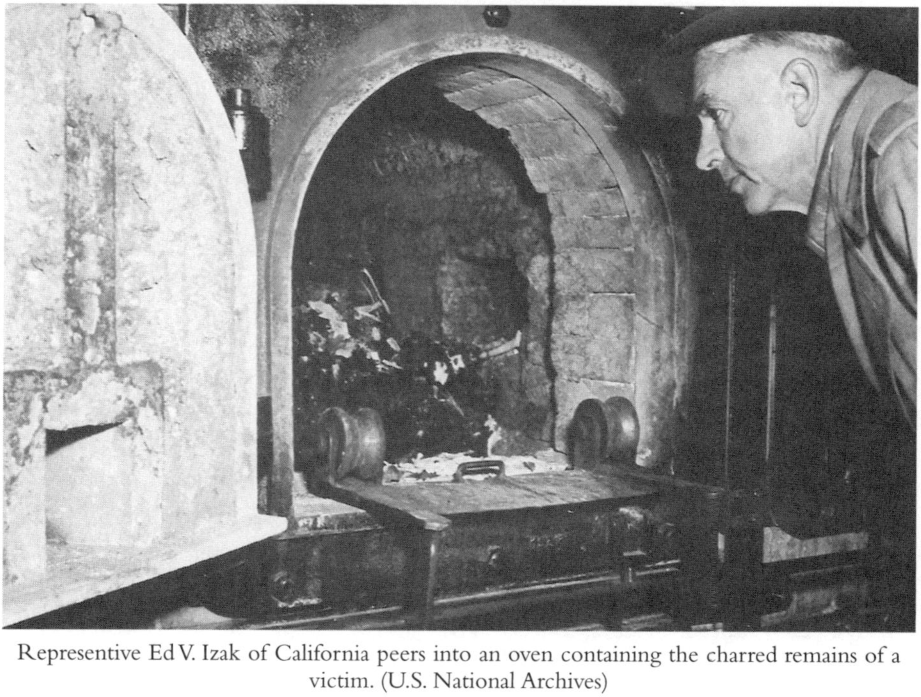

Representive Ed V. Izak of California peers into an oven containing the charred remains of a victim. (U.S. National Archives)

remarked, "We heard atrocity stories from the last war that were not verified, but now we have seen them with our own eyes and they are the most sordid I have ever imagined." Carter Manasco added, "This is the most horrible thing anyone could conceive."[8] Clare Booth Luce commented, "No one wants to believe these things, but it is important that people know they're true."[9]

After the delegation returned to Washington, D.C., Representative Short said in an independent report to Congress, "Every bona fide member of the Gestapo and SS…should be liquidated. Rub them out."[10]

The full report issued by the committee contained the following conclusions: "While the above three camps which were visited by the joint committee differed in some details, they were all of the same general pattern and design and administered for the same purpose. Although different in size, they all carried into effect the same pattern of death by hard labor, starvation, hanging, strangulation, disease, brutality, gas chambers,* gallows, and filthy and unsanitary conditions, which meant inevitable death eventually to every imprisoned person.

"We found that this entire program constituted a systematic form of torture and death administered to intellectuals, political leaders, and others who would not embrace and support the Nazi philosophy and program. We found the extent, devices, methods, and conditions of torture almost beyond the power of words to describe….

"It is the opinion of your committee that these practices constituted no less than organized crime against civilization and humanity and that those who were responsible for them should have meted out to them swift, certain, and adequate punishment."[11]

No word, of course, was mentioned about all the years of official indifference and outright obstructionism by the U.S. State Department and the Roosevelt Administration regarding the plight of the Jews and other persecuted minorities in Europe.

ON APRIL 24 came a delegation of newsmen. Among the editorial entourage were Julius Adler of the *New York Times*; John Randolph Hearst of Hearst Newspapers; Norman Chandler, publisher of the *Los Angeles Times*; Joseph Pulitzer III, publisher of the *St. Louis Post-Dispatch*; Walker Stone, Scripps-Howard

* There were no gas chambers at Buchenwald or Nordhausen; there is still controversy as to whether or not the small gas chamber at Dachau was used to kill inmates.

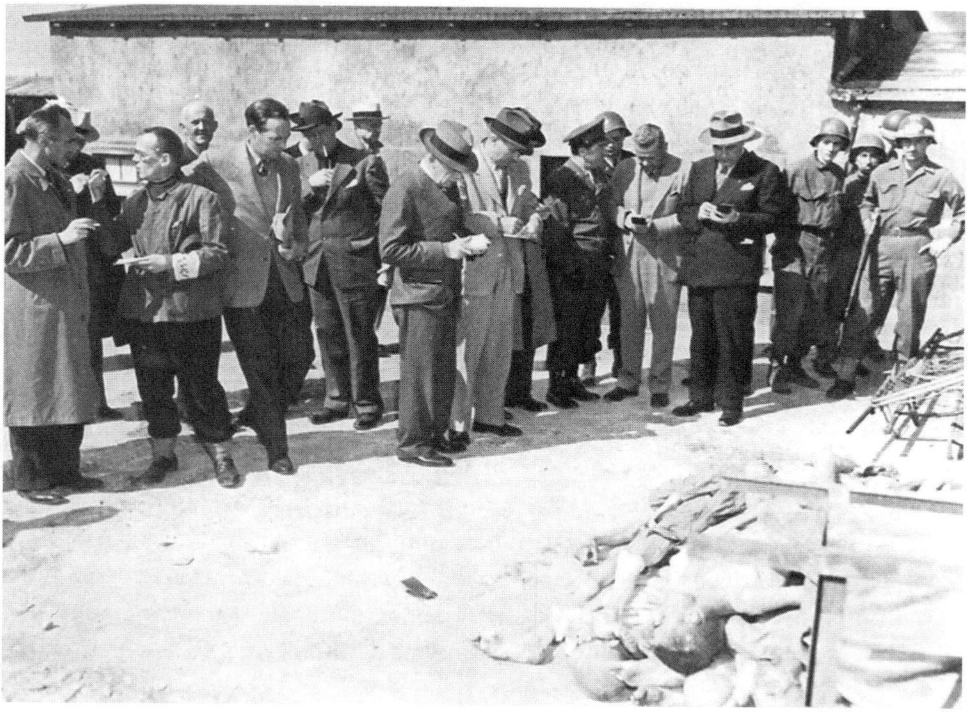

American editors and publishers take notes outside the crematorium, April 25, 1945. (U.S. National Archives)

Newspaper Alliance; E. Z. Dimitman, *Chicago Sun*; and magazine editors William Chenery, *Colliers*; Stanley High, *Reader's Digest*; and Ben Hibbs, *Saturday Evening Post.*[12] *LIFE* magazine photographer Margaret Bourke-White, as well as Army Signal Corps lensmen, arrived to permanently record the scenes of horror.[13]

The *Stars and Stripes* reported that Joseph Pulitzer III "said that he had gone to Europe in a skeptical frame of mind, expecting to find many of the terrible reports already relayed by war correspondents exaggerations and largely propaganda. 'It is my grim duty to report,' Pulitzer wrote, 'that the descriptions of the horrors...have given *less* than the whole truth. The fiendishness of these operations defies description.'"[14]

So filled with revulsion was Pulitzer by what he had seen at the camps that, even two weeks after returning from Germany, he told a rally at New York's Carnegie Hall that all of Germany's surviving members of the general staff, Gestapo, SS, and industrialists should be executed "with Army bullets through their heads"—even if it meant killing a million-and-a-half Germans.[15]

Norman Chandler, the *Los Angeles Times'* publisher, felt the persons responsible should be punished to the full extent of the law: "I'd say it couldn't be too severe," he said. Stanley High, the associate editor of *Reader's Digest*, noted bluntly, "We found no feeling of remorse among the Germans."*[16]

But any retribution was in the future. For the visitors to Buchenwald in April 1945 and beyond, the reality of the scene was still overwhelming. Robert Reid, a correspondent with the BBC who had been tagging along with Patton's Third Army, arrived in a jeep marked "BBC Recording Unit" and, shocked by the condition of hundreds of children, described them as "pathetic, ragged waifs, looking like little old men with yellow faces and shrunken cheeks."[17]

Another of the journalists, a radio reporter named James T. Quirk, told his wife in a letter, "They visited Buchenwald today and found it so bad that they stayed about three minutes and left. I'll admit that it is the most horrible spectacle ever seen by men, but they are supposed to be reporters and should be able to take it without turning pale and gasping like goldfish."[18]

Edward R. Murrow, the esteemed radio correspondent, was also there and was unsparing in his descriptions of what he encountered. At the conclusion of his broadcast, he told his listeners, "As I entered, I was surrounded by men who tried to lift me up on their shoulders.... They were too weak. Many of them could not even get out of bed. I was told that this building had once accommodated eighty horses; now there were 1,200 human beings in it, five to every sleeping space. The stench was beyond imagination.... As I went through to the end of the barrack, I was applauded by the men who were too weak to get up. It sounded like the clapping of babies' hands, they were so weak.[19] I pray you to believe what I have said about Buchenwald. I have reported what I saw, but only part of it. For most of it I have no words.... If I've offended you by this rather mild account of Buchenwald, I'm not the least sorry. I was there."[20]

On April 26, the last official delegation, a combined American-British entourage known as the United Nations War Crimes Commission, toured the camp and were just as horrified as the previous groups.[21]

Published photographs of Buchenwald provided a powerful visual confirmation of the written reports. The writer of an article in the April 30, 1945, issue of *Newsweek* expressed the common sentiment: "For the first time, the American and British publics really believed what they had previously thought

---

* Indeed, when a twenty-five-minute film of the atrocities taken at some of the camps was later shown to German POWs at the Halloran General Hospital on Staten Island as part of a "reorientation program," most of the former Wehrmacht men seemed silent and stoic, their faces betraying no emotion. Some refused to look at the screen and a few kept their hands clapped over their ears to blot out the English soundtrack. When questioned by reporters as to their reaction to the film, some of the POWs said that the ordinary German soldier had no part in such brutality, which they placed solely on the "higher ups." (*New York Times*, June 27, 1945)

impossible: That the Nazis had practiced murder and torture on a gigantic scale. There were the photographs—perhaps the most shocking pictures ever to receive widespread publication."

Finally, once the official visitors had taken their turn at being horrified, the corpses were removed from the camp and buried at the top of the hill near the Bismarckturm, where the Americans also forced some 200 Germans to dig seven large mass graves, disinter 500 decomposed corpses, and rebury them. An American officer overseeing the burial detail had little pity on the Germans, who were complaining of the heat and the stench. "Dig, you sons of bitches," is all he said to them.[22]

ALTHOUGH THE WAR in Europe was not yet over and bitter combat was still taking place north, south, and east of Weimar, Buchenwald became a showcase of Nazi depravity for GIs in Germany. At Eisenhower's insistence, the U.S. Army directed as many units visit Buchenwald as could be spared from their regular operational duties. As at Ohrdruf, American soldiers were baffled and

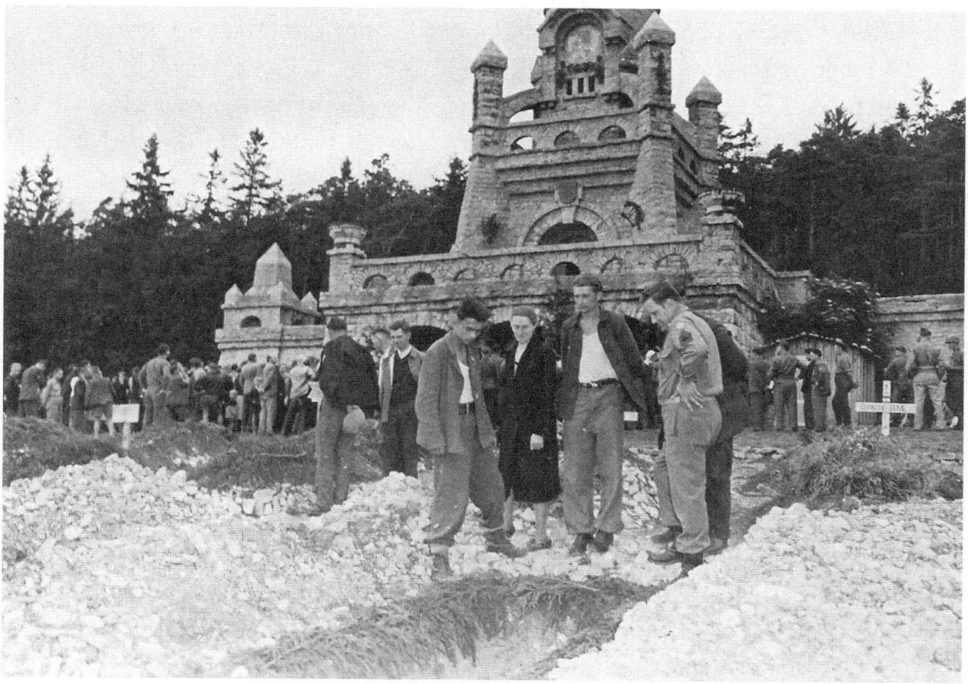

American soldiers and townspeople attend the burial of the ashes of 1,286 victims at the Bismarckturm on the Ettersberg hill, April 1945. (U.S. National Archives)

horrified by what they encountered atop the Ettersberg. First Lieutenant Lewis R. Bird of the 6th Armored Division said that his visit to Buchenwald left him "shocked and angry." Sergeant Charles A. Hogg, Sr., Company D, 69th Tank Battalion, related that Buchenwald left him filled with "utter revulsion and disgust." Private first class John A. Deeney, 146th Signal Company, 6th Armored Division, expressed disbelief "that such things could take place." Staff Sergeant Charles Froelichen, a member of the 6th Armored Division's prisoner interrogation team, confessed that he had to "resist the inclination for revenge." Major Gordon M. Manring, Headquarters Battery, 128th Armored Field Artillery Battalion, said, "By this time we were conditioned to the horrors of war, but this camp was extreme. I had never seen anything to match this."[23]

Michael Bilder, a 5th Infantry Division soldier, said that Buchenwald "was a horror beyond words. The camp had been designed for slave labor, not mass extermination, but we would never have known that from the looks of it. More than two weeks after the liberation, bodies were still stacked in the open as attempts to identify the dead were made. Others were being exhumed from shallow graves. Those inmates who survived bore a closer resemblance to the dead than to the living. The inhumanity almost defies description.... Despite those who claim the Holocaust never happened, or that it was not as bad as reported, I can say definitely that it did indeed happen, and that it was every bit as bad as it has been described!"[24]

As he entered the camp with another soldier, twenty-three-year-old Harry Snodgrass said, "I had never seen anything like this before." He noted that the other GI with him was flabbergasted. "There isn't a God in heaven...no God at all," uttered the other soldier. Snodgrass said he then visited the commandant's office. "There were lampshades made from the skin of Jews. In the crematorium they used the ashes of the inmates to fertilize the fields—the ashes of dead people. After an hour, it just became too much. I was stunned...just stunned. We don't even treat dogs like this."[25]

An unnamed sergeant told a *Newsweek* reporter, "Before this, you would have said all these stories [of atrocities] were propaganda, but now you know they aren't. There are the bodies, and all these guys are dead."[26]

Victor B. Geller, a corporal in the 87th Infantry Division, who first visited Buchenwald on June 7, 1945, had heard that the people of Weimar protested "*Ich habe nicht gewust*"—that they had known nothing about the existence of the camp, a claim that he found hard to believe. "They knew, because some of them said that the location of Weimar was such that when the wind would blow in a certain direction they would have the odor. The answer was they knew, they knew....

"And, of course, every German that I came across later insisted that he was not a Nazi, that he was a very good man, and that he had a cousin in Milwaukee.... The ones I had contact with were out to persuade us that they were the best."[27]

Surgical technician Warren Priest noted, "You have to understand that no one in our unit knew what a concentration camp was. What we learned was so shocking, it traumatized many of us." He told a newspaper reporter in 2007, "I met a man who spoke broken English. He was a minister of bridges and highways in Belgium—a political prisoner. He had found a model boat, and he gave it to me. On the face, it said *Santa Maria*. On the back was a painting of the virgin and the baby Jesus. There were crosses on the sails. The man who gave it to me said the sails were made of human skin." (Priest later donated the sailboat to the U.S. Holocaust Memorial Museum in Washington, D.C.)

In a letter to his mother in April 1945, Priest wrote: "I saw what and why we were fighting. Never, never permit yourself to feel any trace of pity whatsoever for the German people, Mum. They've jeopardized their right to call themselves standing members of our world of civilization." They are certainly no better than the Japs, and in some respects worse. Tell your friends about this. I know it's true because I've seen it."[28]

MANY OF THE GIs pouring into Thuringia no doubt wondered why General Eisenhower, the Supreme Allied Commander himself, had told their commanders—barring operational requirements—to haul as many of their soldiers as possible to Weimar in order to witness the sights and smells of newly liberated Buchenwald. Most of them, like Technician fifth grade Merrill C. Burgstahler of Glencoe, Minnesota, had never heard of Buchenwald.

Bergstahler, a member of the 6th Armored Division's 777th Anti-Aircraft Battalion, recalled that by the time he arrived at Buchenwald, the bodies had been removed and buried, but evidence of the terrible conditions remained. "We had a twenty-four-year-old Dutchman, who had once been a wrestler in the U.S., escort us around," said Burgstahler. "He spoke good English. He showed us a pyramid of bones and ashes six feet high out back of the crematorium. We also visited some of the barracks; they looked like a Midwest hog house. Talk about smell." Burgstahler was shocked beyond belief, as he said he had no prior knowledge of the atrocities that were being committed. "It came out of the blue," he said.[29]

Once he had mentally processed the experience, Burgstahler wrote a letter to his mother, describing some of the things he had seen during his visit: "Saw things that would give a civilian the 'willies' and nightmares for weeks. Can truthfully say anything I had read was an understatement of things I saw with my own eyes. Our guide...was a former prisoner in the camp. He told us things that are impossible for anyone except eyewitnesses to believe. We heard things, took a few pictures, saw things, yes, even smelled things to convince us of German brutality.

"This was not a murder factory but a slow, grinding, agonizing, starvation and torture death—where the actual killing when it finally came was a blessing and a privilege. This was a place where a man was worth at most 5 marks as a bowl of cremated ashes to some loved one who requested the remains (and these were shoveled from a pile of as high as 3,000 people's ashes and sent representing a certain person)—where a man's life was only worth his gold teeth when he died and torture and starvation when he lived.

"This was a place where men were experimented on as human rats though they had 95 to 5 chances of surviving, and men actually volunteered as guinea pigs for an extra slice of bread a day. A place where one inmate killed a buddy for the slice of bread he might have in his hand.

"This was a hall where 800 men slept in a one-story wooden, windowless barracks 80 ft. long—where from two to seven died of suffocation every night during winter. Here was German thoroughness constructed a crematory that would burn a dozen corpses every 14 minutes and which ran 24 hours a day 7 days a week without stopping for long periods. Where one doctor killed 7,000 in three years with only a needle, giving deadly shots to the cripples and maimed who came for help. When the drug took effect they were shoved to fall in a bin and stacked like so much wood. I saw a 25-year-old Dutch man who weighed only 90 pounds—his souvenir was 10 amputated toes, frozen in a march from eastern Germany last winter.

"There were Polish boys as young as 8 years—almost 50,000 prisoners at times in an area half as large as Hutch [Hutchinson, Minnesota] fairgrounds. I saw all this—and more, too much more! I'm not sorry I went, though, as such things make you convinced our dead did not die in vain."[30]

In an interview with the author, Burgstahler concluded, "My background is three-quarters German. When I came home after the war and told the family about Buchenwald, my dad's younger brother refused to believe me when I told him about what I had seen. 'I don't believe you,' he would tell me —'Germans wouldn't do that to other Germans.'"[31]

As troubling as all this is, a question as large as a barrage balloon still hangs in the air: Why was the average American soldier kept in the dark about what he would find when he finally, inevitably, stumbled across the concentration camps?

27
UNPREPARED

"There had never been the slightest bit of training in what a concentration camp was, let alone what to do if you liberated one."

Bernard Kahn
45th U.S. Infantry Division
Dachau liberator

AMERICANS WHO WERE born in the years after World War II may be forgiven for thinking that the saving of the Jews was a primary goal of their government and the Allied armies. Yet—as becomes evident with a study of history—a noble undertaking such as the salvation of millions of people was not the primary, nor even a secondary, reason for the invasion of Europe and the crushing of the totalitarian Nazi regime. The fact that the important, albeit accidental, discovery of the camps, and the freeing of the grateful inmates—one of the great humanitarian acts of all time—does not rate a single sentence or paragraph in U.S. Army Chief of Staff George C. Marshall's *Biennial Reports of the Chief of Staff to the Secretary of War, July 1, 1943, to June 30, 1945* is, to this author at least, astonishing, especially given the tremendous amount of attention and publicity the Holocaust and the discovery of the camps received at the time.

The strange absence of reference to the concentration camps, death camps, Holocaust, and the persecution of Europe's "unwanted" people haunts Marshall's report. The report speaks eloquently of the grand sweep of armies across the seas and continents of the world; the capture of towns, cities, and enemy troops; the crossing of great rivers, plains, and mountain ranges; the valorous deeds of generals and the units they commanded; the problems encountered (logistics, weather, terrain, etc.) and overcome; the crumbling of enemy resistance and the eventual surrender of enemy forces. Within the report, however, not one word—not even a footnote—mentions the existence of the camps and the Army's role in their liberation, nor do the words "concentration camps," "slave-labor camps," "Jews," "genocide," "Auschwitz," "Dachau," "Buchenwald," or "Holocaust" appear anywhere in the text.

No mention is made by the highest-ranking American military officer of the greatest man-made humanitarian disaster ever to befall Europe. Perhaps as a result of this official disinterest, when the soldiers *did* reach the camps, they were profoundly unprepared from almost every standpoint to understand the scope of what they had uncovered—and what to do about it.[1]

Even as esteemed an author/historian as Basil H. Liddell Hart has downplayed the war Hitler waged against the Jews to the point of invisibility. In his epic *History of the Second World War,* he ignores the concentration and death camps; the index does not even contain a single reference to "Jews," "death camps," or "concentration camps." In Liddell-Hart's mind, as no doubt in the minds of many others, the military aspect of the war was separate and distinct from the political (i.e., humanitarian) aspect, and never must the two be considered as two sides of the same coin.

Similarly puzzling is the fact that the armed forces of the United States were generous in recognizing the achievements of individual soldiers through the awarding of medals. There are medals for distinguished service and bravery above and beyond the call of duty. There are medals for meritorious service. There is a medal for wounds received in battle, even one for good conduct. There are victory medals and campaign ribbons issued to troops who served in various theaters of war and who even performed post-war occupation duty in Germany and

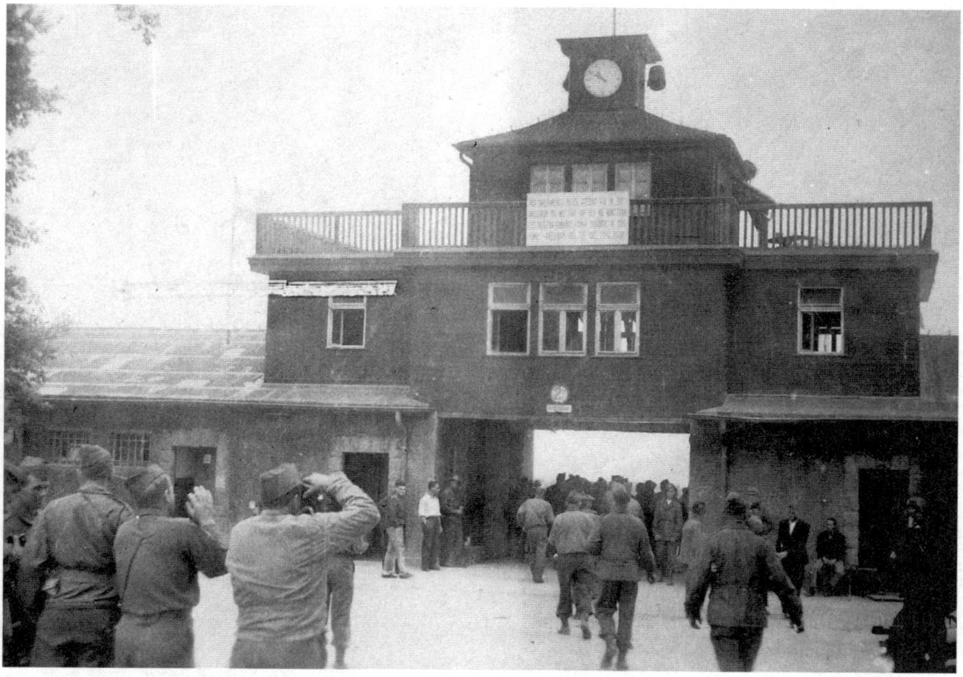

American soldiers, on the orders of General Eisenhower, visited Buchenwald in droves from April through June 1945. Major Louis Fausset, operations officer of the 809th Tank Destroyer Battalion, photographed GIs entering the camp. (Photo by Louis Fausset, courtesy Neal Fausset)

Japan. There is not, however, any ribbon or medal or even a government-issued certificate for any unit or soldier involved in the liberation of a concentration camp. The Center for Military History has a list of Army units that are credited with liberating the various camps, but that is all the "official" recognition that has been doled out.

What can explain General Marshall's and Liddell Hart's lack of mention of one of the most important events in history—the deliberate and calculated slaughter of millions of innocent people? The answer is still unknown.

Why American soldiers were not prepared for the horrors of the concentration camps also remains a major unknown—and should be a major scandal. Why had the Army not used the information about concentration camps that newspapers had been reporting for twelve years and at least considered the *possibility* that concentration camps *might* be encountered by advancing units—and issued guidelines about what to do if that should occur? Why had the Army not psychologically readied its troops for at least the *possibility* that some of them

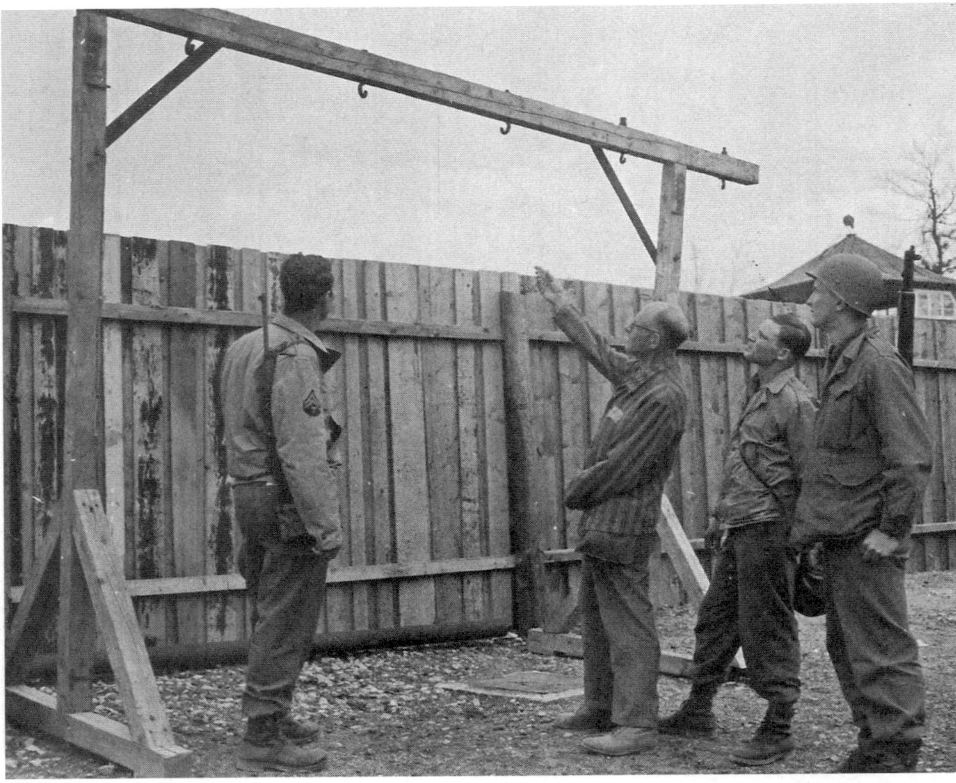

Joseph Brau, a French political prisoner and chief doctor at the camp after Buchenwald was liberated, shows three American soldiers the gallows behind the crematorium. (U.S. National Archives)

might come across scenes of brutality the likes of which they had never seen before and could not comprehend?

One answer may lie in the fact that higher command also did not psychologically prepare soldiers to deal with the effects of seeing their buddies killed in combat or coming across mass casualties killed and wounded by bombing, strafing, artillery, etc. After all, exactly how does a military organization prepare troops for the horrifying sight of disemboweled, decapitated, dismembered, burned, and mangled human bodies? Doctors and some front-line medics (but not all) were given medical instruction that presumably prepared them to deal with treating grievously wounded soldiers and civilians. And a handful of Quartermaster Graves Registration Unit personnel likely had been employed in the funeral industry before entering the military and were presumably accustomed to working with the deceased. The average soldier or junior officer in a line infantry or armor company, however, probably had no more ability or training to cope with scenes of mass death than did the average housewife in Sioux City or a banker in Birmingham. As Michael Hirsh noted in the Introduction to *The Liberators*, "The GIs had received no warning as to what they might find, but that may not have mattered, for as one of them said to me, 'What if we had? How do you prepare to see *that*?'"[2]

Bernard Kahn, a Munich-born American soldier in the 45th Infantry Division who took part in the liberation of Dachau, recalled, "Our GIs were trained in how to spot a German plane, a German uniform, a German weapon, and they were trained to fight, but they were not trained in what to do if they came across a scene such as this. There had never been the slightest bit of training in what a concentration camp was, let alone what to do if you liberated one."[3]

Jan Elvin, an author who wrote about her father's unit unexpectedly coming across the Ebensee slave-labor camp in Austria, echoed that statement when she noted, "While the anti-Semitic nature of the Nazi regime was well known, American troops were too preoccupied with their own piece of the war to give much thought to the concentration camps. Many had heard of them but believed them to be more like the German POW camps they'd encountered, which were unhealthy and punitive but not the unimaginable horrors the soldiers later saw at places like Ebensee and Buchenwald."[4]

Had the soldiers who encountered the camps been presented only with the sight of corpses, even large numbers of corpses discarded like trash, the psychological effect would have been devastating enough. But the camps presented the additional horror of the "living dead"—non-combatants reduced to little more than skin stretched over bones, and that skin often covered by sores, rashes, lice, excrement, and festering wounds. Virtually everyone who entered a camp was immediately struck by the overpowering stench of filth and decomposition, which no doubt added to the distress of the liberators.

And then there was the added component of human suffering, the begging for food, the pleading for water, the abject fear and utter hopelessness written in the eyes and on the faces of the liberated. A normal human being naturally wants to help in the event he or she comes across the victim of an accident or a crime; the sheer, staggering number of people in dire need in the camps simply overwhelmed the average GI who stumbled without warning into these places of death and degradation—places where he was subjected without warning to human organs floating in formaldehyde-filled containers, to shrunken heads, to iron hooks set into blood-stained walls that still bore the marks of heels kicking against the plaster in the last moments of life, to cold ovens filled with burnt skeletons, to artifacts made from human skin.

This aspect of the Holocaust—the reaction of soldiers of the liberating armies—has been too little studied. One of the few to look into it in any depth is Dr. Theresa Lynn Ast, a professor of history at Reinhardt University. In her doctoral dissertation at Emory University, she noted: "American soldiers were not prepared emotionally or psychologically for the enormous human suffering and degradation they witnessed. Viewing the camp atrocities and being exposed to the full extent of Nazi barbarism was a watershed experience for many soldiers. Many developed an all-consuming hatred for Germans, particularly the SS, which occasionally culminated in a 'take no more prisoners' approach to warfare. Conversely, American GIs responded to the malnourished and filthy survivors but, with few exceptions, did not ignore or reject them. They assisted the survivors in every way possible, often grief-stricken that they could not do more."

Of the Americans' apparent lack of information about the persecution of the Jews and other ethnic European minorities, Dr. Ast wrote: "Although information about [concentration] camps was available [in newspapers and magazines], it is difficult to determine whether GIs in Germany in 1945 would have been old enough or interested enough to have taken note of these reports. Just over half of the GIs who viewed the camps in April and May 1945 would have been quite young in 1937, 1938, 1939, anywhere from 10 to 18 years old.... It is unlikely that many 10-18-year-old boys followed the progress and actions of the Nazi regime in detail, unless their families were Jewish or particularly politically aware for either humanitarian, religious, or ethnic reasons."[5]

And yet, the Hollywood film *Casablanca* won the Oscar for Best Picture in 1942 and contains not one but *two* references to concentration camps. However, these references must have flown over the heads of most of the millions of people who saw the movie. How else to explain the later statements by liberators who claimed not to have known about the camps? As Dr. Ast also pointed out that, in the early 1940s, while a great many young American men were in military service, news reports of the increasing murders and mistreatment of Jews by the Nazis were quite frequent, but "many of these news items were written with a skeptical or incredulous tone, as were some reports in the European press."

Combining this almost constant flow of information about Nazi crimes, New York City's well-publicized "Stop Hitler Now" rally and "We Will Never Die" pageants, along with forty anti-Nazi rallies sponsored by a coalition of Jewish groups and held in twenty states, American soldiers should have been armed with plenty of righteous anger and a burning desire "to pay the Nazis back" for their crimes.[6]

However, some Americans *were* paying attention. Victor B. Geller, a student at Cornell University, said he joined the Army's enlisted reserve in March 1943 specifically because of what the Nazis were doing to his fellow religionists. He said, "I knew what I had read before going overseas as a teenager about, of course, the Jewish persecution by the Nazis." Even though he, as a college student, was exempt from being drafted at the time, "I volunteered and joined the army because I felt that it was a Jewish war. So I was aware of this. I knew enough to know that I had to be careful, for example, as a Jew, if I was taken prisoner."[7]

It is a sad fact that the majority of white, Anglo-Saxon Americans who formed the power base and bulk of society at the time, had no great love of Jews, just as they had none for persons of color. "Just as Americans were conscious of their ties to Europe," wrote Ast, "many had no ties to or sympathy for Jews, certainly not for the strange Jews of Eastern Europe. A generally quiescent version of anti-Semitism was pervasive in American society, and influenced beliefs, public behavior, and eventually national policy."[8] It is understandable then that "Remember the Jews!" was not a rallying cry that would have inspired millions of non-Jewish youths to suddenly rush to military recruiting centers.

Then, too, there is the matter of skepticism. As mentioned earlier, the American public was wary of too many "over the top" stories of Nazis abusing civilians, for the flood of false reporting of German atrocities that had taken place during World War I had hardened the public to "falling for" any more tales about German soldiers committing foul deeds, such as murder on a massive scale.

American newspapers, as a consequence, usually refrained from printing such articles on their front pages, even when the news was confirmed by unimpeachable sources.

Because most Americans at that time were of European heritage, there also existed a sense of disbelief when it came to accepting the notion that Europeans—Germans—could do these sorts of things to other Europeans. Germany had always been considered to be a highly advanced, educated, cultured, and civilized nation; how could such barbarities be perpetrated by a society that had spawned a Goethe, a Beethoven, a Brahms? No, such implausible tales must be the work of sick minds or governmental efforts to stir up feeling of hatred toward the enemy. There could be no other explanation.

REPORTS OF WHAT the Nazis were doing to the Jews continued to fill the newspapers and airwaves in the United States and Britain. According to Dr. Ast, after the Soviets overran the Maidanek camp in July 1944, they allowed American officers and reporters to inspect it the next month. Presumably these officers wrote reports to the War Department and General Marshall about their findings. Yet, somehow, that information was not filtered down to the commanders and troops in the field who might come across camps in their zones of operation.

Dr. Ast added that, besides soldiers, "Americans (and citizens of many other nations) often found the reports of concentration camps and atrocities unbelievable. They did not assume they were being lied to or misled; they simply could not comprehend or accept that such terrible events could occur on so massive a scale." It was not until American units began overrunning the camps and seeing for themselves what had taken place there that they finally realized that, not only were the stories true, they were far beyond anything they could have imagined.

Apparently some official reports *did* reach the field. An Army major named George King recalled reading intelligence reports about concentration camps early in 1945, but he wrote them off as being nothing more than rumors. As Dr. Ast wrote, Major King noted, "Upon finally viewing a camp, [the troops] found themselves 'totally unprepared...the actual experience was almost unbelievable.'"

Even those soldiers who had read articles about concentration camps did not possess the means for understanding what the term meant. For many, a "concentration camp" was just another term for "jail" or "prison." Soldiers from the American South had no doubt seen chain gangs of prisoners working on road projects, but nothing in the life experiences of the typical GI could have prepared him to comprehend the reality of the camps.

Dr. Ast also noted, "SHAEF (Supreme Headquarters Allied Expeditionary Force) and Army Group headquarters had enormous amounts of detailed military information to guide their decision-making, but it seems Washington relayed little information about the camps until just prior to their discovery. [However] Rabbi Judah Nadich, as 'advisor on Jewish Affairs to the command general of the European Theater of Operations,' had access to directives, orders, and regulation papers. Rabbi Nadich stated that nowhere was the possible capture of concentration camps mentioned."

Dr. Ast also said that a personal aide to General George Patton, Major Marshall J. Mantler, "had access to a broad array of intelligence information. Assigned to G-2, Mantler interviewed escaped prisoners who testified about concentration camps and the atrocities committed there; however, this information was not distributed to lower level commanders who were approaching the camps. It is Major Mantler's contention that the Army Commanders and General Staff never felt this information was accurate enough to rely upon. Or it is possible this information was considered unimportant, ancillary to the goal of the military, which was to defeat Hitler and his armies?"[9]

The uncomfortable question needs to be asked: If the German people can be indicted for claiming not to know about what was happening at the camps in their own back yards, should not the American military establishment be held accountable for not better informing the soldiers and preparing them for what they were about to encounter?

IT IS CONVENIENT to point to the Germans living near the concentration and death camps and express disbelief at their post-war protestations that they "did not know" about the horrors being perpetrated in the camps. The truth of the matter is that German civilians (and some German soldiers, too) naturally did not want to know what crimes their government was committing, for would not their silence make them complicit in the crimes? If they could remain consciously unaware of the murders and atrocities, then they could deny being a part of them.

Helping the Germans "not to know" were the local newspapers that carried no stories or exposés about the inhuman conditions in which inmates of the concentration camps were held or the mass slaughter of Jews. After all, with even most German clergymen afraid and/or unwilling to speak out against the Nazis' excesses, who could average civilians report such atrocities to without also risking their own arrest and even possible execution? If they went to the local police, they would be reported to the Gestapo or *Sicherheitsdienst*. So complete was the Nazi government's control of its own population that the average German feared that he would simply end up in Buchenwald or some other camp alongside the same people about whom he had expressed concern.

In examining the writings of the American generals such as Eisenhower, Bradley, Patton, and others, and questioning those GIs who came across the camps, it appears that all were ignorant as to what was happening in the camps they uncovered. For example, although he recalled reading countless stories in New York newspapers about the Nazi persecution of the Jews, Captain Mel Rappaport, Combat Command B, 6th Armored Division, who arrived at Buchenwald on or about April 16, insisted that neither he nor the Army "knew in advance about the concentration camps, the killing centers, the gas chambers, the ovens, the hanging bars, the shooting grounds, etc. The big brass hats never told us that we would someday overrun these camps. Not even Patton knew."[10]

U.S. Navy Ensign Robert Beir, stationed in Scotland, also recalled being in the dark about Nazi atrocities at the time. "What did servicemen in Great Britain know about the Holocaust during this time?" he asked, rhetorically. "The answer, simply, was nothing. We did not have access to the *New York Times*. If I read the *London Times*, I don't recall. Certainly, I didn't read about any Jewish massacres. We read *Stars and Stripes*. We worried about our future. We hated the Germans because they were our enemy on the battlefield. Meanwhile, the Nazis were trying to keep the Holocaust as secret as possible."[11]

The reason why most American soldiers have professed an ignorance of the persecutions being heaped upon the Jews and other minorities of Europe may seem puzzling at first, but the answer is really quite simple, and Robert Beir touched on it. Millions of young men who may have been accustomed to reading a daily newspaper in their hometowns were suddenly plucked, either by the draft boards or by their own enlistment, from those hometowns and transported hundreds or thousands of miles away to a military base. A young man from, say, Brooklyn, who regularly read the *New York Times*, might have found himself in 1942 or 1943 at Camp Swift, outside of Bastrop, Texas, where the *New York Times* was not readily available. The local newspaper, the *Bastrop Advertiser*, likely did not carry many stories about the treatment of European Jews and, in any case, the average soldier, even if he had been aware of the situation overseas before entering the military, was too busy with his training duties and too concerned about his possible upcoming deployment to a combat zone to spend much time reading newspapers and attempting to educate himself on the larger picture and the plight of others. His primary focus was on preparing himself for battle.

In addition to intense physical training that was hardening his body for the rigors of combat, the average American soldier was kept busy from dawn to dark with a variety of tasks and duties: improving his marksmanship skills on the rifle range; learning how to disassemble, clean, and reassemble his weapon; learning how to properly throw a grenade; or being instructed on the most effective ways to kill another man, be it with bullet, bayonet, or bare hands.

Despite all this training to prepare young men to enter the belly of the beast and do battle with the enemy, there is no evidence that the average American soldier received any official Army instruction, either in basic training, advanced infantry training, or at briefings in the field once deployed to the European combat zone that would have educated him about concentration camps or readied him for the possibility of encountering such places. Members of specialized military government units *were* schooled in how to govern towns and cities captured from the enemy, and how to deal with large numbers of civilian refugees—but not concentration camps and concentration-camp inmates. And, although the average American soldier was issued numerous training and field manuals on scores of subjects, there were no manuals that told him what to expect or how to conduct himself should he unexpectedly come across a camp filled with tens of thousands of sick and starving persons, or mountains of skeletal corpses of human beings who had been systematically slaughtered.

David Israel, from Brooklyn, New York, was a member of the 320th Military Intelligence Detachment—one of the units that entered Dachau shortly after its liberation on April 29, 1945. He professed that little or nothing was known of the camps before they were reached by American units. "I would think that maybe the guys who went through the Ritchie program* might have had some preparation," he said, "but I'm not at all sure of that. My team had four Ritchie boys. All of us were Jewish except for the captain, who was of Prussian background,

* The "Ritchie Program" was a language and intelligence school set up at Camp Ritchie, Cascade, Maryland, at which soldiers—many of whom were European Jews fluent in German—were trained in the art and science of intelligence gathering, interrogation techniques, and psychological warfare. One of the soldiers, Henry Schwab, said, "I was fully committed to helping my new country win the war against the tyranny of Nazi Germany." Schwab later learned that an uncle and his future father-in-law, Rudolf Marx, had both been held at Buchenwald. Marx managed to buy his way out of Koch's camp but the fate of his uncle and several other relatives is unknown. (Schwab, "The Richie Boys," *The Israel Philatelist*, April 2005)

but I don't remember ever discussing anything about the camps with them. "Articles [in the *New York Times*] pertaining to what went on in Germany were always buried deep because the paper's [Jewish] owners went overboard in trying to show that the paper didn't dwell on Jewish themes."[12]

Even the acclaimed documentary film series, *Why We Fight,* by Frank Capra, which was shown to all U.S. Army inductees as indoctrination, did not dwell on the plight of European Jewry. In fact, in the entire seven hours of films, the Jews are mentioned only once. In the first film, "Prelude to War," over a montage of images of churches and a synagogue, the announcer intones, "Thousands of other men of God— Protestant, Catholic, Jewish—were persecuted, arrested, confined in concentration camps." The scene takes less than fifteen seconds—fifteen seconds out of seven hours. There is not a single mention of *Kristallnacht,* ghettoes, boycotts of Jewish-owned businesses, medical experiments, euthanasia, gas chambers, or any explanation of what the narrator's off-hand reference to "concentration camps" meant. It is no wonder, then, that the average American soldier in 1945 was totally unprepared to come face to face with the shocking reality of the camps. All of that changed, of course, after the discovery of Buchenwald.

As Donald McKale noted, "Today, the Holocaust has become in the West, in the words of a recent writer [Tim Cole, *Selling the Holocaust*], the single 'most talked about and oft-represented event of the twentieth century.' A series of public opinion surveys in the early 1990s in the United States concluded that approximately 95 percent of Americans had heard the term *Holocaust,* and almost as many believed they knew what it meant."[13]

28
MARCHING TO OBLIVION

"What was in store for us? Is this the manner in which it will all end?"
William Shapiro
American prisoner at Berga-an-der-Elster

EVEN WHILE GIs were touring Buchenwald, the death marches from many of the other camps were still continuing. For example, day after day, for three weeks, the plodding procession of prisoners from the Buchenwald sub-camp of Berga-an-der-Elster continued on through the cities of Greiz, Plauen, Hof, Selb, and many more.

To add to the marchers' misery, the German guards did everything in their perverse power to prevent the human herd from being liberated by the advancing

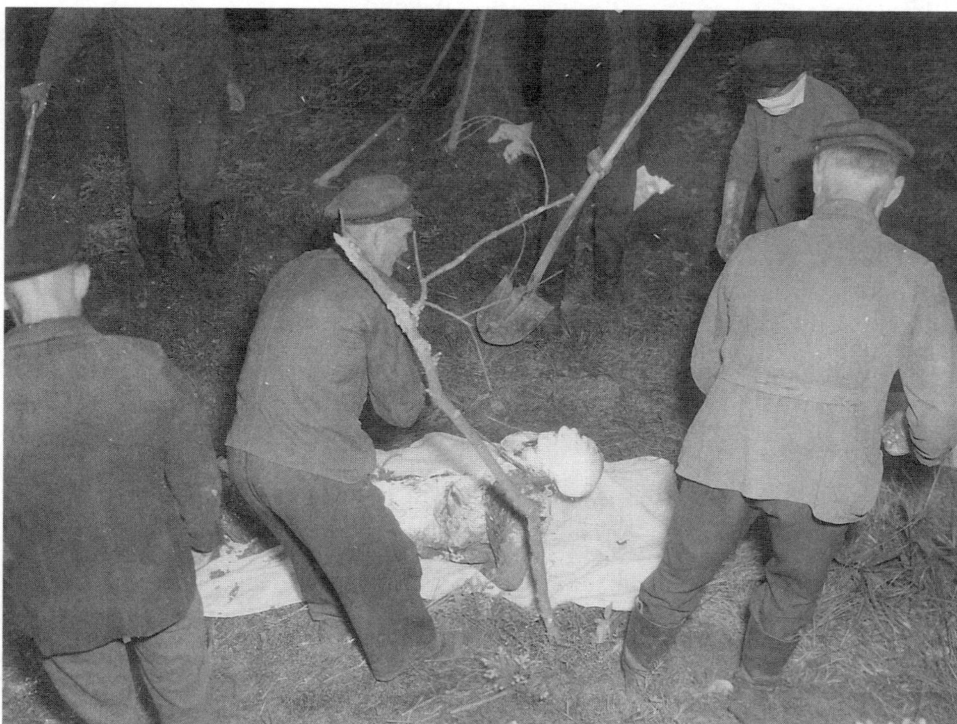

A group of German civilians dig up a victim of one of the death marches. (U.S. National Archives)

Allied armies or being fed and helped by sympathetic farmers and townspeople along the route. And each day more and more Americans fell victim to the pace of the march, to their illnesses and infirmities, to the cruelty of their guards. If a man could not keep up, and if his buddies had not the strength to carry him, he was dispatched by the side of the road with a bullet to the brain.

Medic William Shapiro recalled, "None of us...had any idea how destructive this march would be to our group—all debilitated, exhausted, emaciated, sick, maimed, and cowered soldiers. It was simply walking—no strenuous work. We were totally unprepared for the horrors we would encounter—the profound despair, the inability to continue to take another step forward, the discovery of dead buddies each morning, and the wanton, gross murder along the roads."

Shapiro was horrified by what was taking place along the route. "During my five months of front-line combat," he said, "I had witnessed many instances of gore—dismembered and blown-apart bodies. Dead soldiers were a common sight. But this scene on the 'Death-March Road' was significantly different.... As we approached a steep hill, I saw some of the most gruesome, cruel, barbarous, inhumane acts that I have ever seen in my entire life. As we climbed the hill and caught up to where we had seen the political prisoners in the distance, we saw on each side of the road hundreds of dead Jews. Most of them were in the kneeling position, many on their sides in the fetal position, and all were dead by obvious gunshots behind the head. Many heads were blown open by the force of the shot, and the brains were splattered about.

"It was ghastly. It was indescribably frightening. It was unspeakable. It was so shocking to look at the very recent, awesome destruction of human beings. The murder was, presumably, because they could not continue the march up the inclined road.... What was in store for us? Is this the manner in which it will all end?"[1]

THE MARCH FROM Berga continued southward. Along the way, a few—very few—kindly villagers tried to give the Americans food but were rebuffed by the guards. In all, the GIs from Berga were marched some 125 miles. On April 23, at the village of Rötz, about fifty miles northwest of Cham, a city on the Regen River in Bavaria, the march came to an unexpected end. The famished, utterly exhausted GIs were all herded into a barn for a night of fitful rest. In the morning, the sound of tanks moving closer captured the attention of the

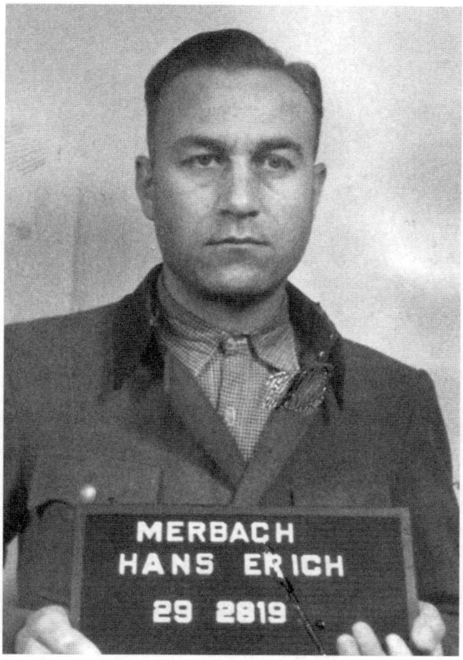

Hans Merbach was in charge of the "death train" that ended up at Dachau at the end of April (U.S. National Archives)

Americans, and those with enough strength crawled to the door of the barn to witness a glorious sight: dozens of tanks and jeeps bearing the white stars of the U.S. Army!

It was Combat Command A of Major General Holmes Dager's 11th Armored Division. The Germans fled at the sight of the tanks. The Americans in the barn, many too weak to stand, wept with joy at the moment of their liberation.[2]

WHILE MOST OF the prisoners from Buchenwald had set out on foot, a special freight train of fifty-nine open and closed freight cars left Weimar for Flossenbürg, some 125 miles to the south, on April 7 with 4,500 inmates. In charge of this shipment was thirty-five-year-old *SS-Obersturmführer* Hans Erich Merbach, who had commanded the guard-dog unit at Buchenwald. As a grim prelude of things to come, on the five-mile march from the camp to the Weimar railroad depot, Martin Rosenfeld, a witness at Merbach's war-crimes trial, said that some 350 inmates were shot and killed, several of them by Merbach personally.[3]

Instead of traveling the expected 125 miles, Merbach's train was continually re-routed. Michael Hirsh, author of *The Liberators*, noted, "The actual trip covered 471 miles over twenty-two days as the train meandered north to Leipzig, then east through Dresden and south into Czechoslovakia, passing through Pilsen, then into Austria, and back west through Munich, all to avoid bomb-damaged tracks and advancing Allied forces."[4]

The witness Rosenfeld also testified that when the train was re-routed through Pilsen, Merbach opened fire on a group of civilians who approached the train with food for the prisoners, killing several of the good Samaritans. At another stop, Merbach allegedly went from one sealed boxcar to another, firing

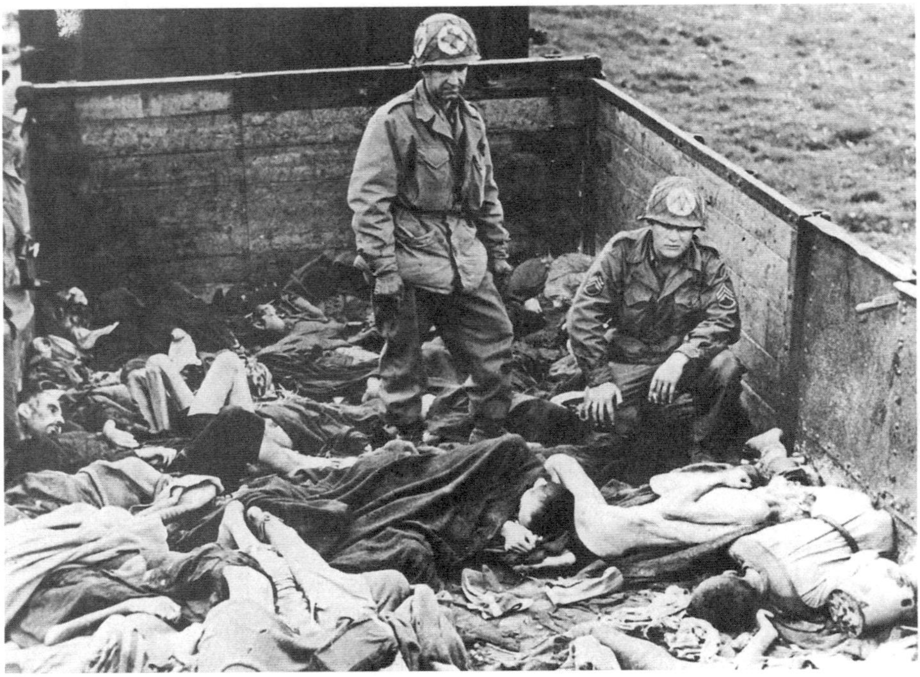

More than 2,300 inmates from Buchenwald were found dead outside Dachau. Here two medics look for signs of life. (U.S. National Archives)

into the packed masses; Rosenfeld said that twenty men in his boxcar were either killed or wounded. Another time, according to Rosenfeld, Merbach ordered all of the French prisoners out of the cars, lined them up, and then gunned them down.*[5]

With all possibility of the train reaching Flossenbürg now gone, the transport was shunted toward Dachau. American pilots spotted the train and, not realizing that it held human cargo, dived on it with machine guns blazing, killing an unknown number of prisoners. On April 26, nearly three weeks after leaving Weimar, the train finally reached Dachau, where it was left on a siding outside the camp's railroad gate; by now almost all the prisoners on board were dead.[6]

One of the first Americans on the scene, Private first class John Lee of the 45th, recalled, "These people were stuffed in these [railroad] cars. The cars had bullet holes all over them, evidently from strafing on the way to Dachau. Most of the GIs just stood there in silence and disbelief. We had seen men in battle blown apart, burnt to death, and die in many ways, but we were never prepared

* Despite denying all the accusations against him, and after presenting witnesses on his behalf, Merbach was found guilty at the tribunal of Buchenwald personnel held at Dachau in 1947; he was hanged at Landsberg Prison on January 14, 1949. (Greene, p. 315; www.jewsihvirtuallibrary.org/jsource/Holocaust/WarCrime10)

for this. Several of the dead lay there with their eyes open, a picture I will never get out of my mind. It seems they were looking at us and saying, 'What took you so long?'"[7]

EVEN WHILE THE Third Reich crumbled, the awful contents of more camps continued to be exposed to the world, and it seemed as though nearly every U.S. Army division in the European Theater of Operations stumbled across at least one camp or sub-camp—many of which had connections to Buchenwald.

Relieving the 6th Armored Division atop the Ettersberg was Major General Horace McBride's 80th Infantry Division. (McBride's infantrymen also went on to liberate Ebensee, a sub-camp of Mauthausen, on May 6.) The 2nd Infantry Division liberated the Buchenwald sub-camp of Leipzig-Schönefeld and the town of Hadamar, where euthanasia programs were carried out. While battling to take Leipzig, the 69th Infantry Division discovered the Leipzig-Thekla camp, another Buchenwald sub-camp, which had been torched by the fleeing SS; hundreds of burnt bodies of inmates were found in the rubble. Another Buchenwald sub-camp, Langenstein, whose 5,000 slaves worked in an underground aircraft factory in the Harz Mountains, was discovered by the 83rd Infantry Division. Another 5,000 slave workers from Buchenwald's Halberstadt-Zweiberge (Malachit) slave-labor camp, also digging underground industrial facilities in the Harz Mountains, were discovered and freed by the 8th Armored Division.[8]

In mid-April the 84th Infantry Division uncovered two Neuengamme sub-camps: Salzwedel and Hannover-Ahlem, while the slave-labor camp of Attendorn, in the Ruhr area, was liberated by the 86th Infantry Division. On April 23, the 95th Infantry Division came across a German prison and labor camp at the town of Werl, and also freed over 5,000 French soldiers in a POW camp. A veteran unit of the Battle of the Bulge, the 99th Infantry Division drove deep into Bavaria, where it discovered and liberated a Dachau sub-camp at Mühldorf. As mentioned earlier, the 104th Infantry Division, along with the 3rd Armored Division, liberated Mittlebau-Dora at Nordhausen.[9]

Also on April 23, the 90th and 97th Infantry Divisions freed the 1,500 remaining prisoners at the Flossenbürg main camp. Greeting them were Léon Blum, the former Prime Minister of France, who had spent time in Buchenwald; Kurt von Schuschnigg, the ex-Chancellor of Austria; and Pastor Martin Niemöller, the former leader of the Confessional Church in Germany, who had been a political prisoner for seven years.* The liberation came too late to save Dietrich Bonhoeffer, a Lutheran pastor and one of the founders of the Confessional Church; he had been executed on April 9, 1945. Admiral Wilhelm Canaris, former head of the *Abwehr* and implicated in plots to kill Hitler; and approximately 30,000 other inmates, along with two unknown American pilots, also perished at Flossenbürg.[10]

At Dachau on April 29, 1945, lead elements of the 45th Infantry Division reached the outer walls of the camp and found the train that had left Buchenwald on April 7 with 4,500 persons aboard sitting abandoned on the tracks outside the railroad gate. The bodies of 2,310 persons were piled into the cars.

Enraged at the discovery of such cruelty, the men of the 3rd Battalion of the 157th Infantry Regiment, under the command of Lieutenant Colonel Felix L. Sparks, broke into the camp at the railroad gate, rounded up whatever SS personnel they could find and, when the SS personnel gave the slightest indication that they might try to resist or escape, shot them down.** Over 20,000 sick and starving people still inside the enclosure at Dachau were forever grateful at the arrival of the 45th and, almost simultaneously, advance elements from the 42nd Infantry Division.[11]

The first week of May brought further revelations of Nazi tyranny. On May 2, the 4th Infantry Division liberated Haunstetten, a Dachau sub-camp, while the 8th Infantry and 82nd Airborne Divisions came upon Wöbbelin, near Ludwigslust, part of the Neuengamme system, and freed 2,500 inmates; another thousand had already been freed by death. The 82nd's commander, Major General James Gavin, ordered all of Ludwiglust's residents above the age of ten to visit the camp and view the evidence of the atrocities committed there. He then went even further than Patton. According to Richard Bessel, author of *Germany 1945*, under Gavin's orders the town's leading citizens "were made to re-bury the dead at a park in front

---

* An ardent anti-Nazi, Niemöller is perhaps best remembered for his statements, "First they came for the communists, but I was not a communist, so I didn't speak up. Then they came for the trade unionists, but I was not a trade unionist, so I didn't speak up. Then they camp for the Jews, but I was not a Jew, so I didn't speak up. Then they came for me and there was no one left to speak for me." (Harold Marcuse, speech, "Martin Niemöller's Famous Quotation," University of California at Santa Barbara, September 12, 2000)

** Shortly after Sparks' men arrived, a patrol from the 42nd Division pulled up at the main gate, where an SS lieutenant was waiting to surrender the camp to the first Americans who came along. Neither Sparks nor Brigadier General Henning Linden, the 42nd's Assistant Division Commander who was leading the patrol, knew that the other unit was there until they met by accident inside the compound. The two units nearly came to blows.

General Patton, in whose Third Army the 45th was then a part, buried an Inspector General's report on the shooting of the SS guards; the only surviving copy of the report was not rediscovered until 1997 at the National Archives. Portions of it were first made public in the author's 1998 book, *The Rock of Anzio.* (Whitlock, *The Rock of Anzio*, passim)

of Ludwiglust's palace in the presence of the town's population."[12]

In some places, the approach of Allied forces compelled some Germans to continue the slaughter. On May 3, 1945, as British troops were bearing down on the harbor of Lübeck, the Germans attempted to transfer 850 Jewish women, formerly at Stutthof, by small boat onto three ships in the harbor, but were refused permission to board; the ships were already overcrowded. As the small boats returned to shore, they were fired upon by SS men, Hitler Youth, and German Marines; over 500 women were killed.[13]

On May 4, the 71st Infantry Division discovered 15,000 prisoners abandoned by their guards at Gunskirchen, a sub-camp of Mauthausen. The main Mauthausen camp—filled with over 110,000 survivors, 28,000 of them Jews—was taken by the 11th Armored Division two days later; Mauthausen's sub-camps, known as Gusen I, II, and III, were opened by the 11th Armored on the same day; a mass grave at Mauthausen contained the remains of nearly 10,000 persons.[14]

Also on May 4, British troops reached Neuengamme, near Hamburg, freeing tens of thousands of inmates in the process. Unfortunately, they were too late to save thousands of others; some 10,000 inmates had already been death-marched toward Lübeck, while thousands more were tranferred to Bergen-Belsen. Another 6,500 prisoners were loaded aboard two ships—the *Thielbeck* and *Cap Arcona*—in a harbor near Hamburg. Without realizing that concentration-camp inmates were aboard, British aircraft strafed and bombed the vessels. The *Thielbeck* sank quickly, carrying most of her cargo of 2,000 inmates to their deaths; the *Cap Arcona*, with 4,500 prisoners aboard, caught fire and capsized. Only about 600 prisoners from both ships survived.[15]

On May 5 at Ebensee, a slave-labor camp in the mountains near Mauthausen, the camp commandant, Anton Ganz, formed up all 18,000 prisoners on the *Appellplatz*. He was flanked by armed SS men and told the group that the Allies were coming and he had orders to surrender the prisoners to them when they arrived. Ganz was also faced with the fact that the previous night half of the SS guard detachment had deserted. According to an inmate, Solomon Salat, Ganz told the inmates that the camp "was not safe, because the Allies might think that it was an army installation and bomb it. But, to ensure the prisoners' safety, [Ganz] proposed that we go to the tunnels and wait there. He would bring all the food to the tunnels."

But the inmates weren't convinced; a rumor making the rounds had it that the prisoner-built tunnels were mined and that the SS was planning on killing them all, then escaping into the countryside. When one of the prisoners screamed out, "No one must go! They will kill us!" the group of inmates hesitated. Soon everyone was screaming "No!"

Ganz was taken aback by this reaction, then said, "All right, if you don't want to go, stay here at your own risk." He and the SS then departed the camp. The following day, before any mass slaughter could be carried out, the U.S. 3rd Cavalry Reconnaissance Squadron arrived to take control of the camp.[16]

On May 6, the 26th Infantry Division freed hundreds of inmates at Gusen. After battling its way up the Italian peninsula and into Austria, the 36th Infantry Division came across Kaufering, a Dachau sub-camp, near Landsberg, Germany. The 63rd and 103rd Infantry Divisions, along with the 101st Airborne and 12th Armored Divisions, also liberated a number of smaller camps associated with Kaufering.[17]

The concentration camp of Theresienstadt, inside occupied Czechoslovakia, was liberated by Soviet forces on May 8, 1945. Of an estimated 140,000 persons who either were incarcerated at, or passed through this concentration camp "showplace," only 17,320 were still alive on May 8; the rest had either died of disease or had been shipped off to the death camps and killed. On that same day, units of the 1st Infantry Division liberated two sub-camps of Flossenbürg: Zwodau and Falkenau-an-der-Eger, both in Czechoslovakia. When the division arrived, Zwodau held 900-1,000 starving female prisoners; Falkenau had just a handful. The men of the 1st Division provided food and badly needed medical attention to the survivors.[18]

AS THE NEWS of what was being discovered at the concentration camps began to be reported, it was greeted with howls of outrage in the U.S. The May 7, 1945, issue of *Life* magazine, for example, contained a spread of gruesome photos of victims who had died at Buchenwald and Gardelegen—photos which prompted several readers to voice their opinions: "May I suggest that *Life* have its atrocity photographs blown up to mural size and that they be used to adorn the walls of the room in which the peace conferences which shall determine the fate of Germany are held?" wrote Jane C. Fales of Rochester, New York.

Robert M. Rosse, a sailor from Hutchinson, Kansas, said, "I for one do not want to see races able to commit such horrible deeds go without their just reward, so I take my hat off to *Life* for bringing the cold truth to the American public regardless of how nauseating it may seem."

A mother, Geane Sutherland of Oakland, California, who had lost her teen-aged soldier son in a German prisoner-of-war camp, said, "These things have got to be shown. The world has to know that these things were not dreamed up by newsmen but actually happened.... These pictures are hard to take—they tear your heart out. I know, and make you so mad you can't see. That's what they're supposed to do, to keep us in there pitching until the end of this war. If my son could stand a German [POW] camp for three months, I can stand looking at pictures which tell the truth, so that his death may be avenged properly.... I'd hate to think that Billy's tormentors escaped what was coming to them."[19]

And yet, no matter how heartfelt these and other expressions of disgust and outrage at the Nazis' excesses were, the nagging question remains—with the American public well informed of concentration camps, mass murder, and inhuman brutality since 1933, why was the situation ignored by the United States government for so long? Why was so little done to save the Jews and other unfortunate populations of Europe?

It is an inescapable question that still hovers like a ghostly specter above the remains of Buchenwald, Dachau, Mauthausen, Auschwitz, and all the other camps that have been preserved as monuments to the depravity of the Nazi regime and mankind.*

---

* It is impossible within the scope of this book to list all of the concentration and death camps and their sub-camps and describe their liberation. Martin Gilbert's exhaustive documentation, *Atlas of the Holocaust,* lists hundreds of camps run by the Nazis and describes their liberation by Allied forces. The United States Holocaust Memorial Museum estimates that, according to SS figures, more than 700,000 prisoners still populated the camps as late as January 1945. It is further estimated that nearly half of the total number of concentration-camp deaths between 1933 and 1945 occurred during the last year of the war. (Gilbert, *Atlas of the Holocaust*, passim)

29
JUSTICE?

"May the demons of the Holocaust be forever shunned as moral misfits from our midst."

Rabbi Murray Kohn
Ohrdruf survivor

AT 3:30 P.M. on April 30, with no chance of victory, and with his regime's crimes laid bare to the world, Adolf Hitler and his bride, the former Eva Braun (they were married a few hours earlier), committed suicide in the command bunker deep beneath the shattered Chancellery and the burning, bombed-out streets of Berlin. They were joined in death by Joseph and Magda Goebbels, who first poisoned six of their seven children—Helmut, Hedda, Heidi, Holde, Helga, and Hilde. (An older son, Harald Quandt, from Magda's first marriage, was a lieutenant in the Luftwaffe and was in an Allied POW compound in North Africa.)[1]

Like rats deserting a sinking ship, the rest of Hitler's entourage fled the bunker in hopes of escaping the wrath of the Russians. Before he died, Hitler had named Grand Admiral Karl Dönitz his successor as Führer and commanded him to carry on the war but, as there was no Third Reich left to lead, Dönitz disobeyed orders and surrendered to the Allies on May 8, 1945. The European phase of World War II was at last over, but the dying and the suffering were not.[2] An empire that Hitler boasted would exist for a thousand years expired after only twelve. Defeat was total; the country was a shambles, a condition from which many predicted would take Germany a century or more to recover. As Dagmar Barnouw, author of *Germany 1945: Views of War and Violence*, noted, "German cities were reduced to rubble; a highly evolved culture had regressed to stone-age living conditions; chaotic, large-scale migrations pushing in different directions seemed to mark the final loss of all order, security, and civility. And, perhaps the most difficult to understand, the revelation of German 'atrocities' signified what might be called a rewinding of civilization back to barbarism."[3]

U.S. Army historian Charles MacDonald wrote, "As the last offensive came to an end, few if any who fought in it could have entertained any doubts as to the right of their cause—they had seen at Buchenwald, Dachau, and at a dozen other places, including little Ohrdruf, what awful tyranny man can practice on his fellow man. To erase those cruel monuments to evil was reason enough for it all, from bloody Omaha Beach to that bridgehead to nowhere over the Elbe."[4]

Predictably, Heinrich Himmler's earlier efforts to secretly bring about a truce with the British and Americans and get them to start a war with the Russians failed. Now a wanted man with a price on his head, on May 8 he attempted to avoid recognition and arrest by shaving off his moustache, donning an eye patch, putting on the uniform of an ordinary member of the German Secret Field Police, and heading north with a small entourage. Stopped at British Army checkpoint on May 23 near the mouth of the Elbe River, Himmler was taken into custody, interrogated, confessed as to his real identity, and demanded to be taken to meet with either Eisenhower or Montgomery; his demands were rebuffed. To escape the justice he saw coming, however, Himmler bit down on a cyanide capsule hidden in his mouth and died within seconds. He was secretly buried by the British in an unmarked grave in a forest on the Lüneburg Heath.[5]

THE MOST DESTRUCTIVE war in history was at last over, but not the suffering or the dying, especially in the camps.

The U.S. Army's official history noted, "A particular problem for [1st Lt. Walter F.] Emmons and his detachment was the multitude of visitors that descended upon them and their charges. The tactical troops, as always, moved on quickly, but after them came newspaper reporters and visitors from other headquarters and from Allied governments and armies. Buchenwald had been an international camp, and among the thirty-one nationalities represented there were men prominent in various fields in their own countries. The prisoners' desire to be away from the place and the visitors' eagerness to do something for them resulted in numerous unauthorized departures; before long, reports were coming back of cases in which former inmates died before reaching home. Finally, 12th Army Group [Omar Bradley] had to prohibit visits to liberated concentration camps without approval of the army commanders."[6]

After more than five-and-a-half years of total, merciless war in Europe—and the deaths of some six million human beings in the concentration and extermination camps—the carnage and destruction in Europe had finally come to an end. It was time for the criminals to be rounded up and brought to justice; finding them would be a major campaign in itself.

Meanwhile, the sick and traumatized liberated survivors of the camps needed to be cared for. Dealing with the tremendous number of freed prisoners suddenly became a major priority for the U.S. Army. Many of them had lost their homes, their fortunes, and their family members. Many who had lived in countries now controlled by the Soviet Union did not want to return.

The refugees and survivors could not simply be turned loose and allowed to wander the roads of Germany, Poland, Czechoslovakia, Belgium, France, Norway, Denmark, Luxembourg, the Netherlands, etc. They had to be cared for medically, fed, clothed, and housed. For many, it meant remaining in the concentration camps for an unknown length of time, no matter how marginal the conditions might be. The enormous task of determining what to do with the survivors was turned over to the United Nations Displaced Persons Branch.[7]

Germany, too, had been completely flattened—socially, economically, and spiritually—and left without a functioning government, economy, infrastructure, or a means to take care of millions of its own citizens. Although some in the U.S. and Soviet governments advocated turning Germany into a purely agrarian nation with no means to ever be able to rearm, realists knew this was neither possible nor desirable. The victors would need to put the vanquished back on their feet. The destroyed infrastructure would need to be rebuilt; basic water, sanitation, and utility services restored; businesses, schools, hospitals, police, courts, and other institutions reconstituted; a government reestablished; and those guilty of Nazi Germany's crimes rounded up and put on trial.[8]

IN MAY 1945, not long after Germany surrendered, Ilse Koch was taking a walk with little Artwin and Gisele through the rubble-strewn streets of Ludwigsburg, near Stuttgart, when she was spotted by a former prisoner from Buchenwald. He went to the municipal authorities, who brought her in for questioning.

"They asked me about the camp," she said, "and I was to tell them all that had happened. I said that I didn't know anything about it and that I could not help them by testifying about the officers, non-coms, and men, not knowing about all the things that had been announced over the radio and press."

She remained free for several more weeks, and then the Americans returned for her on the last day of June 1945.[9] Ilse's turn at justice would have to wait. First, a war-crimes tribunal of the leading Nazis began in the autumn of 1945 in Courtroom 600 at the bomb-scarred Palace of Justice in Nürnberg—the city which had hosted the massive, emotionally powerful Nazi Party rallies in the 1930s.

Nazi Germany's crimes were so enormous that there was no precedent for such trials. Although some have criticized the proceedings as "victors' justice" and akin to writing the rules after the game had already been played, the "London Agreement" of August 8, 1945, signed by representatives from Great Britain, France, the Soviet Union, and the United States, established the authority for the four powers to create international law and conduct tribunals for those accused of committing war crimes, or "crimes against humanity."

Earlier, Adolf Hitler, Josef Goebbels, and Heinrich Himmler had all escaped justice by committing suicide, but there were a number of other high-ranking Nazis and military officers who had been captured and whose ultimate fate would be decided by an international court of law. Twenty-two of the Third Reich's most notorious still-living figures became the focal point of the first, and most famous, of the war-crimes tribunals, which began in Nürnberg on Monday, November 19, 1945.

In the prisoners' dock, guarded by members of the U.S. 1st Infantry Division in white helmet liners and Class A uniforms, was a broad cross-section of the former Nazi hierarchy. Military leaders included Reichsmarschal Hermann Göring, once the commander of the Luftwaffe; Feldmarschal Wilhelm Keitel, former Chief of the High Command of the Armed Forces; his Chief of the Operations Staff, General Alfred Jodl; and Grand Admirals Karl Dönitz and Erich Raeder.

The accused who had been a part of the Nazi government included Deputy Führer Rudolf Hess (deemed by many to be mentally ill); former Foreign Minister Joachim von Ribbentrop; Wilhelm Frick, ex-Minister of the Interior; and Walther Funk and Hjalmar Schacht, both of whom had served as Minister of Economics and President of the Reichsbank.

Those on trial who were implicated in the program to oppress or exterminate the Jews were Gestapo chief Ernst Kaltenbrunner; Nazi Party ideologist Alfred Rosenberg; and Julius Streicher, editor of the viciously anti-Semitic newspaper *Der Sturmer.* They were joined in the dock by Fritz Sauckel, in charge of exploiting concentration camp slave labor, and two Nazi goons who had brutally governed captured territories: Hans Frank, the Governor-General of Poland, and Arthur Seyss-Inquart, the Reich Commissioner of the Netherlands.

There was also an odd assortment of former diplomats and politicians: Baldur von Schirach, who once headed the Hitler Youth movement and later became Gauleiter of Vienna; pre-Hitler Chancellor Franz von Papen; Hans Fritzsche, a high-ranking official in the German Propaganda Ministry; and Konstantin Freiherr von Neurath, German Foreign Minister from 1932 to 1938, and then Heydrich's predecessor as Reich Protector of Bohemia and Moravia from 1939 to 1941.

The tribunal lasted 218 days. By the time the verdicts were read on October 1, 1946, eleven of the accused were condemned to death, seven were sentenced to long prison terms, and three were acquitted. Martin Bormann, Hitler's secretary, who had been tried in absentia, was sentenced to death.*[10]

Those sentenced to death were Frank, Frick, Göring, Jodl, Kaltenbrunner, Keitel, Ribbentrop, Rosenberg, Sauckel, Seyss-Inquart, and Streicher. (Göring, however, would cheat the hangman at the end of the trial by swallowing smuggled-in poison in his cell.) Seven men were given prison terms: Dönitz (ten years); Hess (life in prison); Funk (life); Neurath (fifteen years); Raeder (life); von Shirach (twenty years); and Speer (twenty years). The three men acquitted were Fritsche, von Papen, and Schacht.[11]

Numerous additional cases were heard by Allied tribunals at Nürnberg. These included the "Doctors' (or Medical) Case" (December 9, 1946, to August 20, 1947); the "Erhard Milch Case" (January 2, 1947, to April 16, 1947); the "Justices' (or Judges') Case" (March 5, 1947, to December 4, 1947); the "Pohl/WVHA Case" (April 8, 1947, to November 3, 1947); the "Flick Industrial Case" (April 19, 1947, to December 22, 1947); the "I. G. Farben Case" (August 27, 1947, to July 30, 1948); the "Hostage Case" (July 15, 1947, to February 19, 1948); the "Race and Resettlement Case" (October 20, 1947, to March 10, 1948); the "*Einsatzgruppen* Case" (September 29, 1947, to April 9, 1948); the "Krupp Case" (December 8, 1947, to July 31, 1948); and the "Ministries' Case" (January 6, 1948, to April 13, 1949).

Even today, many Americans assume that the Nürnberg trials wrote the final chapter to the twelve-year nightmare that was the Third Reich. Such was not the case. A series of less-publicized American military tribunals also took place. Out of an initial number of 3,887 accused war criminals, 1,672 of them went on trial at the former concentration camp of Dachau. A tribunal for concentration-camp administrators and guards was conducted there from November 1945 through August 1948. It seems cruelly perverse that, out of the tens of thousands of camp

* The fate of Martin Bormann has long been a matter of intense speculation. While some believe that he escaped Berlin and slipped away to South America, a 1972 discovery and a 1998 investigation shed new light on what actually happened to him. Following Hitler's suicide, while attempting to escape the Russian cordon around Berlin, Bormann was caught up in a fierce battle at the Weidendamm Bridge, then barely avoided capture on May 1, 1945, by Russian troops swarming near the Humboldthafen area of Berlin. Shortly thereafter, Bormann and his companion, SS Dr. Ludwig Stumpfegger, probably decided that escape was impossible and apparently committed suicide by taking cyanide. On May 2, their bodies were seen near the Lehrter Stadtbahnhof station by Reich Youth Leader Artur Axmann and buried in shallow graves. During construction in the area in December 1972, two bodies were unearthed. They were identified at the time by dental records as those of Bormann and (likely) Dr. Stumpfegger. In 1998, the Bormann family requested that DNA tests be performed on the remains. A match with a Bormann relative proved that the body was indeed that of Martin Bormann. (BBC News, May 3, 1998)

guards, administrators, and *Kapos* who were involved in the systematic slaughter and persecution of innocent victims of Nazism for twelve years, the victorious Allies could bring to trial less than 4,000 to face justice for their crimes.

Other trials were held at the former KL Dachau. These included: "U.S. v. Josias Waldeck-Pyrmont, et al" (the "Buchenwald trial"); "U.S. v. Martin Gottfried Weiss, et al;" "U.S. v. Dr. Klaus Karl Schilling;" "U.S. v. Alex Bernhard Piorkowski;" "U.S. v. Hans Altfuldisch, et al" (the "Mauthausen trial"); U.S. v. Lauriano Navas, et a (the "Spanish *Kapos* trial"); U.S. v. Erhart Brauny (the "Gardelegen Massacre trial"); and "U.S. v. Valentin Bersin," et al (the "Malmedy Massacre trial").[12]

The trials at Dachau did not conform to customary civilian judicial procedures as practiced in the U.S. and Britain, and were, in fact, akin to military courts-martial, even though not all the accused, such as Ilse Koch, were (or had been) military personnel. Hearsay testimony was allowed, witnesses for the prosecution were paid for their time, and affidavits (written testimony) were permitted, which precluded defense attorneys from cross-examining those who had submitted the affidavits. Further, those on trial were referred to as the "accused" and not "defendants," and there was no presumption of innocence. It was up to

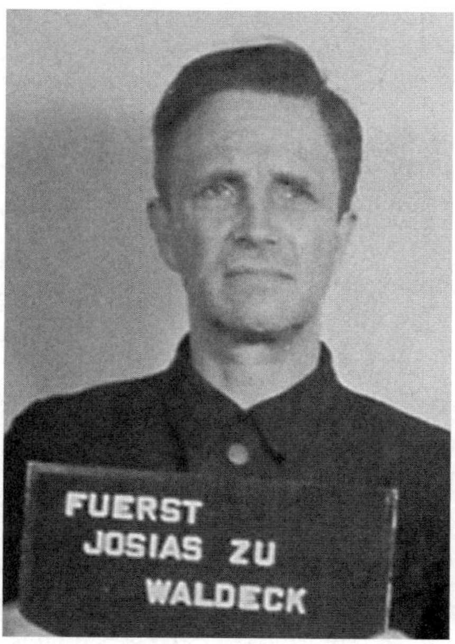

Karl Otto Koch's superior, Josias Erbprinz Waldeck und Pyrmont, the Senior SS and Police Commander for the Fulda-Werra Main SS Territorial Division, whose district included Weimar and Buchenwald (U.S. National Archives)

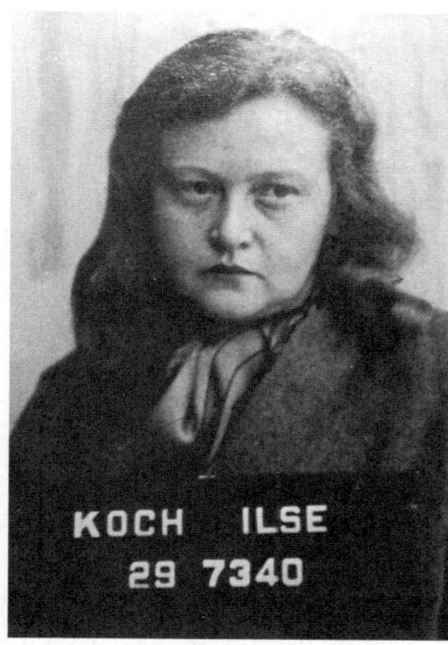

Ilse Koch's "mug shot" (U.S. National Archives)

the accused to prove their innocence, not the duty of the prosecution to prove their guilt. All that was required to prove an accused was guilty was showing that he or she was part of a "common plan," and that he or she had some connection with the place where crimes had been committed.

On April 11, 1947, exactly two years after KL Buchenwald had been liberated, the most sensational of the Dachau trials began. Known officially as *United States v. Josias Erbprinz zu Waldeck-Pyrmont, Case No. 000-50-9* (named for the highest-ranking person on trial, *SS-Obergruppenführer und General der Waffen-SS* Josias Erbprinz zu Waldeck und Pyrmont, the senior SS and police commander for the Fulda-Werra Main Territorial District in whose jurisdiction KL Buchenwald lay), this case brought to court thirty-one defendants who had some association with Buchenwald, including the by-now-notorious Ilse Koch, widow of the first commandant.

The court president was fifty-two-year-old U.S. Army Air Corps Brigadier General Emil Charles Kiel, from Wisconsin; he had previously served as court president of the Dachau war-crimes tribunal. A panel of American military officers, led by Lieutenant Colonel John S. Dwinnell, served as both judge and jury. The prosecutor was William Denson, a former lieutenant colonel.[13]

Only thirty-four, Denson was a seasoned veteran of such tribunals, having previously prosecuted three of them. His conviction rate was one hundred percent. When first assigned to prosecute the atrocious crimes, Denson, a soft-spoken West Point and Harvard Law School graduate from Alabama, was nearly overwhelmed with the duty. "The most difficult part of the trial was trying to present a case that the court would believe," he said, "because the court certainly entertained the same incredulity when they heard my witnesses as I did when I first heard those witnesses. It was absolutely incredible. I didn't believe it. Truthfully, when I was first exposed to this thing, I thought, 'Shucks, innocent people had been mistreated and now they want to come back with a little vengeance.' These stories were just too fantastic, too far out of line for normal behavior.... But when you listen to one witness recite the facts about what happened, and then the next witness testified to the same event, and they didn't have a chance to get together ahead of time and fabricate the stories...you couldn't have gotten two minds to come up with a fantastic set of circumstance that each of them had described separately."

Denson had already served as prosecutor in three war-crimes trials. The first took place in November 1945 with the trial of forty accused former KL Dachau personnel, followed by a trial of sixty-one from Mauthausen (known as the "Altfuldisch trial") then forty-five from Flossenbürg. Although he was on the verge of nervous exhaustion after the Flossenbürg trial, Denson, who had received his discharge from the Army in July 1946 and was working as a civilian prosecutor, was asked if he would prosecute the Buchenwald accused. Despite his mental and physical exhaustion, he agreed.[14]

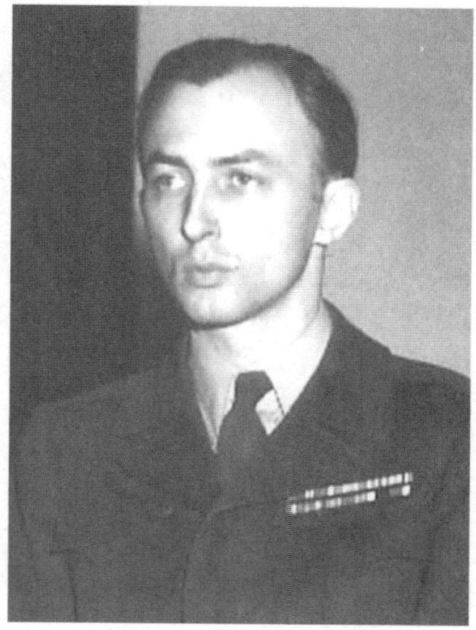

William Denson, war-crimes prosecutor of the accused personnel from KL Buchenwald (U.S. National Archives)

Representing the Buchenwald accused as defense counsel were Major Carl Whitney and Captain Emanuel Lewis. Like all of the tribunal defense attorneys appointed to defend their clients, they had the impossible task of proving that their clients, affiliated with the most evil regime

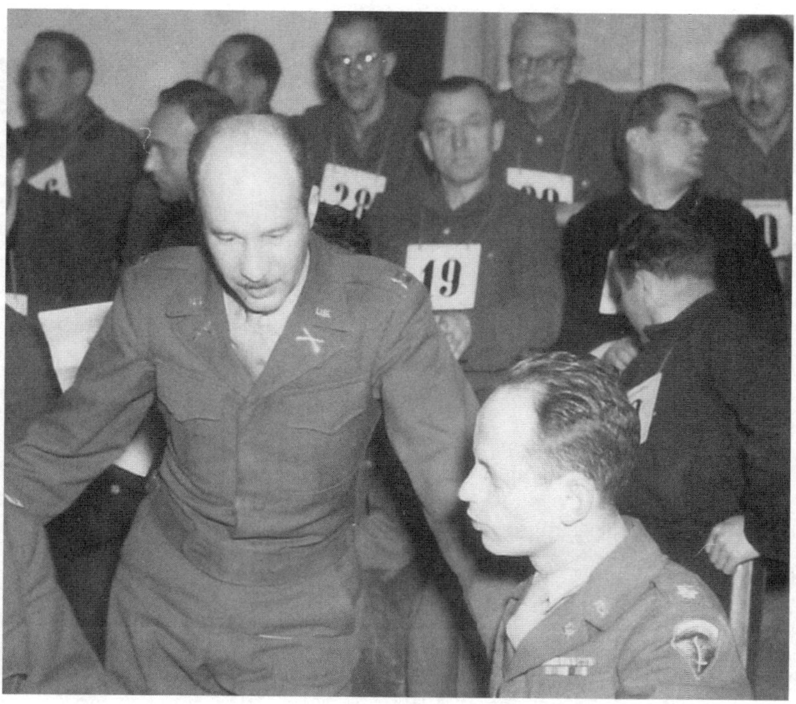

The defense team: Captain Emanuel Lewis (standing) and Major Carl Whitney (U.S. National Archives)

known to recent history and accused of participating in some of the most heinous acts imaginable, were innocent or, at the very least, should be shown leniency by the court.[15]

THE TRIAL OF the Buchenwald accused is covered in considerable detail in the author's *The Beasts of Buchenwald*, so it is unnecessary to go into much detail here. It is sufficient to say that gruesome evidence (a shrunken head, pieces of tattooed human skin, etc.) and a parade of former inmates took the witness stand and, with Denson's expert questioning, all delivered damning testimony about the abuses they saw, heard about, and experienced first-hand that connected the accused to crimes. Lewis and Whitney did their best to poke holes in the testimony, but theirs was a losing battle.

The part of the tribunal that packed the courtroom with reporters and observers was, not surprisingly, Ilse Koch's testimony, for everyone wanted to see and hear the woman whose name had been associated with such horrific crimes. Several months pregnant (she had had a sexual liaison with a fellow prisoner, Fritz Schaffer, at Dachau),[16] she coolly deflected every attempt by

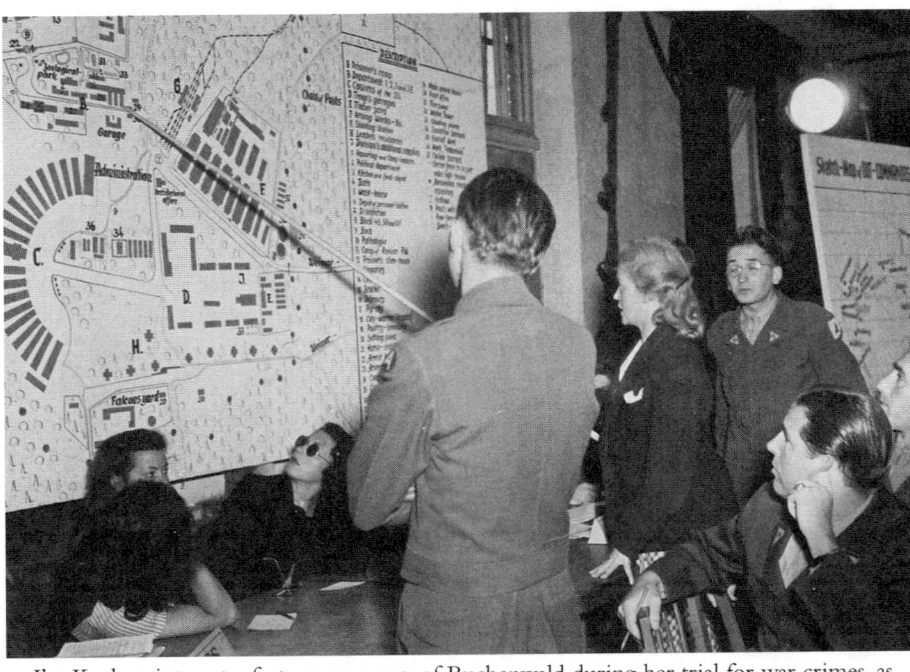

Ilse Koch points out a feature on a map of Buchenwald during her trial for war crimes, as prosecutor William Denson (back to the camera) looks on. (U.S. National Archives)

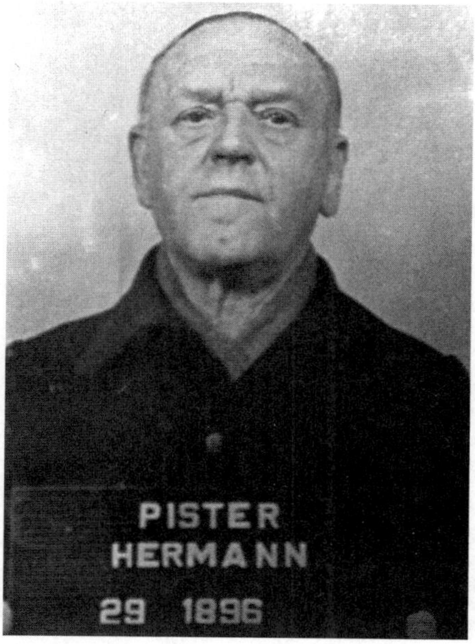

Hermann Pister cheated the hangman by dying of a heart attack. (U.S. National Archives)

Denson to place her at the center of the prisoner abuses, adamantly claiming that she knew nothing about what her husband and the other SS personnel at the camp might have done to the inmates, had never instructed anyone to hurt or humiliate any prisoner, and had never requested that any prisoners with tattoos be killed so that their skin could be turned into objects such as lampshades. She was, she tried to convince the court, nothing more than an innocent wife and mother whose sole duty in life was to look after her little children twenty-four hours a day, seven days a week.[17]

In the end, however, her protestations fell on deaf ears; the testimony of former inmates was just too overwhelming and she, along with the other thirty accused, were found guilty. Many were sentenced to death, and a few even executed, but Ilse was spared the hangman's rope and given life behind bars.*[18]

ON APRIL 23, 1995, Andrew Rosner, a survivor of the Buchenwald sub-camp at Ohrdruf, said to the assembled veterans of the 89th Infantry Division in a ceremony in Wichita, Kansas: "There are those who would tell you World War Two veterans of the 89th Division that what you saw at Ohrdruf and at other camps never happened the way you said it did. The atrocities never happened. The tortures. The hangings. The starvation. The brutality. It never happened and *you never saw it.* They would take your fight for goodness and freedom and call it futile, worthless. Your sacrifices would have no meaning if all that you fought for was

* Due to Cold War politics, in 1948 Ilse's life sentence was commuted by U.S. military authorities to the time already served. Upon her release on October 17, 1949, however, she was arrested by West German authorities and tried for crimes against German citizens. She was again found guilty and sentenced to life. She committed suicide in prison in 1967. (See *The Beasts of Buchenwald*, pp. 252-261)

nothing more than a tale of someone's imaginings. But—we were there. I, the victim. You, the liberators. I, the survivor. You, the witnesses. And together we must, in our golden years on this earth, again do battle with the forces of man's worst evil so that what I saw and you lived through fifty years ago—what we saw—will not be tossed aside as insignificant in the annals of man's history. It *must* be made so important that no one can ever say it didn't happen that way, and therefore they could be allowed to repeat it.

"What you, my liberators, did in 1945 represented all that was good and kind in the world. Had it not been for you, goodness and kindness and compassion would have died. I would have died. A world would have died."[19]

Addressing the same group, Rabbi Murray Kohn, also a survivor of Ohrduf, said: "Fifty years ago, you began the greatest of battles—the battle against the enemies of mankind. You destroyed the Nazi power. You freed the victims of the Nazis. You liberated the world from Fascism.... May God bless you and all of us to secure the final victory over hatred and, as one generation of victims and liberators is slowly fading into eternity, may you as liberators and we, the liberated, be remembered for the price we paid. And may the demons of the Holocaust be forever shunned as moral misfits from our midst and the perpetrators of Nazi tactics today never be forgiven. God bless you all. We shall always remember you for your kindness and humanness."[20]

AS SURPRISING AS it may seem, not all physical traces of the Third Reich have been erased from Europe. It is still possible to visit many places associated with the Hitler regime: the Olympic Stadium in Berlin; the house outside of Berlin where the Wannsee Conference took place; the derelict remains of the huge stadium in Nürnberg where Nazi Party Day rallies were held; the Obersalzburg complex and Hitler's "Tea House" atop the Kehlstein at the Eagle's Nest in Bavaria; Himmler's SS castle known as Wewelsburg outside Paderborn; various military *Kasernen* around the country; flak towers (anti-aircraft gun platforms)—even Hitler's boyhood home and the graves of his parents in Leonding, Austria.

Nor did the camp atop the Ettersberg disappear following the liberation. Once the "zones of occupation" of Germany went into effect, and Weimar found itself on the east side of the "Iron Curtain," the Soviet government turned the camp into a ready-made place for the incarceration, from 1945 to

1950, "of persons who had served the National Socialist regime in an official capacity, but also included victims of arbitrary arrest. Of the approximately 28,000 internees, more than 7,000 died, chiefly as a result of neglect and malnutrition." For all intents and purposes, KL Buchenwald was still alive, although now under new management and in the guise of "Special Camp No. 2."

In 1951, over half of the existing structures at Buchenwald were demolished, and in September 1958, the National Buchenwald Memorial (*Nationale Mahn- und Gedenkstätte Buchenwald*) was established under the auspices of the East German government.

In 1955, a new monumental memorial complex dedicated to the victims of National Socialism replaced the old Bismarckturm on the south slope of the Ettersberg. Below the bell tower, a series of stone pylons along an "Avenue of the Nations" leads visitors to the mass graves and a sculpture of liberated prisoners.[21]

In addition to the Buchenwald Memorial, other remnants of the camps and other places of suffering have been preserved as memorials and as places to remind future generations about the dangers of extremism: Auschwitz-Birkenau, Dachau, Mauthausen, Sachsenhausen, Flossenbürg, Ravensbrück, Theresienstadt, Bergen-Belsen, Natzweiler-Struthof, and Mittelbau-Dora, to name a few. At the sites of other camps that have been torn down, many are marked by a simple memorial.

They are painful places to visit, for one can *almost* see the ranks of abused prisoners standing, terrified, at roll call in their striped uniforms; *almost* hear the shouts of the guards and *kapos* and the barking of dogs; *almost* smell the foul odors of unwashed bodies and decomposing flesh and the stench of the crematorium; *almost* feel the fear in the air. Not everyone can bear the heavy weight of memory, and many a tear has been shed in the parking lots of these places. For those who have the fortitude, however, they are *important* places to visit, for Buchenwald, and the other camps, represent the best and worst of humankind. On one hand they symbolize the depths of depravity to which human beings—guided by a twisted ideology or unrestrained by a moral compass—can sink. On the other hand, they give hope by proving that people can endure the unendurable and triumph over the concerted efforts of others to destroy them.

Buchenwald survivor, author, and recipient of the 1986 Nobel Peace Prize Elie Wiesel has said that only those who actually lived through the Holocaust have the right to represent it in films, books, and plays. We beg to differ, for once the rapidly diminishing ranks of Holocaust survivors are gone, who will carry on and tell the story for future generations?[22]

Sadly, the lessons of history and the Holocaust have been forgotten in the ensuing years as mankind seems bent on its own self-destruction. One need only look at the genocides that have taken place in Cambodia during the Pol Pot regime; the mass murder of the Kurds in Saddam Hussein's Iraq; the "ethnic cleansing" that went on in Serbia-Bosnia-Herzegovina in the mid-1990s; and the mass killings in Darfur and other parts of Africa to realize that humanity has a hard time absorbing the lessons of the past—or doing much to prevent them in the future.

Perhaps, by bringing to light the details of such horrendous examples of "man's inhumanity to man" as perpetrated at Buchenwald and elsewhere, the world can begin to understand how such terrible things can happen and do everything possible—including pre-emptive war—to ensure that they will not happen again.

Like a candle in the wind, however, it is a flickering hope.

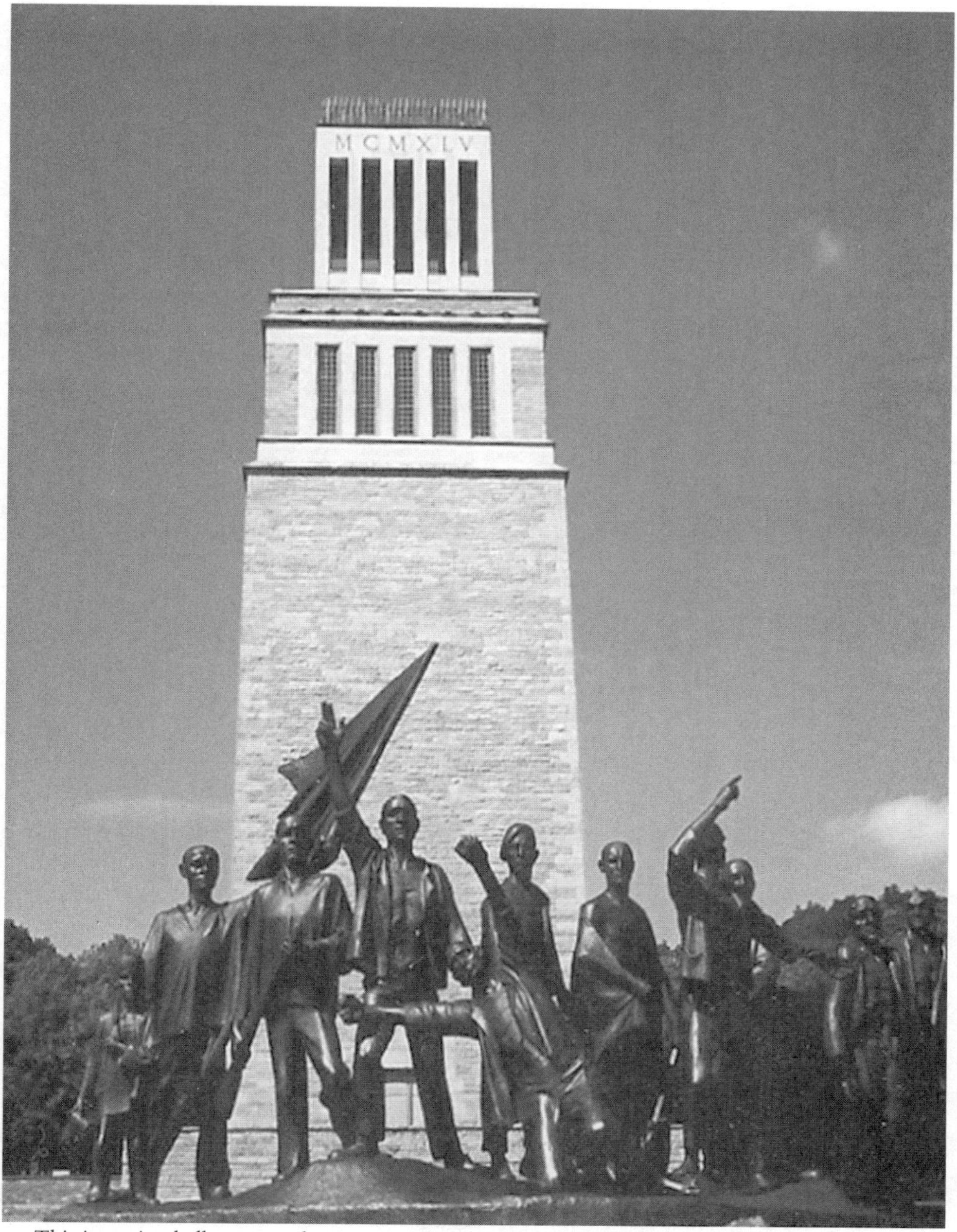

This imposing bell tower and monumental sculpture overlooking the mass graves replaced the Bismarckturm on the south slope of the Ettersberg in 1955. (Author photo)

EPILOGUE

The long line of men and women trudging down the Ettersberg toward their homes in Weimar on April 16, 1945, was uncharacteristically silent with each deep in their own thoughts, yet sharing the same thoughts. What was there to say? No communication was necessary. Occasionally someone sniffled, unable to exorcise the still-too-fresh memories. Then a man half coughed, stifling a groan. Was he regretting his decision to have voluntarily joined in the walk up the Ettersberg earlier that day? At the time, it had seemed like the perfect excuse to finally see how Hitler's Third Reich enemies had been incarcerated.

This day, their senses had been overloaded—brutally bombarded, actually—with too much beyond their perceived realities. Yes, they had all seen the emaciated prisoners wearing their striped pajamas in Weimar, but that was not surprising. They were at war, and food was scarce. They had expected a harsh environment at the Buchenwald Concentration Camp. Instead, they had been inundated with a horror show.

They had begun their journey in an almost festive atmosphere, walking in small groups, with most eager to see their Buchenwald, their beech forest, that had been off-limits for almost eight years. But as they walked closer to the camp they had all known existed, a sense of foreboding slowly washed over them. Some tried to turn back to Weimar but were prodded forward by impatient, unfriendly American soldiers.

Where was the lush forest they remembered? All they could see was barren ground upon which stood ominous buildings, barbed wire, and an imposing gate. And as they approached closer, now walking more hesitantly, a thick, unpleasant smell blanketed everything.

Near the entrance, American soldiers stared at them, their fury barely contained, and thin—horribly thin—inmates with hate-filled eyes watched their every move. Then they were ushered through the gate.

Once inside, there was no escape. Some looked away from the piles of decaying naked corpses, the shrunken heads, the artifacts made from tattooed human skin, the now-cold ovens containing half-burned skeletons, and the ghastly blood-spattered room with the hanging-hooks on the wall, trying to convince themselves that what was on display was nothing more than American propaganda. But even if they refused to look—and believe—they could not escape the groans of dying human beings too ill to climb from their beds. Those groans touched their very souls. Nor could they escape the smell, that terrible smell of blood, feces, rotting flesh, and death… The smell that filled their nostrils and penetrated every pore in their body and every fiber of their clothing.

And their oak! Their beautiful Goethe Oak was now nothing but a blackened stump. *Was it true that Germany would exist only as long as the Goethe Oak stood?*

Their Ettersberg had become a nightmare beyond imagination and many wondered, on that long silent journey back to Weimar, if the Americans would implicate them for what they had just experienced. There were more than a few shudders.

Meals would go untouched that night, and many burned their clothing, but no matter how often they bathed or how vigorously they scrubbed, they could not wash from their bodies—or their memories—the sights, sounds, and smells of Buchenwald. The horror show would never end.

ACKNOWLEDGMENTS

There are so many people to be thanked for their assistance and guidance with this project that I barely know where to begin. Probably the person deserving the most appreciation is someone, per his request, whom I can't name. He asked me to use the pseudonym "Red Triangle" to denote the color of the badge he wore as a political prisoner at Buchenwald. He has spent more than thirty years meticulously researching the concentration camps, specifically Buchenwald and Dachau, correcting the historical record, and exposing persons who have lied or distorted the facts about their involvement in the liberation of the two camps. It is he who started me on this journey over two decades ago with the admonition to tell, as accurately as possible, the story of Buchenwald and its liberation; I have tried to be true to his vision but my only regret is that he wants to avoid the spotlight, which means he won't get the credit he so richly deserves for all his years of exacting, painstaking work.

After Red Triangle comes a long line of others who have contributed in one way or another, and I risk offending them by inadvertently omitting their names. At the head of that line are the liberators and the liberated who allowed me to interview them and/or borrow from their memoirs and letters, or who otherwise provided me with important information—people such as J. Leavitt Anderson, Merrill C. Burgstahler, Don Byers, Joseph J. Geraldi, Leo Laufer, David Israel, Arthur Kinnis, John Ranz, and Mel Rappaport—and all the authors and publishers who permitted me to quote from their works. Words are inadequate to express my gratitude to them, for without their willingness to share their knowledge and experiences, this would be a slim volume indeed.

Many of the photos in this and the other two volumes of the Buchenwald Trilogy came from private sources and have never before been published. For these I thank Alan Bonde, Bernd Schmidt, Louis Gros, Dr. Neal Kahn, John Ranz, Arthur Kinnis, and Neil Fausset. Leslie Keffer Rego, daughter of the first American soldier to set foot in the camp on April 11, 1945, has been extremely gracious in loaning me her late father's photos and letters.

Next I must thank Sabine Stein and everyone at the Buchenwald Memorial archives—which I visited on several occasions—and who, over the years, have been most helpful in my research. Assisting in that effort is my good friend Bernd Schmidt in Weimar who has devoted much of his adult life to doing his own in-depth research about the camp. His friendship and generous help have truly been invaluable, and he has never failed to go out of his way to find and share some arcane piece of information.

Another good friend, Dr. Richard Sommers, recently retired as chief archivist at the U.S. Army Military History Institute in Carlisle, Pennsylvania, and he, too, has been ever ready, willing, and able to guide me through the MHI's vast holdings in search of the photos and documents I needed to help tell the Buchenwald liberation story.

The staff at the National Archives and Records Administration in College Park, Maryland, too, have been extraordinarily helpful over the years during my many research trips there, as were Adair Klein and all the kind people at the Simon Wiesenthal Center and Museum of Tolerance in Los Angeles.

I would also like to thank Cable Publishing's intern, Amanda Brown, for a great job of proofreading.

Of course, Nan Wisherd, my publisher and editor, is owed a lifetime supply of dark chocolate in gratitude for her unflagging enthusiasm for this project.

Finally, the loving support of my wife, Dr. Mary Ann Watson, has never waivered—making it possible for me to fulfill my dream of a career as an author and historian.

Flint Whitlock
Denver, Colorado

SOURCE NOTES

Introduction

1. William L. Shirer, *The Rise and Fall of the Third Reich: A History of Nazi Germany*, New York: Crest, 1964, passim.
2. Eugen Kogon (tr. by Heinz Norden), *The Theory and Practice of Hell: The German Concentration Camps and the System Behind Them*, New York: Berkley, 1984, pp. 60-61.
3. United States Holocaust Memorial Museum, *Historical Atlas of the Holocaust*, New York: Simon & Schuster Macmillian, 1996, passim.

Chapter 1: Hell under Construction

1. *Historical Atlas of the Holocaust*, p. 21; "The Holocaust Just Got More Shocking," *New York Times*, March 1, 2013; Paul Wiseman, "Third Reich's Infrastructure of Horror Far More Widespread Than Thought," *WWII* magazine, July/August 2013, pp. 12-13.
2. Roger Manvell and Heinrich Fraenkel, *Heinrich Himmler: The Sinister Head of the SS and Gestapo*, New York: Skyhorse, 2007, pp. 1-18.
3. Christopher Dillon, "'We'll Meet Again in Dachau': The Early Dachau SS and the Narrative of Civil War." *Journal of Contemporary History*, 45(3), 2010, pp. 535-554.
4. Harry Stein, ed. (tr. Judith Rosenthal), *Buchenwald Concentration Camp 1937-1945: A Guide to the Permanent Historical Exhibition*, Göttingen, Germany: Wallsten Verlag, 2004, p. 25.
5. holocaustresearchproject.org/othercamps/eicke.
6. Erik Larson, *In The Garden of Beasts: Love, Terror, and an American Family in Hitler's Berlin*, New York: Crown, 2011, pp. 211-212.
7. Charles W. Sydnor, Jr., *Soldiers of Destruction: The SS Death's-Head Division, 1933-1945*, Princeton, NJ: Princeton University Press, 1977, p. 23.
8. holocaustresearchproject.org/othercamps/eicke.html.
9. Stein, p. 25.
10. erfurt-web.de/Fritz_Saukel.
11. a.ghearmailt.gd.ogarnig.pl/gd/Weimar.
12. Stein, p. 34.

Chapter 2: The Beasts of Buchenwald

1. Ernst Klee, Willi Dressen, and Volker Riess, eds. *"The Good Old Days": The Holocaust as Seen by Its Perpetrators and Bystanders*. Old Saybrook, CT: Konecky & Konecky, 1988, p. 323; Arthur L. Smith, *Die Hexe von Buchenwald: Der Fall Ilse Koch*. Cologne, Germany: Böhlau Verlag, 1983, pp. 3, 7-18.
2. Flint Whitlock, *The Beasts of Buchenwald: Karl & Ilse Koch, Human-Skin Lampshades, and the War-Crimes Trial of the Century*, Brule, WI: Cable Publishing, 2011, pp. 23-28, 34-40, 49, 54, 67-71.
3. Whitlock, pp. 26-27, 30-32.
4. Stein, p. 92.
5. Jack Van der Geest (with Carol Ordemann), *Was God on Vacation?* self-published, 2002, p. 42.
6. Paul Heinz Victor, *Buchenwald: A Survivor's Memoir*, Tucson, AZ: Wheatmark, 2005, pp. 34-35.
7. *Historical Atlas of the Holocaust*, pp. 22-23; Judith Hemmendinger and Robert Krell. *The Children of Buchenwald: Child Survivors and Their Postwar Lives*, Jerusalem: Gefen Publishing, 2000, p. 48.
8. Van der Geest, p. 42.
9. Sybille Steinbacher, *Auschwitz: A History*, New York: ecco/HarperCollins, 2005, p. 31.
10. Jack Werber, *Saving Children: Diary of a Buchenwald Survivor and Rescuer*, New Brunswick, NJ: Transaction, 1997, p. 49.
11. "United States v. Josias Prince zu Waldeck, et al" ("U.S. v. Waldeck"), trial record, Deputy Judge Advocate's Office, 7708 War Crimes Group, European Command, November 15, 1947, National Archives and Records Administration (NARA), War Crimes Case Files ("Cases Tried") 1945-59, RG-549-000-50-9, Box 437, p. 62.
12. David A. Hackett, ed. and tr., *The Buchenwald Report*. Boulder, CO: Westview, 1995, pp. 338-339; Smith, pp. 36-37; Joshua M. Greene, *Justice at Dachau: The Trials of an American Prosecutor*, New York: Broadway Books, 2003, p. 238.
13. Stein, p. 58; Konrad Morgen testimony, "U.S. v. Waldeck," War Crimes Case Files ("Review and Recommendations of the Deputy Judge Advocate for War Crimes, November 1947"), NARA RG-549-000-50-9, Box 436, p. 2830.
14. Hackett, pp. 62, 217; Smith, p. 39; Stein, pp. 56-57.
15. Whitlock, pp. 67, 100.
16. "U.S. v. Waldeck," War Crimes Case Files ("Cases Tried") 1945-59, NARA, RG-549-000-50-9, Box 437, passim.
17. Stein, pp. 58-59.
18. Paul Grünewald statement, documents related to the Second Trial of Ilse Koch, AG 383 JAG (Lt. Gen. Lucius Clay's report, date missing), NARA RG-549-000-50-9, Box 441.
19. Ilse Koch testimony, "U.S. v. Waldeck," trial transcript, War Crimes Case Files ("Review and Recommendations"), NARA, RG-549-000-50-9, Box 436, pp. 3698-3701, 3724; Smith, pp. 61-62.
20. Kurt Sitte, sworn statement, taken March 9, 1949, "U.S. v. Waldeck," NARA, RG-549-000-50-9, Box 441.
21. Stein, pp. 111-114.
22. Martin Gilbert, *Kristallnacht: Prelude to Destruction*, New York: HarperCollins, 2006, p. 183.
23. Stein, pp. 94-95.
24. Kogon, pp. 91-92.

25. Louis Gros, *Survivor of Buchenwald: My Personal Odyssey through Hell*, Brule, WI: Cable Publishing, 2012, p. 41.
26. Stein, p. 49.

Chapter 3: Chamber of Horrors

1. Stein, p. 37.
2. Sydnor, p. 62.
3. Ibid, p. 30.
4. Sydnor, pp. 37-63; Stein, pp. 37-38; sturmvogel.orbat.com/ss-tk.html.
5. Shirer, pp. 17-823; Martin Gilbert, *The Second World War: A Complete History*, New York: Henry Holt, 1989, pp. 1-30.
6. Shirer, pp. 656-664.
7. Ibid, pp. 791-823.
8. Kogon, 73-80; "U.S. v. Waldeck" ("Review and Recommendations of the Deputy Judge Advocate for War Crimes, November 1947"), Box 436, p. 7.
9. Stein, pp. 93-98.
10. Kogon, pp. 87-88.
11. Werber, p. 71.
12. Kogon, pp. 50-51.
13. Gritz, quoted in Hackett, p. 197.
14. Kogon, p. 106.
15. Stein, pp. 32-33, 95.
16. Kogon, pp. 79-80.
17. Ibid, p. 81.
18. Ibid, p. 109.
19. Gros, pp. 149-151.
20. Kogon, p. 83.

Chapter 4: Turning Men into Monsters

1. Sydnor, p. 23.
2. John P. Sabini and Maury Silver, quoted in Joel E. Dimsdale, *Survivors, Victims, and Perpetrators: Essays on the Nazi Holocaust*, Washington D.C.: Hemisphere, 1980, p. 347.
3. Stein, p. 37.
4. Sydnor, p. 29.
5. Steinbacher, pp. 42-44.
6. Sabini and Silver, quoted in Dimsdale, pp. 329-338.
7. Klee, et al, p. 220.
8. Ibid, pp. 163, 165, 167, 168.
9. Olivia Barbet-Massin, ed., *World War II: The Unseen Visual History*, New York: New Press, 2011, p. 51.
10. Klee, et al, pp. 76-77.
11. Stanley Milgram, *Obedience to Authority: An Experimental View,* New York: Harper & Row, 1974, passim.
12. Philip Zimbardo, "Revisiting the Stanford Prison Experiment: A Lesson in the Power of Situation," *Chronicle of Higher Education*, March 30, 2007.
13. Roger Manvell and Heinrich Fraenkel, *Heinrich Himmler: The Sinister Life of the Head of the SS and Gestapo,* New York: Sky Horse, 2007, pp. 135-137.
14. Peter Padfield, *Himmler: A Full-Scale Biography of One of Hitler's Most Ruthless Executioners*, New York: MjF Books, 1997, p. 551.
15. Ibid p. 300.

Chapter 5: What the World Knew

1. Robert J. Lifton, *The Nazi Doctors: Medical Killing and the Psychology of Genocide*, New York: Basic Books, 2000, p. 131.
2. *Historical Atlas of the Holocaust*, p. 76.
3. Gilbert, *The Second World War,* pp. 198-211.
4. "Slaying of Jews in Galicia Depicted; Deaths Are Put at 15,000," *New York Times*, October 26, 1941.
5. Gilbert, *The Second World War,* p. 226.
6. jewishgen.org/yizkor/Poland/po1001.
7. Gilbert, *The Second World War,* p. 239; history1900s.about.com/od/holocaust/a/babiyar_2.htm.
8. Stein, pp. 43-44, 92.
9. Charles Mullinex, letter to family, April 15, 1945, Bernd Schmidt collection.
10. Mario R. Dederichs, *Heydrich: The Face of Evil*, London: Greenhill, 2006, pp. 134-135; Gilbert, *The Second World War,* p. 292.
11. Gilbert, *The Second World War: A Complete History,* p. 277.
12. Ibid, pp. 273-274.
13. Dederichs, pp. 134-138.
14. Hermann Pister interrogation, "U.S. v. Waldeck," trial transcript, March 4, 1947, NARA, RG-549-000-50-9, Box 437.
15. Stein, p. 43.
16. politische-bildung-rip.de/fileadmin/download/Hinzert-e.
17. "U.S. v. Waldeck," "Review and Recommendations," NARA, RG-549-000-50-9, Box 436, pp. 75-76.
18. "40,000 Here View Memorial to Jews," *New York Times*, March 2, 1942.
19. "Extinction Feared by Jews in Poland," *New York Times,* March 1, 1942.
20. "Over One Million Jews Already Killed by Nazis," *Daily Telegraph* (London), June 25, 1942.
21. Robert Beir (with Brian Josepher), *Roosevelt and the Holocaust*, Fort Lee, NJ: Barricade Books, 2006, pp. 170-174.
22. Jennie Lebel, *The Mufti of Jerusalem: Haj-Amin el-Husseini and National-Socialism*, Belgrade, Serbia: Cigoya Stampa, 2007.
23. Doris Kearns Goodwin, *No Ordinary Time: Franklin and Eleanor Roosevelt—The Home Front in World War II*, New York: Simon & Schuster, 1994, pp. 101-102.
24. Stein, p. 214; Werber, p. 86.
25. Stein, p. 43; *Historical Atlas of the Holocaust*, p. 77.
26. William Manchester, *The Arms of Krupp: 1587-1968*, New York: Bantam, 1982, pp. 545-550.
27. Ibid, p. 558.

28. Benjamin J. Ferencz, *Less than Slaves: Jewish Forced Labor and the Quest for Compensation*, Cambridge, MA: Harvard University Press, 1979, p. 111; Manchester, p. 546.
29. Manchester, p. 567.
30. Ibid, p. 691.
31. "Grim Ghettos," *Newsweek*, August 10, 1942.
32. "Reich Deporting French Jews to 'Polish Silesia,' Report Says." *New York Times*, August 20, 1942.
33. Robert Clary, *From Holocaust to Hogan's Heroes: The Autobiography of Robert Clary*, Lanham, MD: Madison Books, 2001, pp. 61-81.
34. Gilbert, *The Second World War,* pp. 367-371, 374, 377, 398-399.
35. pbs.org/wgbh/amex/holocaust/filmmore/reference/primary/index.html; pbs.org/wgbh/amex/holocaust/peopleevents/pandeAMEX101.html.
36. "Roosevelt Says U.S. Will Join in Investigation of Atrocities," *New York Times*, October 8, 1942; scrapbookpages.com/DachauScrapBook/DachauTrials/Introduction.html.
37. yadvashem.org.il.
38. Gilbert, *The Second World War*, p. 370.
39. Gilbert, *The Second World War*, p. 376.
40. "Himmler Program Kills Polish Jews: Wise Gets Confirmations," *New York Times*, November 25, 1942.
41. Donald McKale, *Hitler's Shadow War: The Holocaust and World War II*, New York: Cooper Square Press, 2002, pp. 394-395.

Chapter 6: The Devil's Doctors

1. Stein, pp. 124-126; Lifton, p. 139.
2. Andre N. Sofair and Lauris C. Kaldjian, "Eugenic Sterilization and a Qualified Nazi Analogy: The United States and Germany, 1930-1945," *Annals of Internal Medicine*, 2000, p. 313.
3. Max Domarus, and Patrick Romane, eds., *The Essential Hitler: Speeches and Commentary*, Wauconda, IL: Bolchazy-Carducci, 2007, pp. 382-383.
4. Shirer, pp. 78, 142-164, 209-210.
5. Lifton, pp. 270-278; Vivien Spitz, *Doctors from Hell: Horrific Account of Nazi Experiments on Humans*, Boulder, CO: Sentient Publications, 2005, pp. 44-45; pbs.org/wgbh/nova/holocaust/experiments.
6. Götz Aly, Peter Chroust, and Christian Pross (tr. by Belinda Cooper), *Cleansing the Fatherland: Nazi Medicine and Racial Hygiene*, Baltimore, MD: Johns Hopkins University Press, 1994, pp. 147-149.
7. pbs.org/wgbh/nova/holocaust/experiments.html.
8. Spitz, pp. 44-45.
9. Lifton, pp. 270-278.
10. Kogon, pp. 153-174; Edwin Black, *War Against the Weak: Eugenics and America's Campaign to Create a Master Race*, New York: Four Walls Eight Windows, 2003, p. 332.
11. Lifton, p. 154.
12. Closing brief, "U.S. v. Karl Brandt, et al.," found at nuremberg.law.harvard.edu.
13. Ibid, Transcript: "U.S. v. Karl Brandt, et al.," found at nuremberg.law.harvard.edu.
14. "Farben is Accused in Typhus Tests: Affidavit from Chief Doctor at Buchenwald Says Concern Knew Prisoners were Used," *New York Times*, November 25, 1947.
15. pbs.org/wgbh/nova/holocaust/experiments.html.
16. Kogon, pp. 149-150.
17. Walter Poller, *Butchers of Buchenwald*, New York: Zebra, 1977, pp. 104-110; Spitz, p. 227.
18. Sydnor, p. 339.
19. "SS Dr. Ding Diary," document 1999-141, date unknown, Simon Wiesenthal Center, Los Angeles.
20. Spitz, pp. 200-201.
21. Kogon, p. 150.
22. Balochowsky testimony, International Military Tribunal, Vol. VI, p. 306, found at avalon.law.yale.edu/imt/o1-29-46.asp.
23. pbs.org/wgbh/nova/holocaust/experiments.html.
24. Poller, pp. 105-105.
25. Spitz, p. 229.
26. Ibid, pp. 227-228.
27. Kogon, p. 144.
28. Closing arguments, "U.S. v. Karl Brandt, et al.," found at nuremberg.law.harvard.edu.
29. Ibid.
30. Ibid.
31. Robert Fisk, "Butcher of Buchenwald in an Egyptian Paradise," *The Independent* (London), August 7, 2010.
32. Kogon, pp. 147-168.
33. Florence Tamagny, *A History of Homosexuality in Europe: Berlin, London, Paris 1919-1939,* New York: Algora, 2004, p. 210.
34. dachaukzblogspot.com/2011/11/Buchenwald-kz-1937-1945-part-1.
35. Tamagny, p. 424; Guenther Grau, *Hidden Holocaust? Gay and Lesbian Persecution in Germany, 1933-1945,* London: Cassell & Cie., 1993, pp. 282-284; Richard Plant, *The Pink Triangle: The Nazi War Against Homosexuals*, New York: Macmillan, 1988, pp. 175-178.
36. pbs.org/wgbh/nova/holocaust/experiments.html; Spitz, pp. 115-134.
37. Transcript: "U.S. v. Karl Brandt, et al.," found at nuremberg.law.harvard.edu.
38. "U.S. v. Waldeck," War Crimes Case Files ("Review and Recommendations"), NARA, RG-549-000-50-9, Box 436, p. 8.
39. "Conduct of the Ilse Koch War Crimes Trials, Hearings Before the Investigations Subcommittee of the Committee on Expenditures in the Executive Departments," NARA, RG-549-000-50-9, Box 426, p. 1070.

Chapter 7: The Demented Doctor

1. Edwin Black, found at hnn.us/articles/1796.
2. Black, pp. 319-335.
3. Kogon, p. 160.

Chapter 8: Super Weapons

1. Manvell and Fraenkel, p. 223.
2. Gilbert, *The Second World War*, pp. 390, 392, 398, 405.
3. Michael J. Neufeld, *Von Braun: Dreamer of Space, Engineer of War*, New York: Knopf, 2007, passim; history.msfc.nasa.gov/vonbraun/bio.html.
4. Yves Béon, *Planet Dora: A Memoir of the Holocaust and the Birth of the Space Age*, Boulder, CO: Westview, 1997, X-XI, Neufeld, pp. 80-114.
5. Neufeld, passim.
6. Zebu.uoregon.edu/~js/space/lectures/lec04.
7. Stein, pp. 134-151.
8. Werber, p. 57.
9. Stein, p. 204.
10. U.S. National Archives news release, January 29, 2000.
11. "V-2 Plant Survivors Publicize Their Story," *Huntsville* (AL) *Times*, February 28, 2000.
12. Neufeld, passim.
13. Norman Davies, *No Simple Victory: World War II in Europe, 1939-1945*, New York: Viking, 2007, pp. 25, 110-112; Gilbert, *The Second World War*, pp. 441-442.
14. Davies, pp. 111-112.
15. Albert Speer. *Inside the Third Reich*, New York: Avon, 1970, pp. 471-472.
16. Pierre Julitte, *Block 26: Sabotage at Buchenwald*. Garden City, NY: Doubleday, 1971, pp. 149-181.
17. Gilbert, *The Second World War*, pp. 446, 448, 451.
18. Ibid, p. 453.
19. Neufeld, pp. 153-156; Gilbert, *The Second World War*, p. 453; astronautix.com/Astros/thialter.htm.
20. Speer, p. 474.
21. Béon, pp. XII-XVI.
22. "V-2 Plant Survivors Publicize Their Story," *Huntsville Times*, February 28, 2000.
23. Béon, pp. V-XII; Julitte, p. 179; Brochure: "The Mittelbau-Dora Concentration Camp," publication no. T-1021.
24. ushmm.org/wlc/en/?ModuleId=10005143.
25. Speer, p. 467.
26. Béon, pp. XIV-XV.
27. perso.orange.fr/d-d.natanson/dora.
28. Stein, p. 212.
29. 80th Infantry Division G-1 Journal, April 1945; lodging-germany.com/info/ Weimar.
30. Bill Yenne, *Big Week: Six Days that Changed the Course of World War II*. New York: Berkley Caliber, 2012, passim.
31. Béon, p. XII.
32. Ernst Stuhlinger and Frederick I. Ordway III, *Wernher von Braun, Crusader for Space: A Biographical Memoir*. Malabar, FL: Krieger, 1994, p. 44.

Chapter 9: Official Indifference

1. Beir, p. 201.
2. "Action—Not Pity—Can Save Millions Now!" (Advertisement), *New York Times*, February 8, 1943.
3. "Save Doomed Jews, Huge Rally Pleads," *New York Times*, March 2, 1943.
4. Editorial, "Sanctuary for Europe's Jews," *New York Times*, March 3, 1943.
5. "40,000 Here View Memorial to Jews," *New York Times*, March 10, 1943; David S. Wyman, *The Abandonment of the Jews: America and the Holocaust, 1941-1945*, New York: The New Press, 1998, p. 91; Beir, pp. 201-202.
6. Beir, pp. 201-204.
7. Doris Kearns Goodwin, p. 173.
8. pbs.org/wgbh/amex/holocaust/Peopleevents/pandeAMEX101.html.

Chapter 10: Buchenwald, Inc.

1. S. Jonathan Wiesen, "German Industry and the Third Reich: Fifty Years of Forgetting and Remembering," *Dimensions: A Journal of Holocaust Studies*, Vol. 13, No. 2, Braun Holocaust Institute.
2. ushmm.org/wlc/article.php?lang=en&Moduleld.
3. "Trials of the War Criminals before the Nurnberg Military Tribunals under Control Council Law No. 10," Nurnberg, October 1946-April 1949, Col. V (Oswald Pohl trial).
4. Shirer, p. 1258.
5. Michael Thad Allen, *The Business of Genocide: The SS, Slave Labor, and the Concentration Camps*, Chapel Hill, NC: University of North Carolina Press, 2002, p. 1.
6. M.T. Allen, pp. 1-2; Stein, p. 145.
7. "Nazi Conspiracy and Aggression, Vol. IV," Document No. 2171-PS.
8. Stein, pp. 144-145.
9. Werber, pp. 71-72.
10. Stein, p. 140.
11. Ibid, pp. 141-142.
12. "U.S. v. Waldeck," War Crimes Case Files ("Review and Recommendations"), NARA, RG-549-000-50-9, Box 436, p. 5.
13. Julitte, pp. 214-215.
14. Stephen E. Ambrose, *D-Day, June 6, 1944: The Climactic Battle of World War II*. New York: Simon and Schuster, 1994, passim.
15. Basil Liddell Hart, *History of the Second World War*, New York: G.P. Putnam's Sons, 1970, p. 550.
16. Gros, pp. 36-37.
17. Ibid, p. 95.
18. Ibid, pp. 98-99.
19. Ferencz, pp. 110-111.

20. "Ford Motor Co. Charged in Nazi Secret Profits on Slave Labor," *The Daily Republican*, March 18, 1998.

21. Stein, p. 204.

22. Julitte, pp. 198-252.

23. Hackett, pp. 322-323; Stein, pp. 215, 227; Red Triangle monograph, "Mystery of the Buchenwald S.O.S. Message."

24. Stein, pp. 207-216; Kogon, pp. 255-273, 278.

25. Stein, pp. 213-214; Red Triangle letters to author, May 25, 1998, September 4, 1998, September 14, 1998, January 20, 1999.

26. Stein, pp. 210-216.

27. Ibid, pp. 212-213.

28. Stein, p. 212; Gros, pp. 95-101.

Chapter 11: The Little Children Suffer

1. Werber, pp. 95, 99.
2. Gilbert, *The Boys: The Untold Story of 732 Young Concentration Camp Survivors.* New York: Henry Holt, 1996, p. 186.
3. Ibid, pp. 189-190.
4. Werber, pp. 95-104.
5. Gros, p. 101.
6. Manchester, pp. 607, 613; Ferencz, pp. 94-96.

Chapter 12: The End Nears

1. "Jewish Rally Urges Gas Attacks on Nazis," *New York Times*, June 20, 1942.
2. Julitte, p. 271.
3. Gros, pp. 56-57.
4. David Glantz (tr.), and Harold Orenstein (tr.), *Belorussia 1944: The Soviet General Staff Study.* London: Routledge, 2001, p. 176.
5. Ian Kershaw, *The End: The Defiance and Destruction of Hitler's Germany, 1944-1945*, New York: Penguin, 2011, p. 92.
6. *Historical Atlas of the Holocaust*, p. 208.
7. Shirer, pp. 1356-1402.
8. Domarus, p. 14; Shirer, pp. 1316-1405; Stein, pp. 195-198; Gilbert, *The Second World War*, pp. 555-559.
9. Stein, pp. 168-169; Domarus, p. 14; Julitte, p. 291; "Nazi Conspiracy and Aggression," Vol. IV, Document No. 2171-PS.
10. Flint Whitlock, *Given Up for Dead: American GIs in the Nazi Concentration Camp at Berga*, Boulder, CO: Westview, 2005, pp. 131-149.

Chapter 13: No Place for a Princess

1. Stein, pp. 195-198.
2. "U.S. v. Waldeck," War Crimes Case Files ("Review and Recommendations"), Box, 436, p. 4.
3. Stein, pp. 196-198.
4. "Princess Mafalda Reported Killed," *New York Times*, April 25, 1945.
5. S. Gelichi, "Remembrance of Otto of Hesse," *Journal of Archaeology*, 1997, pp. 3-4.
6. "Princess Mafalda Reported Killed," *New York Times*, April 25, 1945.
7. "[Pulitzer] Urges Executions of 1,500,000 Nazis," *New York Times*, May 23, 1945.
8. "Princess Mafalda Reported Killed," *New York Times*, April 25, 1945; answers.com/topic/princess-mafalda-of-savoy; themrsastor.blogspot.com /2006/08/reflective-Sundays.html; reference.com/ browse/wiki/Prince_Philip_of_Hesse-Kassel.

Chapter 14: Fallen to Earth

1. Arthur G. Kinnis and Stanley A. Booker, *168 Jump into Hell*, Victoria, Canada: self-published, 1999, pp. 2-28.
2. Justin Skinner, "Remembering Buchenwald: Forest Hill Collegiate students hear a survivor's story," insidetoronto.com, November 10, 2010.
3. Kinnis, p. 42; Hackett, p. 123.
4. M.R.D. Foote, *SOE: The Special Operations Executive 1940-1946.* London: Greenwood/BBC Books, 1984, passim.
5. Christopher Burney, *The Dungeon Democracy,* New York: Duell, Sloan and Pearce, 1946, p. 83.
6. Kinnis, p. 42.
7. Hackett, p. 123.
8. Kinnis, p. 175; David Stafford, *Endgame, 1945: The Missing Final Chapter of World War II,* New York: Little, Brown and Company, 2007, pp. 56-57.

Chapter 15: Mission 132

1. Joseph J. Geraldi, interview by author, November 15, 2011; wymaninstitute.org/letters/2002-12-24-failure.
2. Geraldi, interview by author, November 15, 2011.
3. "Report of Operational Day Mission No. 132, 24 August 1944, 94th Combat Bomb Wing, 401st Bombardment Group (H)," provided to author by Don Byers.
4. Geraldi, interview by author, November 15, 2011.
5. Kinnis, p. 34.
6. Gros, pp. 111-113.
7. Kinnis, pp. 34-35.
8. Gros, pp. 114-115.
9. Rolf Kralovitz (trans. by Eva R. Cohn), *TenZeroNinety in Buchenwald: A Jewish Prisoner Tells His Story,* Cologne, Germany: Walter-Meckauer-Kreis, 1998, pp. 56-57.
10. Gilbert, *The Boys*, p. 189.
11. Benedict D'Agostini Papers, 615th Bomb Squadron Collection, Army Air Force Section, World War II Survey, Archives, USAMHI.
12. Kinnis, p. 65.
13. Gros, pp. 115-116.
14. Kinnis, p. 85.

15. Ibid, p. 36.
16. Ibid, p. 120.
17. Kogon, p. 278.
18. scrapbookpages.com/BuchenwaldResistance.
19. "Princess Mafalda Reported Killed," *New York Times*, April 25, 1945; "Nazis Killed Boris, Princess Related," *New York Times*, May 23, 1945; answers.com/topic/princess-mafalda-of-savoy; themrsastor.blogspot.com/2006/08/reflective-Sundays.html.
21. Stein, p. 205.
22. *Thüringer Gauzeitung*, August 27, 1944.
23. Julitte, p. 189.

Chapter 16: Life in the Ruins

1. Stein, p. 227.
2. vcalc.net/cu-bckup.
3. Speer, p. 472; v2rocket.com.
4. Kinnis, p. 34.
5. Ibid, p. 124.
6. Ibid, pp. 37-39.
7. Ibid, p. 33.
8. Ibid, p. 41.
9. Stein, pp. 174-175.
10. Kinnis, p. 43.
11. Padfield, p. 547.
12. *Historical Atlas of the Holocaust*, pp. 200-201.
13. Kinnis, p. 93; Joe Moser and Gerald Baron, *A Fighter Pilot in Buchenwald,* Bellingham, WA: Edens Veil Media, 2009, pp. 123-124.
14. Ibid, pp. 45-46.

Chapter 17:
The Beginning of the End

1. Gilbert, *The Second World War*, pp. 570, 576, 593.
2. Manvell and Fraenkel, pp. 78, 100.
3. Ibid, pp. 198-200.
4. Gilbert, *The Second World War*, pp. 590-591; zplac2b.com/464th/sortie.htm.
5. Jack Fishman, *And the Walls Came Tumbling Down: The Secret World War II Allied Operation that Saved D-Day and Unleashed the Greatest Mass Prison Escape in History*, New York: MacMillan, 1983, pp. 250-251; pbs.org/wgbh/amex/holocaust/filmmore/reference/primary/bombjohn.htm.
6. jewishvirtuallibrary.org/jsource/Holocaust/natzweiler.html.
7. "Alsace Nazi Prison Neat and Efficient," *New York Times*, December 5, 1944.
8. "U.S. Board Bares Atrocity Details Told by Witnesses at Polish Camps," *New York Times*, November 26, 1944.
9. Hugh M. Cole, *U.S. Army in World War II: The European Theater of Operations. The Ardennes: Battle of the Bulge*, Washington, DC: Center of Military History, 1995, passim.
10. Stein, p. 137.
11. Daniel Blatman (tr. by Chaya Galai), *The Death Marches: The Final Phase of Nazi Genocide,* Cambridge, MA: Belknap/Harvard, 2011, pp. 1, 137.
12. *Historical Atlas of the Holocaust*, pp. 204-209.
13. Blatman, p. 59.
14. "U.S. v. Waldeck," War Crimes Case Files ("Review and Recommendations"), NARA, RG-549-000-50-9. Box 436, p. 5.
15. Gros, pp. 135-138.
16. Blatman, p. 102.
17. McKale, pp. 258-260.
18. Gilbert, *The Second World War*, p. 633.
19. Ibid, p. 634.
20. Ibid, p. 634.
21. Kershaw, *The End*, passim.
22. Gilbert, *The Second World War*, p. 638; Michael E. Haskew, ed., *The World War II Desk Reference*, New York: HarperCollins, 2004, p. 378; David M. Kennedy, ed., *The Library of Congress World War II Companion,* New York: Simon & Schuster, 2007, pp. 406-407; Kershaw, *The End*, p. 246.
23. Stein, p. 224; Blatman, p. 97.
24. Clary, p. 61.
25. Ibid, pp. 94-96.
26. John Ranz, *Inhumanity: Death March to Buchenwald and the Last Jews of Bendzin*, Bloomington, IN: AuthorHouse, 2007, pp. 47-48.
27. 8thafhs.org/combat1945.htm.
28. 487thbg.org/Stories/JackFishman StanleyLog1945.
29. "U.S. v. Waldeck," War Crimes Case Files ("Review and Recommendations"), NARA, RG-549-000-50-9, Box 436, pp. 12, 20.
30. "*Luft-terror gegen Weimar: Mehr als 330 Tot*," *Thüringer Gauzeitung*, February 15, 1945.
31. Clary, p. 96.
32. Ranz, pp. 50-51.
33. Herbert Hömig (Dietrich Grille and August-Wilhelm Kaiser, eds.), "*Thüringen unter dem Nationalsozialismus*," *Kultur und Geschichte Thüringens*, Stiftung Thüringen, Wiesbaden, Germany: Druckerei am Parkfeld, 1990, p. 19.
34. Stein, p. 253.
35. Blatman, pp. 105, 131-132.
36. Stein, p. 224.
37. Clary, pp. 83-101.
38. Gilbert, *The Boys*, pp. 193-195.
39. Ranz, pp. 60-61.

Chapter 18:
Third Army to the Rescue

1. Charles B. MacDonald, *U.S. Army in World War II: The European Theater of Operations, The Last Offensive*, Washington, DC: Center of Military History, 1993, pp. 322-324.
2. Ibid, pp. 185-220.

3. Kershaw, *The End*, pp. 203-204, 210-211, 250, 270.
4. Blatman, pp. 138-140.
5. Gilbert, *The Second World War*, pp. 649-650.
6. Shelby L. Stanton, *World War II Order of Battle*, New York: Galahad, 1984, passim.
7. MacDonald, *The Last Offensive*, pp. 36-37, 376.
8. *Armored Attacker*, April 4, 1945.
9. Blatman, pp. 144-145.
10. Gilbert, *The Second World War*, p. 651.
11. Gilbert, *The Second World War*, pp. 651-652; MacDonald, *The Last Offensive*, pp. 298-300.
12. Gilbert, *The Second World War*, p. 637-658.
13. Manvell and Fraenkel, p. 224.
14. Manvell and Fraenkel, p. 224, 233-234; Blatman, pp. 139, 166.
15. Manvell and Fraenkel, p. 225.
16. Robert W. Grow, interview by Hollis Alpert, April 23, 1945, USAMHI.
17. Stanton, pp. 159-163.
18. Charles B. MacDonald, *The Mighty Endeavor: American Armed Forces in the European Theater in World War II*, New York: Oxford University Press, 1969, pp. 373-378.
19. George S. Patton Jr., *War As I Knew It*, Boston: Houghton Mifflin, 1947, pp. 279-280; MacDonald, *The Mighty Endeavor*, p. 477.

Chapter 19: Ordeal at Ohrdruf

1. MacDonald, *The Mighty Endeavor*, p. 477; bach-cantatas.com/Tour/Ohrdruf.htm.
2. "Division Finds Underground Nazi HQ," *The Rolling W*, April 12, 1945; Stein, pp. 182-183, 226, 233.
3. greyfalcon.us/Located%20near%20Ohrdruf.htm.
4. Stein, pp. 182-183.
5. Greunuß testimony, U.S. v. War Crimes Case Files ("Review and Recommendations"), trial transcript, NARA, RG-549-000-50-9, Box 436; Stein, p. 254.
6. "*Raketen in Thüringen*," *Frankfurter Allgemeine Zeitung*, October 27, 2002; forum.axishistory.com; werewolf.greyfalcon.us/Ohrdruf.html.
7. Klaus Wiegrefe, "*Wie nah war Hitler an die A-Bombe?*" *Der Spiegel*, March 14, 2005.
8. Robert S. Allen, *Lucky Forward: The History of Patton's Third U.S. Army*, New York: Vanguard Press, 1947, pp. 371-372.
9. Albert Kesselring, *The Memoirs of Field-Marshal Kesselring*, London: Greenhill, 2007, p. 369.
10. gtgj.de.
11. Blatman, pp. 1, 137-138, 143-144, 172-173.
12. Stein, p. 227.
13. Kershaw, p. 331.
14. Stein, p. 229.
15. Ibid, p. 227.
16. Werber, p. 104.
17. Stein, p. 227.
18. Smith, p. 95; Hackett, p. 337.
19. Leo Laufer, interview by author, December 20, 2006.
20. jewishvirtuallibrary.org/jsource/biography/ jabotinsky.html.
21. Leo Laufer, interview by author, December 20, 2006.
22. Ibid.
23. Laufer memoir.
24. Murray Kohn, speech, April 23, 1995, draft in 89th Infantry Division Society folder, WWII-7781, USAMHI.
25. Laufer memoir.
26. Kogon, p. 274.
27. Werner Fricke testimony, April 16, 1947, "U.S. v. Waldeck," War Crimes Case Files ("Review and Recommendations"), NARA, RG-549-000-09-50, Box 435.
28. Blatman, p. 145.
29. Kohn speech, April 23, 1995.
30. Andrew Rosner, speech, April 23, 1995, draft in 89th Infantry Division Society folder, WWII-7781, USAMHI.

Chapter 20: Evacuating Buchenwald

1. Stein, p. 227.
2. Ibid, pp. 227, 230-231.
3. Ibid, p. 227, Werber, pp. 105-107.
4. Ranz, p. 69.
5. Stein, p. 227.
6. Ranz, pp. 69-70.
7. Stein, p. 227.
8. Stein, pp. 227-228; Kogon, p. 284.
9. "Red Triangle," monograph: "The Train Ride into Hell," January 27, 1998.
10. Werber, p. 105.
11. Manvell and Fraenkel, p. 225; Gilbert, *The Boys*, pp. 196-223.
12. Hackett, pp. 322-323.
13. "Red Triangle," monograph: "The Mystery of the Buchenwald S.O.S. Message," May 29, 1998.
14. Stein, p. 227.
15. "Red Triangle," monograph: "The Mystery of the Buchenwald S.O.S. Message," May 29, 1998.

Chapter 21: Overrunning Ohrdruf

1. Patton, p. 284.
2. Jesse Harris memoirs, USAMHI.
3. After-action Report, Combat Command A, 4th Armored Division, April 1945, USAMHI.
4. Harris memoirs; War Diary of the 3rd Battalion, 355th Infantry Regiment, U.S. Army Military History Institute.
5. Rosner speech.
6. Laufer memoir.

7. J. Leavitt Anderson, interview by author, November 7, 2007.
8. Message, G-2, 4th Armored Division to VIII Corps, April 5, 1945, USAMHI.
9. Message, VIII Corps to Third Army, April 5, 1945, USAMHI.
10. Laufer memoir.
11. 89infdivww2.org/ohrdruf/ohrdrufintro.htm.
12. Sol R. Brandell memoir, USAMHI.
13. "The 89th Infantry Division 1942-1945," Washington, DC: *Infantry Journal*, 1947, p. 129.
14. Stanley N. Hodson, letter to the editor, *Lewiston* (ME) *Journal*, April 13, 1945, USAMHI.
15. Bruce Nickols, found at remember.org/witness/ohrdruf.html.
16. Ralph G. Cole memoir, found at 89infdivww2.org/memories/forgottencole.htm.
17. Wencie Higuera questionnaire, USAMHI.
18. William F. Charboneau Jr. questionnaire, USAMHI.
19. remember.org/witness/ohrdruf.html.
20. Bruce Nickols, found at remember.org/witness/ohrdruf.html.
21. Michael Hirsh, *The Liberators: America's Witnesses to the Holocaust*, New York: Bantam, 2010, p. 31.
22. 89infdivww2.org/ohrdruf/gram4.htm.
23. After-action Report, CCA, 4th Armored Division, quoted in Earl F. Ziemke, *U.S. Army Historical Series: The U.S. Army in the Occupation of Germany 1944-1946,* Washington, DC: Center of Military History, 1990, pp. 231-232.
24. Hayden A. Sears report, CCA, 4th Armored Division, April 1945, USAMHI.
25. Ziemke, pp. 231-232.

Chapter 22: The Liberation of Buchenwald

1. "U.S. v. Waldeck," War Crimes Case Files ("Review and Recommendations"), NARA, RG-548-000-09-50, Box 436, p. 36.
2. "21,000 Prisoners are Liberated by Division at Buchenwald," *Armored Attacker*, May 5, 1945; "Red Triangle," monograph: "The Alleged Discovery of Buchenwald by Two French 'GIs,'" June 1, 2000.
3. Ranz, pp. 71-72.
4. buchenwald.de/en/473.
5. Stein, p. 232.
6. Clary, p. 102.
7. "Red Triangle," letters to author, May 25, 1998, September 4, 1998, September 14, 1998, January 20, 1999; Stein, pp. 213-214.
8. library5.gl.lit.edu/frames.asp? page+feuer&ext+_t.
9. "Red Triangle," letters to author, May 25, 1998, September 4, 1998, September 14, 1998, January 20, 1999.
10. Stein, p. 232.
11. Clary, p. 102.
12. "Red Triangle," letters to author, September 4, 1998, January 20, 1999.
13. Eliezer ("Elie") Wiesel, *Night*, New York: Hill and Wang, 1985, pp. 135-136.
14. "Red Triangle," letters to author, May 25, 1998, September 4, 1998, September 14, 1998, January 20, 1999; Stein, pp. 232-233; Gros letter to author, November 15, 2012.
15. "Four 9th AIB Doughs Find Buchenwald," *Armored Attacker*, May 5, 1945.
16. "Red Triangle," letter to author, June 4, 2007.
17. Stein, p. 232
18. "Red Triangle," letter to author, August 3, 2001.
19. "Red Triangle," letters to author, December 19, 1997, May 25, 1998.
20. Operations Report, Combat Team 9, 9th Armored Infantry Battalion, CCA, 6th Armored Division, April 1945, USAMHI.
21. Fredric Keffer, letter to Maurice Bolle, provided to author by his daughter, Leslie Keffer Rego, May 5, 1975.
22. Gros, p. 172.
23. Keffer, letter to Bolle, May 5, 1975.
24. "Red Triangle," letter to author, June 4, 2007; Operations Report, CT 9, 9th Armored Infantry Battalion, 6th Armored Division, April 1945, USAMHI.
25. Ranz, p. 73.
26. "Red Triangle," letter to George P. Hofmann, 6th Armored Division historian, December 7, 1972.
27. Clary, p. 103.
28. Ranz, p. 74.
29. "3,048 French Dead Found in Nazi Camp; 900 Slain Near Weimar," *New York Times*, April 15, 1945.
30. "Nordhausen: A Hell Factory Worked by the Living Dead," *Newsweek*, April 23, 1945.

Chapter 23: The Surrender of Weimar

1. 80th Infantry Division G-3 Journal, April 12, 1945, USAMHI.
2. Howard E. Congdon, memoir, USAMHI.
3. "Prison Camp is Overrun; 20,000 Political Captives are Found at Buchenwald," *New York Times*, April 13, 1945; "Big Prison Camp Uncovered," *New York Herald Tribune*, April 13, 1945.
4. 80th Infantry Division G-3 Journal, April 12, 1945, USAMHI.
5. Michael Korda, *Ike: An American Hero*, New York: HarperCollins, 2007, pp. 567-573; Dwight D. Eisenhower, *Crusade in Europe*, Garden City, NY: Doubleday, 1948, p. 401; George C. Marshall, *The War Reports of General George C. Marshall, General Henry H. Arnold, and Admiral Ernest J. King: Biennial Report of the Chief of Staff of the United States Army to*

the Secretary of War, July 1, 1943-June 30, 1945, Philadelphia: J.B. Lippincott, 1947, p. 194.

6. 3rd [Army] Takes Weimar Without One Shot; 80th Division Leader Brings About Surrender of Historic German City," *New York Times*, April 12, 1945.
7. "Red Triangle," letter to author, December 19, 1997.
8. Hemmendinger and Krell, p. 21.
9. Ibid, p. 116.
10. Ibid, p. 138.
11. "Lau Recalls Liberation as Child at Buchenwald," *Jerusalem Post*, April 10, 1995.
12. 80th Infantry Division G-1 Journal, April 1945, USAMHI.
13. "U.S. v. Waldeck," War Crimes Case Files ("Review and Recommendations"), NARA, RG-549-000-09-50, Box 436, p. 7.

Chapter 24: Ike at Ohrdruf

1. "President Roosevelt is Dead," *New York Times*, April 13, 1945.
2. Mel Rappaport, letter to author, November 17, 2007.
3. Charles R. Codman, *Drive*, Boston: Little, Brown, 1957, p. 281.
4. Patton, pp. 292-294.
5. Codman, pp. 281-283.
6. Carlo D'Este, *Patton: A Genius for War*, New York: HarperCollins, 1995, pp. 720-721.
7. Eisenhower, *Crusade in Europe*, pp. 408-409.
8. Omar N. Bradley, *A Soldier's Story*, Chicago: Rand McNally, 1951, p. 539.
9. Hobart R. Gay papers, USAMHI.
10. Codman, pp. 281-283.
11. Robert H. Abzug, *Inside the Vicious Heart: Americans and the Liberation of Nazi Concentration Camps*, New York: Oxford University Press, 1985, p. 19.
12. Peter Belpulsi, Richard Lukehart, Norman Sue memoirs, USAMHI.
13. Harry C. Butcher, *My Three Years with Eisenhower,* New York: Simon and Schuster, 1946, p. 803.
14. Eisenhower, letter to George C. Marshall, April 14, 1945, Eisenhower Presidential Library, Abilene KS.
15. Eisenhower, *Crusade in Europe*, p. 409.
16. Laufer, memoir.

Chapter 25: Patton at Buchenwald

1. Codman, pp. 283-290.
2. Patton, p. 301.
3. bbc.co.uk/ww2peoplewar/stories/86/a3940986.shtml.
4. Patton, p. 293; Stanley P. Hirshson, *General Patton: A Soldier's Life*, New York: HarperCollins, 2000, p. 628; "Nazi Death Factory Shocks Germans on Forced Tour," *New York Times*, April 18, 1945.
5. Patton, pp. 298-299.
6. Patton, letter to Eisenhower, April 15, 1945, copy in Eisenhower Presidential Library, Abilene, KS.
7. Andrea and Erich Kloss papers, Weimar City Archives, File 54 4-01/1.
8. "Arriving at Buchenwald," *Concord* (NH) *Monitor,* October 25, 2007.
9. Stein, pp. 237-238; Medical Department Activities Report, 120th Evacuation Hospital Semi-Mobile, June 10, 1945, found at buchenwaldandbeyond.com/history/headquarters.htm.
10. Stein, p. 240.
11. Medical Department Activities Report, 120th Evacuation Hospital Semi-Mobile, June 10, 1945, found at buchenwaldandbeyond.com/history/headquarters.htm.
12. Charles Mullinex, letter to family, April 15, 1945, Bernd Schmidt collection.
13. "Horrifying Images are Etched in His Mind Forever," *Minneapolis Star Tribune*, February 12, 2007.
14. "The Liberators," *Minnesota Legionnaire*, March 2007.
15. Andrea and Erich Kloss papers.
16. Harry Herder, memoir.
17. "Horrifying Images are Etched in His Mind Forever," *Minneapolis Star Tribune*, February 12, 2007.
18. Andrea and Erich Kloss papers.
19. "Nazi Death Factory Shocks Germans on Forced Tour," *New York Times*, April 18, 1945.
20. Andrea and Erich Kloss papers.
21. Harry Herder, memoir.
22. Andrea and Erich Kloss papers.
23. Lorenz C. Schmuhl, personal journal, April 16, 1945, U.S. Holocaust Memorial Museum archives.
24. Eric F. Wood, Charles H. Ott, S.M. Dye, "Inspection of German Concentration Camp for Political Prisoners Located at Buckenwald [sic] on the North Edge of Weimar made…on the morning of 16th April 1945," copy at USAMHI.
25. Ziemke, pp. 238.
26. John Toland, *Hitler*, New York: Ballantine, 1976, pp. 1187-1188; John Toland, *The Last Hundred Days*, New York: Bantam, 1967, p. 455; Manvell and Fraenkel, pp. 226-227;
27. Shirer, pp. 1468-1476; Toland, *The Last 100 Days*, pp. 613-614; Toland, *Hitler*, pp. 1187-1188.
28. Günther Morsch, *From Sachsenburg to Sachsenhausen: Pictures from the Photograph Album of a Concentration Camp Commandant*, Berlin: Metropol, 2007, p. 7; jewsihgen.org/forgottencamps/Misc/MainSearchEng.html.
29. Walter Bartel (ed.), *Buchenwald: Mahnung und Verpflichtung—Dokumente und Berichte*, Munich: Kongress Verlag, 1960, pp. pp. 64, 87, 203.

Chapter 26: Tourist Destination

1. Richard Bessel, *Germany 1945: From War to Peace.* New York: Harper, 2009, p. 171.
2. "Buchenwald Tour Shocking to MPs," *New York Times*, April 23, 1945; "Nazi Policy of Organized Murder Blackens Germany for All History," *Newsweek*, April 30, 1945, p. 56.
3. Medical Department Activities Report, 120th Evacuation Hospital, Semi-Mobile, Report, June 10, 1945, found at buchenwaldandbeyond.com/history/headquarters.htm.
4. James R. Stanhope, *Buchenwald Camp: The Report of a Parliamentary Delegation, April 1945.* London: H.M. Stationery Office, 1945, p. 7.
5. Medical Department Activities Report, op cit
6. "Congressmen See Buchenwald," *New York Times*, April 22, 1945.
7. Medical Department Activities Report, ibid.
8. "Atrocity Report Issued by Army: Buchenwald an 'Extermination Factory,' SHAEF is told," *New York Times*, April 29, 1945.
9. "Congressmen See Buchenwald," *New York Times*, April 22, 1945.
10. "National Affairs: To Look at Horror," *Newsweek*, May 28, 1945, pp. 34-35.
11. Alben Barkley, "Atrocities and Other Conditions in Concentration Camps in Germany: Report of the Committee Requested by General Dwight D. Eisenhower to the Chief of Staff, General George C. Marshall, to the Congress of the United States." Senate Document No. 47, 79th Congress, May 15, 1945. Washington, DC: U.S. Government Printing Office, 1945, pp. 14-15.
12. "Editors Condemn Nazis' Brutality," *New York Times*, May 6, 1945.
13. "Atrocity Report Issued by Army: Buchenwald an 'Extermination Factory,' SHAEF is Told," *New York Times*, April 29, 1945.
14. "Editors Take Tour of Nazi Horror Camps," *Stars and Stripes*, May 11, 1945.
15. "[Pulitzer] Urges Execution of 1,500,000 Nazis," *New York Times*, May 23, 1945
16. "U.S. Editors Back, Urge Harsh Peace," *New York Times*, May 9, 1945.
17. David Stafford, pp. 54-56.
18. James T. Quirk, quoted in Hirshson, p. 629.
19. Edward R. Murrow, quoted in Stein, p. 240.
20. Samuel Hynes, et al, *Reporting World War II: American Journalism 1938-1946*, 2 volumes. New York: Library of America, 1995, Vol. II, p. 685.
21. "War Crimes Group to Inspect Camps," *New York Times*, April 26, 1945.
22. "Nazi Policy of Organized Murder Blackens Germany for All History," *Newsweek*, April 30, 1945, p. 57.
23. Lewis R. Bird, Charles A. Hogg, Sr., John A. Deeney, Charles Froelichen, Gordon M. Manring questionnaires, USAMHI.
24. Michael C. Bilder, *A Foot Soldier for Patton: The Story of a "Red Diamond" Infantryman with the U.S. Third Army*, Philadelphia: Casemate, 2008, p. 229.
25. tnholcom.org/bio.php?id=65.
26. "Nazi Policy of Organized Murder Blackens Germany for All History," *Newsweek*, April 30, 1945, p. 57.
27. Victor B. Geller, quoted in *Ours to Fight For: American Jewish Voices from the Second World War*, New York: Museum of Jewish Heritage, 2003, pp. 80, 82.
28. "Arriving at Buchenwald," *Concord* (NH) *Monitor*, October 25, 2007.
29. Merrill C. Burgstahler, interview by author, June 21, 2007.
30. Burgstahler, letter to mother, May 18, 1945.
31. Burgstahler, interview by author, June 21, 2007.

Chapter 27: Unprepared

1. Marshall, pp. 141-208, 247-300.
2. Hirsh, p. xiv.
3. Bernard Kahn (with Neil Kahn and Flint Whitlock), *Fight On: A GI's Odyssey Back to Nazi Germany*, Brule, WI: Cable Publishing, 2013, pp. 236-237.
4. Jan Elvin, *The Box from Braunau: In Search of My Father's War,* New York: Amacom, 2009, p. 156.
5. Theresa L. Ast, doctoral dissertation, "Confronting the Holocaust: American Soldiers Who Liberated the Concentration Camps," Emory University, 2000, pp. i, 55, 58, 59, 61, 62, 75, 76.
6. Ast, p. 58.
7. Geller, quoted in *Ours to Fight For*, pp. 79-80.
8. Ast, pp. 59-62.
9. Ibid, pp. 75-76.
10. Mel Rappaport, interview by author, September 5, 2006.
11. Beir, p. 43.
12. David Israel, correspondence with author, April 21, 2008.
13. McKale, p. 464.

Chapter 28: Marching to Oblivion

1. Whitlock, *Given Up for Dead*, pp. 167-182.
2. Ibid, pp. 136-193.
3. Greene, pp. 257-262.
4. Hirsh, p. 194.
5. Greene, p. 258.
6. Greene, p. 258; Whitlock, *The Rock of Anzio: From Sicily to Dachau—A History of the 45th Infantry Division*, Boulder, CO: Westview, 1998, p. 357.
7. Whitlock, *The Rock of Anzio*, p. 358.
8. ushmm.org/lc_04/focus/pdf
9. Ibid.
10. Gilbert, *The Second World War*, pp. 685-686; oregonstate.edu/dept/holocaust/flossenburg.
11. Whitlock, *The Rock of Anzio*, pp. 351-386.

12. Bessel, p. 171; 508pir.org/odyssey/Germany/germany_16.htm.
13. Gilbert, *The Second World War*, pp. 683-684; Kershaw, p. 234.
14. Gilbert, *The Second World War*, pp. 687-688.
15. Ibid, pp. 683-684.
16. bob.swe.uni-linz.ac.at/Ebensee.
17. ushmm.org/lc_04/focus/pdf.
18. ushmm.org/wlc/media_cm.php?lang+en&ModuleId=10005424&Media=2468.
19. Letters to the editor, *Life*, May 28, 1945.

Chapter 29: Justice?

1. Toland, *The Last 100 Days*, pp. 613-614.
2. Shirer, pp. 1468-1475.
3. Dagmar Barnouw, *Germany 1945: Views of War and Violence*, Bloomington: Indiana University Press, 1996.
4. MacDonald, *The Mighty Endeavor*, p. 481.
5. Manvell and Fraenkel, pp. 228-248; Toland, *The Last 100 Days*, pp. 639-640; "The Gravediggers Return to Lübeck," *After the Battle*, No. 17, 1977, pp. 1-5.
6. Ziemke, p. 239.
7. Albert K. Coles and Harry L. Weinberg, *United States Army in World War II: Special Studies, Civil Affairs; Soldiers Become Governors,* Washington, DC: Office of the Chief of Military History, Department of the Army, 1964, p. 581.
8. Bessel, pp. 1-9.
9. Ilse Koch testimony, "U.S. v. Waldeck," trial transcript, War Crimes Case Files ("Review and Recommendations"), NARA, RG-549-000-50-9, Box 436, p. 3716.
10. Ann and John Tusa, *The Nuremberg Trial*, New York: Skyhorse, 2010, passim.
11. law2.umkc.edu/faculty/projects/ftrials/nuremberg/subsequenttrials.html.
12. scrapbookpages.com/DachauScrapbook/DachauTrials.html.
13. Greene, pp. 243-251.
14. Ibid, passim.
15. Ibid, pp. 308-309.
16. "*Ilse Koch: Lady mit Lampenschirm*," *Der Spiegel*, July 1950; "Ilse Koch Has Baby," *New York Times*, October 30, 1947.
17. Ilse Koch testimony, "U.S. v. Waldeck," trial transcript, War Crimes Case Files ("Review and Recommendations"), NARA, RG-549-000-50-9, Box 436, pp. 3706-3707, 3711, 3721-3722, 3725.
18. "U.S. v. Waldeck," War Crimes Case Files ("Review and Recommendations"), NARA, RG-549-000-09-50, Box 436, pp. 2-3.
19. Rosner speech, April 23, 1995, draft in 89th Infantry Division Society folder, WWII-7781, USAMHI.
20. Kohn speech, April 23, 1995, draft in 89th Infantry Division Society folder, WWII-7781, USAMHI.
21. Pamphlet, "Buchenwald Memorial: Miscellaneous Camp Records," published by Buchenwald Memorial.
22. McKale, p. 468.

BIBLIOGRAPHY

INTERVIEWS and CORRESPONDENCE:

Anderson, J. Leavitt. Interview by author, November 7, 2007.

Burgstahler, Merrill C. Interview by author, June 21, 2007.

_______________. Letter to mother, May 18, 1945.

Corrigan, Cyril John. Interview by University of Minnesota Center for Holocaust and Genocide Studies, found at: chgs.umn.edu/histories/minnesotans/buchenwald.

Geraldi, Joseph J. Interview by author, November 15, 2011.

Grow, Robert W. Interview by Hollis Alpert, April 23, 1945. Copy in U.S. Army Military History Institute (USAMHI), Carlisle, PA.

Herbst, Harold. Interview by United States Holocaust Memorial Museum (date unknown), found at: ushmm.org/wlc/en/media_oi.php?Moduleld=10005198&Mediald=1141.

Israel, David. E-mail to author April 18, 2008.

Laufer, Leo (formerly Shmuel Leib). Interview by author, December 20, 2006.

Mullinex, Charles. Letter to family. April 15, 1945. Bernd Schmidt collection.

Ranz, John, (formerly Johanen Goldkranz). Interview by author, January 8, 2008.

___________. *Inhumanity: Death March to Buchenwald and the Last Jews of Bendzin*, Bloomington, IN: AuthorHouse, 2007.

Rappaport, Mel. Interview by author, September 5, 2006.

___________. Letter to author, November 17, 2007.

"Red Triangle" (former Buchenwald inmate). Correspondence with author. December 19, 1997, May 25, 1998, September 4, 1998, September 14, 1998, January 20, 1999, August 3, 2001, June 4, 2007.

____________. Letter to George P. Hofmann, 6th Armored Division historian, December 7, 1972.

____________. Monograph. "The Alleged Discovery of Buchenwald by Two French 'GIs.' " June 1, 2000.

____________. Monograph. "The Mystery of the Buchenwald SOS Message." May 29, 1998.

____________. Monograph. "The Train Ride Into Hell," January 27, 1998.

Stein, Sabine. Interview by author, November 15, 2006.

ORIGINAL SOURCE MATERIAL, MEMOIRS, SPEECHES, & OFFICIAL DOCUMENTS:

After-action Report, Combat Command A, 4th Armored Division, April 1945, USAMHI.

Balochowsky, Alfred. Testimony, International Military Tribunal, Vol. VI, found at avalon.law.yale.edu/imt/o1-29-46.asp.

Barkley, Alben. "Atrocities and Other Conditions in Concentration Camps in Germany: Report of the Committee Requested by General Dwight D. Eisenhower to the Chief of Staff, General George C. Marshall, to the Congress of the United States." Senate Document No. 47, 79th Congress, May 15, 1945. Washington, DC: U.S. Government Printing Office, 1945.

Bepulsi, Peter A. Memoirs. USAMHI.

Bird, Lewis R. Questionnaire. USAMHI.

Brandell, Sol R. Memoir. USAMHI.

Buchenwald Memorial. Miscellaneous camp records.

Cole, Ralph. Memoir. USAMHI.

Coles, Albert K., and Harry L. Weinberg. *United States Army in World War II: Special Studies, Civil Affairs; Soldiers Become Governors*. Washington, DC: Office of the Chief of Military History, Department of the Army, 1964.

"Conduct of the Ilse Koch War Crimes Trials, Hearings Before the Investigations Subcommittee of the Committee on Expenditures in the Executive Departments," National Archives and Records Administration (NARA), College Park, MD, RG-549-000-50-9, Box 426.

Congdon, Howard E. Memoir. USAMHI.

D'Agostini, Benedict. D'Agostini papers, 615th Bomb Squadron Collection, Army Air Force Section, World War II Survey, Archives, USAMHI.

Deeney, John A. Questionnaire. USAMHI.

"Eighth Air Force Mission Report for Operation 568, 24 August 1944." U.S. Air Force Historical Records Center, file 520.332.

80th Infantry Division G-1 Journal, April 1945. USAMHI.

80th Infantry Division G-3 Journal, April 12, 1945. USAMHI.

Eisenhower, Dwight D. Letter to George Marshall, April 15, 1945. Eisenhower Presidential Library and Archives, Abilene, KS.

Froelichen, Charles. Questionnaire. USAMHI.

Gay, Hobart R. Papers. USAMHI.

Greunuß, Werner. Testimony. "United States v. Josias Prince zu Waldeck, et al," (U.S. v. Waldeck). War Crimes Case Files ("Review and Recommendations"), trial transcript, NARA, RG-549-000-50-9, Box 436.

Grünewald, Paul, statement. Documents related to the Second Trial of Ilse Koch, AG 383 JAG (Lt. Gen. Lucius Clay's report, date missing). NARA RG-549-000-50-9, Box 441.

Harris, Jesse. Memoirs. USAMHI.

Himmler, Heinrich. Speech in International Military Tribunal, Vol. 29 ("*Urkunden und anderes Beweismaterial*"), found at avalon. law.yale.edu.

Hogg, Charles A. Questionnaire. USAMHI.

Horn, Otto. *Buchenwald Lagerbericht Nr. 1,* April 11, 1945.

Keffer, Frederic. Personal journal entries, April 14-19, 1945; letter to grandfather, May 23, 1945; letter to Maurice Bolle, May 5, 1975. (Copies of correspondence provided to author by his daughter Leslie Keffer Rego.)

Kloss, Andrea and Erich Kloss. Papers. Weimar City Archives, File 54 4-01/1.

Koch, Ilse. Testimony, "U.S. v. Waldeck," trial transcript, War Crimes Case Files ("Review and Recommendations"), NARA, RG-549-000-50-9, Box 436.

Kohn, Murray. Speech, April 23, 1995, to the 89th Infantry Division Society. Draft in 89th Infantry Division Society folder, WWII-7781, USAMHI.

Lukehart, Richard C. Memoirs. USAMHI.

Manring, Gordon M. Questionnaire. USAMHI.

Medical Department Activities Report, 120th Evacuation Hospital, Semi-Mobile. Report, June 10, 1945, found at buchenwaldandbeyond.com/history.

Message, G-2, 4th Armored Division to VIII Corps, April 5, 1945, USAMHI.

Message, VIII Corps to Third Army, April 5, 1945, USAMHI.

"Nazi Conspiracy and Aggression." Vol. IV, Document No. 2171-PS.

Operations Report, Combat Team 9, 9th Armored Infantry Battalion, CCA, 6th Armored Division, Period 25 March-17 April 1945. Dated 21 April 1945. NARA, RG 407, Box 24096.

Owens, Edward F. Memoirs. "Report of Operational Day Mission No. 132, 24 August 1944, 94th Combat Bomb Wing, 401st Bombardment Group (H)," provided to author by Don Byers.

Pister, Hermann. Interrogation. "U.S. v. Waldeck," trial transcript, March 4, 1947. NARA, RG-549-000-50-9, Box 437.

Rosner, Andrew. Speech, April 23, 1995, draft in 89th Infantry Division Society folder, WWII-7781, USAMHI.

Schmuhl, Lorenz C. Personal journal, entry for April 16, 1945. Washington, DC: U. S. Holocaust Memorial Museum archives.

Sears, Hayden A. Report, CCA, 4th Armored Division, April 1945, USAMHI.

Sitte, Kurt. Sworn statement taken March 9, 1949, "U.S. v. Waldeck." NARA, RG-549-000-50-9, Box 441.

602nd Tank Destroyer Battalion Morning Reports, April 1945. NARA.

"SS Dr. Ding Diary." Document 1999-141, date unknown. Simon Wiesenthal Center, Los Angeles, CA.

Stanhope, James R. *Buchenwald Camp: The Report of a Parliamentary Delegation, April 1945*. London: H.M. Stationery Office, 1945.

Sue, Norman. Memoirs. USAMHI.

"Trials of the War Criminals before the Nurnberg Military Tribunals under Control Council Law No. 10," Nurnberg, October 1946-April 1949, Col.V (Oswald Pohl trial).

"U.S. v. Waldeck." Trial record. Deputy Judge Advocate's Office, 7708 War Crimes Group, European Command, November 15, 1947. NARA, War Crimes Case Files ("Cases Tried") 1945-59, RG-549-000-50-9, Boxes 436, 437, 438, 441.

War Diary. 3rd Battalion, 355th Infantry Regiment, USAMHI.

Wood, Eric F., Charles H. Ott, S.M. Dye, "Inspection of German Concentration Camp for Political Prisoners Located at Buckenwald [sic] on the North Edge of Weimar made...on the morning of 16th April 1945." Copy in USAMHI and U.S. Holocaust Memorial Museum archives.

BOOKS:

Abzug, Robert H. *Inside the Vicious Heart: Americans and the Liberation of Nazi Concentration Camps*. New York: Oxford University Press, 1985.

Allen, Michael Thad. *The Business of Genocide: The SS, Slave Labor, and the Concentration Camps*. Chapel Hill, NC: University of North Carolina Press, 2002.

Allen, Robert S. *Lucky Forward: The History of Patton's Third U.S. Army*. New York: Vanguard Press, 1947.

Aly, Götz, Peter Chroust, and Christian Pross (tr. by Belinda Cooper). *Cleansing the Fatherland: Nazi Medicine and Racial Hygiene*. Baltimore, MD: Johns Hopkins University Press, 1994.

Ambrose, Stephen E. *Citizen Soldiers: The U.S. Army from the Normandy Beaches to the Bulge to the Surrender of Germany - June 7, 1944-May 7, 1945*. New York: Simon & Schuster, 1997.

______________. *D-Day, June 6, 1944: The Climactic Battle of World War II*. New York: Simon & Schuster, 1994.

Arnold-Forster, Mark. *The World At War*. New York: Stein and Day, 1973.

Baker, Nicholson. *Human Smoke: The Beginnings of World War II, The End of Civilization*. New York: Simon & Schuster, 2008.

Barbet-Massin, Olivia, ed. *World War II: The Unseen Visual History*. New York: New Press, 2011.

Barnouw, Dagmar. *Germany 1945: Views of War and Violence*. Bloomington: Indiana University Press, 1996.

Bartel, Walter (ed.). *Buchenwald: Mahnung und Verpflichtun—Dokumente und Berichte*. Munich: Kongress Verlag, 1960.

Beevor, Antony. *The Second World War*. New York: Little, Brown, 2012

Beir, Robert (with Brian Josepher). *Roosevelt and the Holocaust*. Fort Lee, NJ: Barricade Books, 2006.

Béon, Yves. *Planet Dora: A Memoir of the Holocaust and the Birth of the Space Age*. Boulder, CO: Westview, 1997.

Bessel, Richard. *Germany 1945: From War to Peace*. New York: Harper, 2009.

Bilder, Michael C. *A Foot Soldier for Patton: The Story of a "Red Diamond" Infantryman with the U.S. Third Army*. Philadelphia: Casemate, 2008.

Black, Edwin. *War Against the Weak: Eugenics and America's Campaign to Create a Master Race*. New York: Four Walls Eight Windows, 2003.

Blatman, Daniel (tr. by Chaya Galai). *The Death Marches: The Final Phase of Nazi Genocide*. Cambridge, MA: Belknap/Harvard, 2011.

Bradley, Omar N. *A Soldier's Story*. Chicago: Rand McNally, 1951.

Burney, Christopher. *The Dungeon Democracy*. New York: Duell, Sloan and Pearce, 1946.

Butcher, Harry C. *My Three Years with Eisenhower.* New York: Simon & Schuster, 1946.

Caines, Christopher, tr. *World War II: The Unseen Visual History*. The Caen Memorial. New York: The New Press, 2011.

Clary, Robert. *From Holocaust to Hogan's Heroes: The Autobiography of Robert Clary*. Lanham, MD: Madison Books, 2001.

Codman, Charles R. *Drive*. Boston: Little, Brown and Company, 1957.

Cole, Hugh M. *U.S. Army in World War II: The European Theater of Operations. The Ardennes: Battle for the Bulge*. Washington, DC: Center of Military History, 1995.

Cruikshank, Charles. *Deception in World War II*. Oxford, UK: Oxford University Press, 1979.

Davidson, Susie, ed. *I Refused to Die: Stories of Boston Area Holocaust Survivors and Soldiers Who Liberated the Concentration Camps of World War II*. Somerville, MA: Ibbetson Street Press, 2005.

Davies, Norman. *No Simple Victory: World War II in Europe, 1939-1945*. New York: Viking, 2007.

D'Este, Carlo. *Patton: A Genius for War*. New York: HarperCollins, 1995.

Dederichs, Mario R. *Heydrich: The Face of Evil*. London: Greenhill Books, 2006.

Deschner, Günther. *Reinhard Heydrich: A Biography of the Man Behind the "Final Solution."* New York: Stein and Day, 1981.

Dimsdale, Joel E., ed. *Survivors, Victims, and Perpetrators: Essays on the Nazi Holocaust*. Washington, DC: Hemisphere Publishing, 1980.

Domarus, Max, and Patrick Romane, eds. *The Essential Hitler: Speeches and Commentary*. Wauconda, IL: Bolchazy-Carducci Publishers, 2007.

Eisenhower, Dwight D. *Crusade In Europe*. Garden City, NY: Doubleday, 1948.

Ellis, John. *The Sharp End: The Fighting Man in World War II*. New York: Charles Scribner's Sons, 1980.

Elvin, Jan. *The Box from Braunau: In Search of My Father's War*. New York: Amacom, 2009.

Feig, Konnilyn G. *Hitler's Death Camps: The Sanity of Madness*. New York: Holmes & Meier, 1979.

Ferencz, Benjamin B. *Less than Slaves: Jewish Forced Labor and the Quest for Compensation*. Cambridge, MA: Harvard University Press, 1979.

Fischel, Jack R. *The Holocaust*. Westport, CT: Greenwood Press, 1998.

Fishman, Jack. *And the Walls Came Tumbling Down: The Secret World War II Allied Operation that Saved D-Day and Unleashed the Greatest Mass Prison Escape in History.* New York: MacMillan, 1983.

Foote, M.R.D. *SOE: The Special Operations Executive 1940-1946*. London: Greenwood/BBC Books, 1984.

Garson, Paul. *New Images of Nazi Germany: A Photographic Collection*. Jefferson, NC: McFarland, 2012.

Geest, Jack van der (with Carol Ordemann). *Was God on Vacation?* Self-published, 2002.

Gilbert, Martin. *The Boys: The Untold Story of 732 Young Concentration Camp Survivors.* New York: Henry Holt, 1996.

____________. *The First World War: A Complete History*. New York: Henry Holt, 1994.

____________. *The Holocaust: The Jewish Tragedy,* Glasgow: William Collins, 1990.

____________. *Kristallnacht: Prelude to Destruction*. New York: HarperCollins, 2006.

____________. *The Second World War: A Complete History*. New York: Henry Holt, 1989.

Glantz, David (tr.), and Harold Orenstein (tr.), *Belorussia 1944: The Soviet General Staff Study*. London: Routledge, 2001.

Goldhagen, Daniel J. *Hitler's Willing Executioners: Ordinary Germans and the Holocaust*. New York: Alfred A. Knopf, 1996.

Goodwin, Doris K. *No Ordinary Time: Franklin and Eleanor Roosevelt—The Home Front in World War II*. New York: Simon & Schuster, 1994.

Graber, G. S. *The History of the SS*. New York: David McKay Co., 1978.

Grau, Guenther. *Hidden Holocaust? Gay and Lesbian Persecution in Germany, 1933-1945*. London: Cassell & Cie., 1993.

Greene, Joshua M. *Justice at Dachau: The Trials of an American Prosecutor*. New York: Broadway Books, 2003.

Grille, Dietrich, and August-Wilhelm Kaiser, eds. *Kultur und Geschichte Thüringens: Thüringen Unter Dem Sternenbanner, April bis Juni 1945*. Mainz: Stiftung Thüringen, 1989.

Gros, Louis, *Survivor of Buchenwald: My Personal Odyssey Through Hell*. Brule, WI: Cable Publishing, 2012.

Gurewitsch, Bonnie, William L. O'Neill, and Jay M. Eidelman, eds. Victor B. Geller in *Ours to Fight For: American Jewish Voices from the Second World War.* New York: Museum of Jewish Heritage, 2003.

Hackett, David A., ed. and tr. *The Buchenwald Report*. Boulder, CO: Westview Press, 1995.

Haskew, Michael E. ed. *The World War II Desk Reference*. New York: HarperCollins, 2004.

Heiber, Helmut, and David Glantz. *Hitler and his Generals: Military Conferences 1942-1945*. New York: Enigma Books, 2003.

Hemmendinger, Judith, and Robert Krell. *The Children of Buchenwald: Child Survivors and Their Postwar Lives.* Jerusalem: Gefen, 2000.

Hirsh, Michael. *The Liberators: America's Witnesses to the Holocaust*. New York: Bantam Books, 2010.

Hirshson, Stanley P. *General Patton: A Soldier's Life*. New York: HarperCollins, 2002.

Historical Atlas of the Holocaust. New York: Simon & Schuster/Macmillan, 1996.

Hömig, Herbert, (Dietrich Grill and August-Wilhelm Kaiser, eds.). "*Thüringen unter dem Nationalsozialismus,*" *Kultur und Geschichte Thüringens*. Stiftung Thüringen, Wiesbaden, Germany: Druckerei am Parkfeld, 1990.

Hynes, Samuel, et. al., *Reporting World War II: American Journalism 1938-1946*. 2 vols. New York: Library of America, 1995.

Julitte, Pierre. *Block 26: Sabotage at Buchenwald.* Garden City, NY: Doubleday, 1971.

Kahler, Erich. *The Germans.* Princeton, NJ: Princeton University Press, 1974.

Kahn, Bernard, with Neil Kahn and Flint Whitlock. *Fight On: A GI's Odyssey Back to Nazi Germany.* Brule, WI: Cable Publishing, 2013.

Kennedy, David M. *The Library of Congress World War II Companion.* New York: Simon & Schuster, 2007.

Kershaw, Ian. *Hitler: A Biography.* New York: W. W. Norton 2008.

___________. *The End: The Defiance and Destruction of Hitler's Germany, 1944-1945.* New York: Penguin, 2011.

Kesselring, Albert. *The Memoirs of Field-Marshal Kesselring.* London: Greenhill, 2007.

Kinnis, Arthur G. and Stanley A. Booker. *168 Jump into Hell.* Victoria, Canada: self-published, 1999.

Klee, Ernst, Willi Dressen, and Volker Riess, eds. *"The Good Old Days:" The Holocaust as Seen by Its Perpetrators and Bystanders.* Old Saybrook, CT: Konecky & Konecky, 1988.

Kogon, Eugen (tr. by Heinz Norden). *The Theory and Practice of Hell: The German Concentration Camps and the System Behind Them.* New York: Berkley, 1984.

Korda, Michael. *Ike: An American Hero.* New York: HarperCollins, 2007.

Kralovitz, Rolf (tr. by Eva R. Cohn). *TenZeroNinety in Buchenwald: A Jewish Prisoner Tells His Story.* Cologne, Germany: Walter-Meckauer-Kreis, 1998.

Laquer, Walter. *The Terrible Secret: Suppression of the Truth about Hitler's "Final Solution."* Boston: Little, Brown and Company, 1980.

Larson, Erik. *In the Garden of Beasts.* New York: Crown, 2011.

Lebel, Jennie. *The Mufti of Jerusalem: Haj-Amin el-Husseini and National-Socialism.* Belgrade, Serbia: Cigoya Stampa, 2007.

Liddell Hart, Basil. *History of the Second World War.* New York: G.P. Putnam's Sons, 1970.

Lifton, Robert J. *The Nazi Doctors: Medical Killing and the Psychology of Genocide.* New York: Basic Books, 2000.

Lochner, Louis P., ed. *The Goebbels Diaries.* Garden City, NY: Doubleday, 1948.

MacDonald, Charles B. *The Mighty Endeavor: American Armed Forces in the European Theater in World War II.* New York: Oxford University Press, 1969.

___________ *U.S. Army in World War II: The European Theater of Operations. The Last Offensive.* Washington, DC: Center of Military History, 1993.

Magliveras, Konstantinos D. *Exclusion from Participation in International Organisations: The Law and Practice behind Member States' Expulsion and Suspension of Membership.* Leiden, Holland: Martinus Nijhoff Publishers, 1999.

Manchester, William. *The Arms of Krupp: 1587-1968.* New York: Bantam, 1982.

Manvell, Roger, and Heinrich Fraenkel. *Heinrich Himmler: The Sinister Life of the Head of the SS and Gestapo.* New York: Sky Horse, 2007.

Marshall, George C. *The War Reports of General George C. Marshall, General Henry H. Arnold, and Admiral Ernest J. King: Biennial Report of the Chief of Staff of the United States Army to the Secretary of War, July 1, 1943-June 30, 1945.* Philadelphia: J.B. Lippincott, 1947.

McKale, Donald M. *Hitler's Shadow War: The Holocaust and World War II.* New York: Cooper Square Press, 2002.

Milgram, Stanley. *Obedience to Authority: An Experimental View.* New York: Harper & Row, 1974.

Morsch, Günther. *From Sachsenburg to Sachsenhausen: Pictures from the Photograph Album of a Concentration Camp Commandant.* Berlin: Metropol, 2007.

Moser, Joe, and Gerald Baron. *A Fighter Pilot in Buchenwald.* Bellingham, WA: Edens Veil Media, 2009.

Mosse, George L. *Nazi Culture: Intellectual, Cultural and Social Life in the Third Reich.* New York: Grosset & Dunlap, 1966.

Neufeld, Michael J. *Von Braun: Dreamer of Space, Engineer of War.* New York: Knopf, 2007.

Northedge, F.S. *The League of Nations: Its Life and Times, 1920–1946.* New York: Holmes & Meier, 1986.

Padfield, Peter. *Himmler: A Full-Scale Biography of One of Hitler's Most Ruthless Executioners.* New York: MjF Books, 1997.

Patton, George S., Jr. *War as I Knew It.* Boston: Houghton Mifflin, 1947.

Plant, Richard. *The Pink Triangle: The Nazi War Against Homosexuals,* New York: Macmillan, 1988.

Poller, Walter. *Butchers of Buchenwald.* New York: Zebra, 1977.

Poprzeczny, Joseph. *Odilo Globocnik: Hitler's Man in the East.* Jefferson, NC: McFarland, 2004.

Ranz, John. *Inhumanity: Death March to Buchenwald and the Last Jews of Bendzin.* Bloomington, IN: AuthorHouse, 2007.

Reitlinger, Gerald. *The SS: Alibi of a Nation, 1922-1945.* New York: Penguin, 1968.

Roth, Artur. *Unter den Augen der SS: Otto Roth und der bewaffnete Aufstand im KZ Buchenwald.* Bonn, Germany: Pahl-Rugenstein Verlag, 1995.

Schellenberg, Walter. *The Labyrinth.* New York: Harper & Brothers, 1956.

Shephard, Ben. *After Daybreak: The Liberation of Belsen, 1945.* London: Random House, 2006.

Shirer, William L. *The Rise and Fall of the Third Reich: A History of Nazi Germany.* Greenwich, CT: Crest/Fawcett, 1964.

Smith, Arthur L. *Die Hexe von Buchenwald: Der Fall Ilse Koch.* Cologne, Germany: Böhlau Verlag, 1983.

Sterilization and a Qualified Nazi Analogy: The United States and Germany, 1930-1945." *Annals of Internal Medicine,* 2000.

Speer, Albert. *Inside The Third Reich.* New York: Avon, 1970.

Spitz, Vivien. *Doctors from Hell: Horrific Account of Nazi Experiments on Humans.* Boulder, CO: Sentient Publications, 2005.

Stafford, David. *Endgame, 1945: The Missing Final Chapter of World War II.* New York: Little, Brown and Company, 2007.

Stanton, Shelby L. *World War II Order of Battle.* New York: Galahad, 1984.

Stein, George H. *The Waffen SS: Hitler's Elite Guard at War, 1939-1945.* Ithaca, NY: Cornell University Press, 1966.

Stein, Harry, ed. (tr. Judith Rosenthal). *Buchenwald Concentration Camp 1937-1945: A Guide to the Permanent Historical Exhibition.* Gottingen, Germany: Wallstein Verlag, 2004.

Steinbacher, Sybille. *Auschwitz: A History.* New York: ecco/HarperCollins, 2005.

Stuhlinger, Ernst, and Frederick I. Ordway III. *Wernher von Braun, Crusader for Space: A Biographical Memoir.* Malabar, FL: Krieger, 1994.

Sydnor, Charles W., Jr. *Soldiers of Destruction: The SS Death's-Head Division, 1933-1945.* Princeton, NJ: Princeton University Press, 1977.

Tamagny, Florence. *A History of Homosexuality in Europe: Berlin, London, Paris 1919-1939.* New York: Algora, 2004.

Toland, John. *Hitler.* New York: Ballantine, 1976.

____________. *The Last 100 Days.* New York: Bantam, 1967.

Trunk, Isaiah. *Judenrat: The Jewish Councils in Eastern Europe Under Nazi Occupation.* New York: Macmillan, 1972.

Tusa, Ann and John. *The Nuremberg Trial,* New York: Skyhorse, 2010.

United States Holocaust Memorial Museum. *Historical Atlas of the Holocaust.* New York: Simon & Schuster Macmillian, 1996.

Victor, Paul Heinz. *Buchenwald: A Survivor's Memoir.* Tucson, AZ: Wheatmark, 2005.

Werber, Jack. *Saving Children: Diary of a Buchenwald Survivor and Rescuer.* New Brunswick, NJ: Transaction, 1997.

Whitlock, Flint. *The Beasts of Buchenwald: Karl & Ilse Koch, Human-Skin Lampshades, and the War-Crimes Trial of the Century.* Brule, WI: Cable Publishing, 2011.

_________. *Given Up for Dead: American GIs in the Nazi Concentration Camp at Berga.* Boulder, CO: Westview Press, 2005.

_________. *The Rock of Anzio: From Sicily to Dachau—A History of the 45th Infantry Division.* Boulder, CO: Westview Press, 1998.

Wiesel, Eliezer ("Elie"). *Night.* New York: Hill and Wang, 1985.

Wyman, David S. *The Abandonment of the Jews: America and the Holocaust, 1941-1945.* New York: The New Press, 1998.

Yenne, Bill. *Big Week: Six Days that Changed the Course of World War II.* New York: Berkley Caliber, 2012.

Ziemke, Earl F. *U.S. Army Historical Series: The U.S. Army in the Occupation of Germany 1944-1946.* Washington, DC: Center of Military History, 1990.

Zipfel, Friedrich. *Gestapo und Sicherheitsdienst.* Berlin: Arani Verlag, 1960.

PAMPHLETS/BROCHURES:

Buchenwald Memorial. Weimar: Gedenkstätten Buchenwald und Mittelbau-Dora, 2005.

Cemetery at the Bismarck Tower, The. Weimar: Gedenkstätten Buchenwald und Mittelbau-Dora, n.d.

Der Ehemalige Postenweg Der SS: Ein Rundgang Um Das Lager. Weimar: Gedenkstätten Buchenwald und Mittelbau-Dora, 2005.

Geheime Staatspolizei/Staatspolizeistelle Weimar. Weimar: Gedenkstätten Buchenwald und Mittelbau-Dora, 1996.

Lageplan des KZ Buchenwald und Karte der Außenkommandos. Weimar: Gedenkstätten Buchenwald und Mittelbau-Dora, 2002.

The Little Camp. Weimar: Gedenkstätten Buchenwald und Mittelbau-Dora, 2004.

The Mittelbau-Dora Concentration Camp. Weimar: Gedenkstätten Buchenwald und Mittelbau-Dora, 2002. Publication no.1021.

NEWSPAPERS, MAGAZINES, PERIODICALS:

"Action—Not Pity—Can Save Millions Now!" (Advertisement), *New York Times,* February 8, 1943.

"All-Europe Purge of Jews Reported." *New York Times,* October 8, 1943.

"All Reich to See Camp Atrocities." *New York Times,* April 25, 1945.

"Allies Round Up War Criminals." *Life,* May 28, 1945.

"Alsace Nazi Prison Neat and Efficient," *New York Times,* December 5, 1944.

"Arriving at Buchenwald" (Warren Priest's account). *Concord* (NH) *Monitor.* October 25, 2007.

"At Liberated Prison Camps in Germany: Nazi Tormentors Fall into Hands of the Allies." *New York Times,* April 26, 1945.

"Atrocities: Capture of the German Concentration Camps Piles Up Evidence of Barbarism that Reaches the Low Point of Human Degradation." *Life,* May 7, 1945.

"Atrocity Report Issued by Army: Buchenwald an 'Extermination Factory,' SHAEF is told." *New York Times,* April 29, 1945.

"Berlin Ousts Last Jews." *New York Times,* April 15, 1943.

"Big Prison Camp Uncovered." *New York Herald Tribune,* April 13, 1945.

Brinkley, Alan. "Minister Without Portfolio" *Harpers.* February 1983.

"Buchenwald." (Editorial) *New York Times,* April 19, 1945.

"Buchenwald Guards to be Tried April 11." *New York Times,* March 9, 1947.

"Buchenwald Tour Shocking to MPs." *New York Times,* April 23, 1945.

"Buchenwald Worse than Battlefield." *New York Times,* April 28, 1945.

"Butcher of Buchenwald in an Egyptian Paradise," *Independent, The.* (London, England), August 7, 2010.

"Case of Ilse Koch, The." (Editorial) *New York Times,* Deember 28, 1948.

"Congressmen and Army Chiefs Get a Firsthand View of Nazi Horror Camps." *New York Times,* April 27, 1945.

"Congressmen See Buchenwald." *New York Times,* April 22, 1945.

"Congressmen See War Camp Horror." *New York Times*, April 26, 1945.

"Czech Official Cites Buchenwald Crimes." *New York Times*, April 15, 1947.

"[Rabbi Wise] Demands Jews Be Saved." *New York Times*, December 27, 1942.

Denny, Harold. "The World Must Not Forget: What Was Done in the German Prison Camps Emphasized the Problem of What to Do with a People Who Are Morally Sick." *New York Times*, June 6, 1945.

"Despair Blankets Buchenwald Camp." *New York Times*, April 20, 1945.

Dillon, Christopher. "'We'll Meet Again in Dachau': The Early Dachau SS and the Narrative of Civil War." *Journal of Contemporary History*, 45(3), 2010.

"Division Finds Underground Nazi HQ." *The Rolling W*, April 12, 1945.

"Editors Condemn Nazis' Brutality." *New York Times*, May 6, 1945.

"Editors Take Tour of Nazi Horror Camps." *Stars and Stripes*, May 11, 1945.

"89th Infantry Division, The," *1942-1945*. Washington, DC: *Infantry Journal,* 1947.

"Ex-Prisoner Tells Of Reich 'Cruelty;' Hungarian Says Beatings in Concentration Camps Made Conditions 'Terrible.' " *New York Times*, July 25, 1933.

"Excerpts from Senate Inquiry Report in Ilse Koch Case." *New York Times,* December 27, 1948.

"Extinction Feared by Jews in Poland." *New York Times,* March 1, 1942.

"Farben is Accused in Typhus Tests: Affidavit from Chief Doctor at Buchenwald Says Concern Knew Prisoners were Used." *New York Times*, November 25, 1947.

"Ford Motor Co. Charged in Nazi Secret Profits on Slave Labor," *The Daily Republican,* March 18, 1998.

"Foreign News: Germany." *Time*, April 30, 1945.

"40,000 Here View Memorial to Jews." *New York Times*, March 2, 1942.

"Four 9th AIB Doughs Find Buchenwald." *Armored Attacker*, May 5, 1945.

"Frau Koch Disavows Buchenwald Crimes." *New York Times*, July 11, 1947.

"Freeing the Survivors." *U.S. News and World Report*. April 3, 1995.

"French Notables Freed in Germany." *New York Times*, April 16, 1945.

Gelichi, S. "Remembrance of Otto of Hesse." *Journal of Archaeology*, 1997.

"Germans are Unmoved by Atrocity Film; Prisoners Lay War Crimes to 'Higher-Ups.' " *New York Times*, June 27, 1945.

"Germans Criticize War Crimes Trial." *New York Times*, November 1, 1945.

"Germans Give Ilse Koch Life Term for Crimes Against Countrymen." *New York Times*, January 16, 1951.

"Germans in Soviet Zone Plan Trial for Ilse Koch." *New York Times*, November 1, 1945.

"Germans Murder 5,000 Prisoners Removed from Buchenwald Camp." *New York Times*, April 30, 1945.

"Germany: Horror." *Time*, April 30, 1945.

"Goebbels Turns Fire on 'Jewish Problem': Nazi Propaganda Chief Looks to Anti-Semitism Among Allies." *New York Times*, May 9, 1943.

"The Gravediggers Return to Lübeck." *After the Battle*, November 17, 1977.

"Grim Ghettos." *Newsweek*, August 10, 1942.

"Head of King Tut Relative Listed in Nazi Art Cache." *New York Times*, April 12, 1945.

"A Hell Factory Worked by the Living Dead." *Newsweek*, April 23, 1945.

"Himmler Program Kills Polish Jews: Wise Gets Confirmations." *New York Times*, November 25, 1942.

"Hitler's Power Over Germany: The Nazi Strength Analyzed." *New York Times*, April 9, 1933.

Hodson, Stanley N. Letter to the editor, *Lewiston* (ME) *Journal*, April 13, 1945.

"The Holocaust Just Got More Shocking." *New York Times*, March 1, 2013.

"Horrifying Images are Etched in His Mind Forever." *Minneapolis Star Tribune*. February 12, 2007.

"Ilse Koch Hangs Herself in Cell." *New York Times*, September 3, 1967.

"Ilse Koch Has Baby." *New York Times*, October 30, 1947.

"Ilse Koch is Transferred to West German Hands." *New York Times*, October 17, 1949.

"Ilse Koch: Lady mit Lampenschirm." *Der Spiegel*, July 1950.

"Ilse Koch Sues Bavaria." *New York Times*, October 18, 1966.

"Ilse Koch Trial Ends in Germany." *New York Times*, January 13, 1951.

"Jewish Rally Urges Gas Attacks on Nazis." *New York Times*, June 20, 1942.

Keiler, Jonathan F. "Revolts in the Death Camps." *WWII History*, January 2008.

"Lack of Evidence Saved Frau Koch." *New York Times*, October 1, 1948.

"Lau Recalls Liberation as Child at Buchenwald." *Jerusalem Post*, April 10, 1995.

"The Liberators." *Minnesota Legionnaire*, March 2007.

"Luft-terror gegen Weimar: Mehr als 330 Tot." *Thüringer Gauzeitung*, February 15, 1945.

"Making of Gas Laid to Farben Leaders." *New York Times*, November 27, 1947.

McKay, Andrew. "Buchenwald: A Survivor's Tale." *Manhattan Spirit*, April 14, 1995.

"Moskowitz Sees End of Reich Jews: Hitler's Program is One of Extermination, He Says on Return from Tour." *New York Times*, June 29, 1933.

"Mrs. Luce Tells Nazi Slave Policy, Aimed to Protect Secret Weapons." *New York Times*, May 4, 1945.

"National Affairs: To Look at Horror." *Newsweek*, May 28, 1945.

"Nazi Cruelty at Buchenwald Concentration Camp." *The Canberra Times*, April 16, 1947.

"Nazi Death Factory Shocks Germans on Forced Tour." *New York Times*, April 18, 1945.

"Nazi Germany Reveals Official Pictures of its Concentration Camps." *Life*, August 21, 1939.

"Nazi Policy of Organized Murder Blackens Germany for All History." *Newsweek*, April 30, 1945.

"Nazis Blame Jews for Big Bombings; Goebbels Says 'Extermination' of All in Europe 'and Perhaps Beyond,' Will Result." *New York Times*, June 13, 1942.

"Nazis Blot Out Czech Village; Kill All Men, Disperse Others." *New York Times*, June 11, 1942.

"Nazis Killed Boris, Princess Related," *New York Times*, May 23, 1945.

"Nazis Round Up 300 Jews in Nuremberg; Business Men Are Paraded Through City." *New York Times*, July 21, 1933.

"New Group Sets Up 'Hebrew Nation.' " *New York Times*, May 19, 1944.

"New Trial for Ilse Koch is Essential." (Editorial) *Philadelphia Inquirer*, December 28, 1948.

"New York Escaped V-2 Rockets by 6-Month Margin, Army Says." *New York Times*, June 14, 1945.

"Nordhausen: A Hell Factory Worked by the Living Dead." *Newsweek*, April 23, 1945.

"Opening of Palestine as Homeland Demanded by Jewish Conference." *New York Times*, September 2, 1943.

"Over One Million Jews Already Killed by Nazis." *Daily Telegraph* (London), June 25, 1942.

"Patton Strikes Gold." *Newsweek*, April 16, 1945.

"Penalty for Ilse Koch Asked." *Newsweek*, January 12, 1951.

"Pister Captured." *Newsweek*, June 14, 1945.

"President Roosevelt is Dead." *New York Times*, April 13, 1945.

"Princess Mafalda Reported Killed." *New York Times*, April 25, 1945.

"Prison Camp is Overrun; 20,000 Political Captives are Found at Buchenwald." *New York Times*, April 13, 1945.

"Prosecution Finishes Evidence on Farben." *New York Times*, November 26, 1947.

"[Pulitzer] Urges Execution of 1,500,000 Nazis." *New York Times*, May 23, 1945.

"Raketen in Thüringen," *Frankfurter Allgemeine Zeitung*, October 27, 2002.

Rees, Laurence. "A Fond Look Back." *World War II*. July/August 2013.

"Reich Deporting French Jews to 'Polish Silesia,' Report Says." *New York Times*, August 20, 1942.

Riley, Neal J. "Frederick Lea, 95; helped care for Buchenwald's freed prisoners." (Frederick Lea obituary). *Boston Globe*, March 14, 2011.

"Roosevelt Death Encourages Nazis." *New York Times*, April 14, 1945.

"Roosevelt Says U.S. Will Join in Investigation of Atrocities." *New York Times*, October 8, 1942.

"Sanctuary for Europe's Jews." (Editorial) *New York Times*, March 3, 1943.

"Save Doomed Jews, Huge Rally Pleads." *New York Times*, March 2, 1943.

"Senators Propose 'Bestial' Ilse Koch Stand New Trial." *New York Times*, December 27, 1948.

Sidney Gritz obituary. *Palm Beach* (FL) *Post*. December 29, 2005.

"Slain Polish Jews Put at a Million." *New York Times*, November 26, 1942.

"Slaying of Jews in Galicia Depicted; Deaths Are Put at 15,000." *New York Times*, Oct. 26, 1941.

Sofair, Andre N. and Lauris C. Kaldjian, "Eugenic

"Soviet Wants Ilse Koch; East Zone of Germany Would Try 'Beast of Buchenwald.' " *New York Times*, March 24, 1949.

"Tests on Prisoners by Nazis Described; Burns Inflicted on Buchenwald Inmates in Quest for Remedy, 3 Frenchmen Declare." *New York Times*, June 28, 1945.

"31 of Buchenwald Placed on Trial." *New York Times*, April 12, 1947.

"3 Czechs Testify at Koch Hearing." *New York Times*, December 9, 1948.

"3,048 French Dead Found in Nazi Camp; 900 Slain Near Weimar," *New York Times*, April 15, 1945.

"3rd [Army] Takes Weimar Without 1 Shot; 80th Division Leader Brings About Surrender of Historic German City." *New York Times*, April 12, 1945.

Thüringer Gauzeitung, August 27, 1944.

"Toscanini Refuses to Go to Baireuth [sic]; Won't Conduct at Wagnerian Festival Because of Persecution of Jews." *New York Times*, June 6, 1933.

"21,000 Prisoners Are Liberated by Division at Buchenwald." *Armored Attacker*, May 5, 1945.

"22 Nazis Will Die for War Crimes." *New York Times*, August 15, 1947.

"2,000,000 Murders by Nazis Charged" *New York Times*, August 8, 1943.

"U.S. Board Bares Atrocity Details Told by Witnesses at Polish Camps." *New York Times*, November 26, 1944.

"U.S. Commutes Term of Nazi Torturer." *New York Times*, September 17, 1948.

"U.S. Editors Back, Urge Harsh Peace." *New York Times*, May 9, 1945.

"V-2 Plant Survivors Publicize Their Story." *Huntsville* (AL) *Times*, February 28, 2000.

"War Crime Report Horrifies Capital." *New York Times*, May 16, 1945.

"War Crimes Group to Inspect Camps." *New York Times*, April 26, 1945.

"War Crimes: Nordhausen." *Life*, May 28, 1945.

"Why Didn't We Bomb Auschwitz?" *Washington Post*, April 17, 1983.

Wiegrefe, Klaus. "Wie nah war Hitler an die A-Bombe?"

Der Spiegel, March 14, 2005.

Wiesen, S. Jonathan. "German Industry and the Third Reich: Fifty Years of Forgetting and Remembering." *Dimensions: A Journal of Holocaust Studies*, Vol. 13, No. 2, Braun Holocaust Institute.

Wiseman, Paul. "Third Reich's Infrastructure of Horror Far More Widespread Than Thought." *World War II*, July/Aug. 2013.

"The Witch of Buchenwald: The Good and the Horrible Were All the Same to Ilse, the Plaything of the SS." *Newsweek*, July 28, 1947.

Zimbardo, Philip. "Revisiting the Stanford Prison Experiment: A Lesson in the Power of Situation," *Chronicle of Higher Education*, March 30, 2007.

MISCELLANY:

Ast, Theresa Lynn. Doctoral dissertation: "Confronting the Holocaust: American Soldiers Who Liberated the Concentration Camps." Emory University, 2000.

Skinner, Justin. "Remembering Buchenwald: Forest Hill Collegiate students hear a survivor's story." insidetoronto.com.

U.S. National Archives news release, January 29, 2000.

a.ghearmailt.gd.ogarnig.pl/gd/Weimar.

answers.com/topic/princess-mafalda-of-savoy.

archives.gov/publications/prologue/1999/spring/nazi-gold-merkers-mine-treasure.html.

astronautix.com/Astros/thialter.

bach-cantatas.com/Tour/Ohrdruf.

bbc.co.uk/ww2peoplewar/stories/86/a3940986.

bob.swe.uni-linz.ac.at/Ebensee.

buchenwald.de/en/473.

dachaukz.blogspot.com/2011/11/buchenwald-kz-1937-1945-part-1.html (provided by Herbert Stolpmann).

dailyrepublican.com/ford_slave_labor.html.

8thafhs.org/combat1945.htm.

89infdivww2.org/ohrdruf/ohrdrufintro.

erfurt-web.de/SaukelFritz.

forum.alexanderpalace.org.

forum.axishistory.com/index.php?id+3317.

487thbg.org/Stories/JackFishmanStanleyLog1945.

greyfalcon.us/Located%20near%20Ohrdruf.htm.

gtgj.de.

history.msfc.nasa.gov/vonbraun/bio.

history1900s.about.com/od/holocaust/a/babiyar_2.htm.

hnn.us/articles/1796.

holocaustresearchproject.othercamps/eicke.

jewishgen.org/yizkor/Poland/po1001.

jewishvirtuallibrary.org/biography/jabotinsky.html.

jewishvirtuallibrary.org/jsource/Holocaust/natzweiler.html.

law.umkc.edu/faculty/projects/ftrials/Nuremberg/subsequenttrials.

library5.gl. lit.edu/frames.asp?page+feuer&ext+_t.

lodging-germany.com/info/Weimar.

motlc.learningcenter.wiesenthal.org/text/x12/xm1996.

nadir.org/nadirperiodika/antifa_nachrichten.

nizkor.org/hweb/camps/Buchenwald.

nuremberg.law.harvard.edu.

oregonstate.edu/dept/holocaust/flossenburg.

pbs.org/wgbh/amex/holocaust/filmmore/reference/primary.

pbs.org/wgbh/amex/holocaust/filmmore/reference/primary/bombjohn.html.

pbs.org/wgbh/amex/holocaust/filmmore/reference/primary/index.html.

pbs.org/wgbh/amex/holocaust/peopleevents/pandeAMEX101.html.

pbs.org/wgbh/nova/holocaust/experiments.html.

peachtree-online.com/Yellow_Star_no_art/Adults/theresienstadt.

perso.orange.fr/d-d.natanson/dora.

politische-bildung-rip.de/fileadmin/download/Hinzert-e.

reference.com/browse/wiki/Prince_Philip_of_Hesse-Kassel.

remember.org/witness/ohrdruf.html.

scrapbookpages.com/BergenBelsen/ConcentrationCamp.html.

scrapbookpages.com/BuchenwaldResistance.html.

scrapbookpages.com/DachauScrapBook/DachauTrials/Introduction.html.

sturmvogel.orbat.com/ss-tk.html.

themoscowtimes.com/stories/2005.

themrsastor.blogspot.com/2006/08/reflective-Sundays.

tnholcom.org/bio.php?id=65.

truthdig.com/report/page3/20061113_growing_up_with_gore_vidal.

ushmm.org/lc_04/focus/pdf.

ushmm.org/wlc/en/?ModuleId=10005143.

ushmm.org/wlc/media_cm.php?lang+en&ModuleId=10005424&Media=2468.

vcalc.net/cu-bckup.

v2rocket.com.

werewolf.greyfalcon.us/Ohrdruf.

wymaninstitute.org/letters/2002-12.24-failure.php.

yadvashem.org.il.

Zebu.uoregon.edu/~js/space/lectures/lec04.

Zhukov.mitsi.com/Kursk.

zplac2b.com/464th/sortie.

INDEX

ILLUSTRATIONS: Bold, italics
PEOPLE: Bold

A

Abwehr, 324
Acevedo, Tony, 219
Adenauer, Konrad, 155
Adler, Julius, 300
Ahr River, 203
Allen, Robert S., 213
Allen, Terry, 258
Allied prisoners at KL Buchenwald, 160-161, 162-163, 178-181, 183-184
Alsace-Lorraine, France, 190, 217
Amery, Jean, 155
Amt D-II, 137
Amt 10, 212
Amalia, Anna, 19-20
American Jewish Congress, 69, 122, 126,
  "Stop Hitler Now" rally, 124-125, 313
American League for a Free Palestine, 148
Amiens, France, 186
Anderson, J. Leavitt, 240
Antelme, Robert, 155
Anti-Semitism, 11, 14, 39, 54, 56, 61-64, 71, 85, 86, 127, 138n
Army Research Center Peenemünde, 107, 109, ***108***, 111, 112, ***112***, 114-115, 116, 117-118, 213n
Arnstadt, Germany, 212
Aschaffenburg, Germany, 205n
Attendorn KL, 323
Augsburg, Germany, 120
Auschwitz KL, 44, 183, 185, 186, 188-189, 194, 198, 219, 224, 227, 308, 327, 339
  Bombing of, 186, 187
  Evacuation of, 190-191
  Liberation of, 193
Austria, 43, 207, 217, 311, 321, 326
Axmann, Artur, 332n

B

Babi Yar, 64-65
Bach, Johann S., 20, 211
Bad Kreuznach, Germany, 206
Bad Langensalza, Germany, 235
Bad Orb, Germany, 217
Balachowsky, Alfred, 91, 154
Baltic Sea, 192
Bandy, Paul, 259
Barkley, Alben W., 298
Bartel, Walter, 142
Bastogne, Belgium, 206
Battle of the Bulge (see also Operation *Wacht-am-Rhein*), 205, 206, 209, 217, 323
Baum, Alex, 112, 117-118
Bayer, 128
Becker, Karl Emil, 105, 107
Beethoven, Ludwig van, 314
Beir, Robert, 126, 316
Belgium, 43, 44, 196, 205, 206, 235, 330
Ben-Ami, Jacob, 126
Bendzin, Poland, 195, 256
Bénès, Edvard, 43-44, 98
Bennett, Robert J., 248, ***248***, 253, 254, 255
Bepulsi, Peter A., 272
Bergson Group, 71, 126-127, 189
Bergson, Peter H., 122-123, 124, ***124***, 125-126, 126-127, 148, 189
Berlin, Germany, 157, 193-194, 207, 213, 240, 263, 293, 294, 328, 332n, 338
Bernadette, Folke, 208
Bernstein, Col., 268
"Big Three" Conference, 194
"Big Week" bombing campaign, 120
Bilder, Michael, 304
Billroda, Germany, 178
Bird, Lewis, 304
Bismarck, Otto von, 3, 20
Bismarckturm, 3, ***3***, 20, 287, 303, ***303***, 339
Blechhammer KL, 195
Blitzkrieg (lightning war), 44
Blockälteste, 28-29, 50, 162, 230, 231
Blum, Léon, 154, 154n, 323
Blutstraße (Blood Road), 48, 275, 287
BMW (Bavarian Motor Works), 128
Bodot, Paul, 254n
Böhlen, Germany, 196
Bonhoeffer, Dietrich, 324
Bonn, Germany, 203
Boris III of Bulgaria, 157
Bormann, Martin, 332
Bourke-White, Margaret, 301
Bracker, Milton, 188
Bradley, Omar N., 193n, 203, 209, 210, 263, 267, ***269***, 270-271, 273, 277, 280, 316, 329
Brahms, Johannes, 314
Brandell, Sol, 242
Brandt, Karl, 87, 88
Braun, Eva, 328
Braun, Wernher von, 106, ***106***, 111n, 107, 109, 112, 113, 116, 121
Bräuning, Edmund, 226n, 227
Breitscheid, Rudolph, 154, 174
Brill, Hermann, 296-297
British Army
  21st Army Group, 203, 207, 325
British Broadcasting Company (BBC), 302
British Parliament delegation visits Buchenwald, 297-298
Brooks, Allison C., 165,
Brooks, C. Wayland (see also *Sturmabteilung*), 298
Brooks, Morton, 218
Brown Shirts, 15-16, 15n

Brunswick, Germany, 120

Buchenwald Concentration Camp, 11-12, 79, 83, 94, 134-139, ***136***, 156, 157, 160, ***166***, 179, 191, 194, 195, 200, 207, 208, 210, 211, 212, 214, 215, 216, 217, 219, 220, 224, 227, 229-230, 232-236, 245, 247, 248-258, 264-266, 271, 275-307, 293-307, ***296***, 308, ***309***, 311, 316, 318-319, 321, 323, 324, 326, 327, 328, 329, 338-339, 340

- *Appell / Appellplatz*), 46-47, 49, 50, 162, ***296***
- Barracks, 30, ***40***, 45-46
- Bombing of, 166, 167-170, 171, ***171***, 172-173, 175, ***175***, 178, 295
- British Parliament delegation visits, 297-298
- Brothel, 131
- Building of, 2, 6, 13, 19, 20-22, ***21***, ***22***, 23-24, ***23***, 27
- Bunker (*Zellerbau*), 23, ***31***
- Children at, 143-146, 144n, 145-146, ***145***, 170-171, 264-265, ***265***
- Crematorium, 6, 23, 49, 118, 133, 149, 161, 163, 164, 170, 174, 175, 178, 181, 192
- Danish policemen at, 182
- DAW (*Deutsche Ausrüstungswerke*), 72, 109, 129, 130-131, 134, 135, 140, 142, 147
- Death registry (*Totesbuch*), 27
- Deaths at, 190, 199, 214, 294-295
- Doctors, 33, 36, ***37***, 82, 86, 87, ***87***, 88, 89-90, ***89***, ***90***, 91, 92, ***92***, 92n, 93, 94, 94n, 95, 97-98, 99, 100-101, ***101***, 101-103, ***103***, 130
- Evacuation of, 216, 250
- *Fichtenhain*, 154, 155, 174
    - Notable inmates, 154-155, ***156***, 157, 174
    - Bombing of, 165-177, ***171***, ***173***, ***176***, ***177***
- Food and meals, 47, 48, 50
- Guards, 42, 43, 51, ***51***, 52-53, ***52***, 53n, 54-55, ***55***, 61, 134, 138, 176, ***176***
- Gustloff-Werk II factory, 4, 109, ***110***, 111, ***111***, 114-115, 130-131, 134, 136, 138-139, 142, 149, 150-151, 161, 165 169, ***173***
- Human-skin artifacts (see also Lampshades), 36-37, ***38***
- Infirmary, 96-97, ***97***, 98
- Inmate population, 190, 194, 214
- Inmates, 27, 36, 38, 40, 42, 48, 49, 50, 62, 80, 91, 92, 96-98, 99, 100-101, ***101***, 101-103, ***103***, 119, 132, 134-137, ***135***, 139, 146, 149, 150-151, 158-161, 162, 163, 167, 168, 169-170, 172-173, 174, 179-181, 188
    - Rented to German industries, 73-74, 74n, 114, 116, 128, 129, 146-147
    - Russian POWs, 93, 294-295
    - SOE (Special Operations Executive) POWs, 163-164
- International Camp Committee, 141
- Liberation of, 251-258, 266, 267
- "Little Camp," 93, 101, 131, 144, 161-162, 164, 167, 168, 172, 179, 180, 181, 182, 198-199, 284
- Medical experiments, 82-98
- Music at, 182
- Naming of, 27
- Plans for rebellion, 72, 139, 140-142, 165
- Processing new inmates, 27-30, 161
- Quarry (*Steinbruch*), 39-41, ***40***
- Sanitary conditions, 47
- Special Camp No. 2, 339
- Tools/methods of torture/killings, 30, ***31***, 48, 49-50, 66, 164n
- U.S. Congressional delegation visit, 298, ***299***
- U.S. editors and publishers visit, 300-303, ***302***
- Work groups (*Arbeitskommando* or *Kommando*), 47, 48, 114-115, 131-132, ***132***
- Zoo, 24

Buchenwald Manifesto, 297-297

Bulgaria, 157

Burgstahler, Merrill C., 305-307

Burke, Edmund, 12

Burkel, Josef, 18

Burney, Christopher, 163, 215

Busse, Ernst, 142

Butcher, Harry C., 272

C

Calloway, Capt., 281, 282, 287

Cambodia, 340

Canaris, Wilhelm, 324

Canfield, Gordon, 298

Cap Arcona (ship), 325

Capra, Frank, 318

Carnegie Hall, 301

Casablanca (film), 313

Chaff, 170, 170n

Cham, Germany, 320

Chamberlain, Houston S., 85

Chamberlain, Neville, 44

Chamberlain, William H., 263

Chandler, Norman, 300, 302

Chandon-Moët, Paul, 154

Charboneau, William F. Jr., 243

Chatenay, Pierre, 264

Chelmno, Poland, 63

Chemnitz, Germany, 233, 234

Chenery, William, 301

Church, Samuel H., 123n

Churchill, Winston, 64, 104, 114, 117, 163, 194

Ciufoli, Domenico, 142

Clauberg, Carl, 86

Clin, M., 154

Coates, Edmund, 256

Codman, Charles R., 5, 268, 270, 271-272, 275-277, 278, 279

Cole, Ralph G., 243

Cologne, Germany, 142n, 203

Combat Box, 166, 166n

Compiègne, France, 191

Concentration/death/slave-labor camps, 9, 10, 11, 87

- Auschwitz-Birkenau, 18, 24, 28, 44, 55, 73, 76, 77, 79, 83, 86, 87, 96, 129, 131n, 141, 183, 185, 186, 187, 188-189, 190, 191, 193, 194, 198
- Bad Sulza, 19
- Belzec, 79
- Berga-an-der-Elster, 153, 217-219, 319, 320
- Bergen-Belsen, 87, 147n, 191, 214, 271, 293-294, 325, 339

Cobelwitz, 195
Columbia-Haus, 25
Dachau, 13, 16, 17, 18, 19, 23, 24, 25, 29, 36, 45, 55, 83, 87, 94, 129, 131n, 154, 155, 188, 191, 219, 229, 232-233, 271, 298, 308, 311, 322, 324, 326, 327, 328, 334, 339
Liberation of, 322-323
War-crimes trials held at, 94, 332-334
Drancy, 76, 76n
Ebensee, 311, 323, 325
Eichendorf, 219, 224
Erla, 271
Espenfeld, 212
Esterwegen, 25
Falkenau-an-der-Eger, 326
Flossenbürg, 83, 155, 157, 191, 229, 230, 232, 321, 322, 323-324, 326, 335, 339
Gardelegen, 326
Groß-Rosen, 39, 83, 191, 194-195, 198, 200
Halberstadt-Zweiberge (Malachit), 323
Hannover-Ahlem, 325
Hohnstein, 25
Kaufering, 326
Langenstein, 323
Le Struthof (See Natzweiler-Struthof)
Leipzig-Schönefeld, 323
Leipzig-Thekla, 271n, 323
Lichtenburg, 25
Leimeritz, 232
Maidanek, 65, 73, 152, 189, 314
Mauthausen, 83, 323, 325, 327, 334-335, 339
Mittelbau-Dora (Nordhausen), 117-118, 119-120, 121, 179, 205, 208, 234, ***257***, 258,
258, 300n, 323, 339
Inmates, 117-119
Workers' revolt, 119-120
Muna, 212
Natzweiler-Struthof, 87, 94, 187-188, 339
Neuengamme, 83, 94, 182, 191, 323, 32
Niederhagen, 83
Nohra, 16, 17, 17n, 266
Ohrdruf, 208, 210, 211-214, 216, 219-220, ***220***, 224-225, 226-227, 228, 232, 237-240, 242-247, 267-274, ***269***, 277, 280, 303, 328, 337, 338
Possible A-bomb test at, 213
Ottmuth, 77
Ravensbrück, 86, 87, 96, 131, 227, 294
Sachsenburg, 6, 21, 25
Sachsenhausen, 13, 21, 25, 45, 79, 83, 87, 89, 129, 155, 212, 219, 294, 339
Salzwedel, 323
Schönebeck, 137-138
Sobibor, 79
Stutthof, 192-193, 212, 325
Theresienstadt, 216, 229, 323, 339
Trassenheide, 112, 166
Treblinka, 79, 87
Wöbbelin, 324
Zwodow, 326
Concerzowo, Margarete, 14
Congden, Howard E., 259-262
Cool, Pieter, 215
Costello, Normand O., 259
Crawinkel, Germany, 212, 224
Culin, Frank L., 209
Czechoslovakia, 43-44, 67, 98, 321, 325, 330

D

D'Agostini, Benedict, 171
Dager, Holmes, 321
Daimler-Benz, 128
Daladier, Édouard, 44, 154
Dalton, Hugh, 163
Daluege, Kurt, 64
Damaszyn, Gwidon, 139
Danzig, Poland, 192
Darfur, 340
Daub, Gerald, 217-218
Dauteuil, Donat "Don," 159
Davidson, Charles, 256
Davies, Norman, 113
DAW (German Armament Works), 129,
Death marches, 190-191, 193, 214, 217-219, 226, 227, 229-230, 231 (fn0, 232-234, 294, 295, 319-323
Debouche, Carl, 94n
Deeney, John A., 304
Degner, Lawrence A., 262-263
Delattre, Lucien, 150
Denmark, 44, 63, 182, 330
Denson, William, 94, 334-337, ***335***, ***336***
Desard, Emmanuel, 254n
Dewey, Thomas, 267
Dietsche, Arthur, 91
Ding, Erwin (Schuler), 87, 89-91, ***90***, 91, 92, 92n, 93, 94
Dimitman, E.Z., 301
Dönitz, Karl, 328, 331
Dornberger, Walter, 113
Dresden, Germany, 194, 321
Dupont, Victor, 62, 182-183
Dutch Underground at Buchenwald, 179
Dwinnel, John S., 334
Dye, S.M., 292

E

Eddy, Manton S., 203, 205, 206, 210, 268, 271
Eden, Anthony, 80
Edwards, Carter, 162, 179
Eichman, Adolf, 192
Eichorn, Franz, 250
Eicke, Theodor, 17-18, ***17***, 19, 25, 29, 42, 83
Eiden, Hans, 250, 252
Einsatzgruppen, 63, 65
Eisele, Hannes, 87, 90, 94, 94n, ***95***
Eisenhower, Dwight D., 79-80, 193n, 208, 263, 267-268, ***269***, 270, 271, 272-273, 277, 279,
303, 305, 316, 329
Elana of Montenegro, 155
Elbe River, 209, 210, 329

Elephant Hotel, 20, 197
Elting, Howard, Jr., 70-71
Emmons, Water F., 293, 329
England, rocket attacks on, 109n, 207, 224
Erft River, 203
Erfurt, Germany, 196, 209, 210, 250, 266
Essen, Germany, 73
Ettersberg (hill), 1, 6, 19, 20, 114, 154, 160, 178, 180, 190, 198, 216, 232, 282, 304, 323, 338-339
Eugenics, 99-100
Euskirchen, Germany, 203
Evacuation of camps (see Death Marches)

F

Falconry, 154
Falkenberg, Anton, 155
Farben, I.G., 128, 186, 332
Fellman, Norman, 218
Feuer, Max, 251
"Final Solution," 66
Finkelstein, Sevek, 145
Finley, Thomas, D., 209
Fisher, Erica, 262
Fleck, Egon, 254
Fleming, Ian, 163
Florstedt, Hermann, 33
Foch, Ferdinand, 292
Ford, Henry, 138n
Ford Werk AG (subsidiary of Ford Motor Company), 128, 138, 138n
France, 43, 44, 63, 161, 163n, 179, 185, 187, 205, 235, 330
Franco, Francisco, 7
Frank, Hans, 331
Frankfurt-am-Main, Germany, 205, 206, 217
Frankfurter, David, 109n
French Army, 187, 188
French Resistance, 159
Freud, Sigmund, 99
Freudenberg, Fritz, 251
Frick, Wilhelm, 331
Fricke, Werner, 226n
Friedenberg, Stanley, 244
Fritzsche, Hans, 331
Froelichen, Charles, 304
Fromm, Friedrich, 152
Funk, Walther, 331

G

Gamelin, Maurice, 154
Ganz, Anton, 325-326
Gavin, James, 324-325
Gay, Hobart R., 271, 279
Gebhardt, Karl, 87
Geller, Victor B., 304, 313
George, Walter F., 298
Gera, Germany, 196, 233
Geraldi, Joseph J., 165-166
German Army (Wehrmacht), 43, 192
Army Group Vistula, 204
German Earth and Stone Works, Inc., 39
German Economic Enterprises, 128
German Marines, 325
Germany, 6-11, 20, 25, 33, 39, 43, 44, 51, 53n, 54, 61, 63, 66, 69, 70, 71, 73-74, 76n, 77, 78, 80, 84, 85, 86, 87, 100, 104, 105-106, 107, 109, 114, 115, 120, 123, 125, 129, 134, 137, 138n, 140, 141, 143, 146, 148, 150, 151-152, 155, 187, 205, 217, 226, 286, 296, 297, 309, 312, 313-314, 330, 331, 338
Gestapo (Secret State Police), 9, 66, 75, 76, 157, 159, 181, 186, 188, 192, 222-223, 294, 301, 316
Geve, Thomas, 250
Gisevius, Hans B., 155
Gladstone, Bill, 159
Glineur, Henri, 142
Gobineau, Joseph A. Comte de, 85
Goebbels children, 328
Goebbels, Josef, 14, 74, 104, 105, 208, 267n, 328
Goebbels, Magda, 328
Goethe, Johann W., 6, 19-20, 314
Goethe Oak, 6, 20, 21, 176, ***177***
Gold, Reich, 268
Goldberg, Moniek, 233
Goldkranz, Johannen (John Ranz), 195-196, 195, 197-198, 202, 230, 231, 249-250, 256, 257
Goldman, Nahum, 127
Gommlich, Hellmuth, 19
Göring, Hermann, 66-67, 107n, 120, 154, 331
Gossel, Germany, 212
Gotha, Germany, 120, 210, 211, 235, 237, 238, 271, 273, 284
Gottschalk, Herbert, 253, 255
Grant, Madison, 85
Grand Mufti of Jerusalem, 72
Great Britain, 44, 159, 179, 187, 316, 331
Greiz, Germany, 319
Gritz, Richard, 42, 48
Greunuß, Werner, 87, 212
Gros, Louis, 134-137, ***135***, 142, 146, 147, 149-151, 167-170, 172-173, 191-192, 252, 255
Groschke, Richard, 27
Grow, Robert W., 206, 209, 248
Grunewald, Paul, 36
Guderian, Heinz, 207
Gugig, Willi, 170
Gusen, Germany, 326
Gustloff, Wilhelm, 109n
Gustloff-Werk I (factory), 197
Gustloff-Werk II (factory), 4, 109, 109n, ***110***, 111, ***111***, 114-115, 130-131, 134, 136, 138-139, 142, 149, 150-151, 154, 160-161, 169, 178, 187, 277
Gypsy (Roma) prisoners, 29, 36, 48, 80, 87, 131, 143, 180

H

Hackmann, Heinrich, 30, 32, ***32***
Hadamar, Germany, 323
Halder, Franz, 155
Halloran General Hospital, 302n
Halloran, Walter, 286, 289

Hamburg, Germany, 325
Hammelburg, Germany, 206n
Handelsman, Jack, 146
Handloser, Siegfried, 87, ***87***, 88
Hardcastle, Bill, 159
Harris, Albert E., 248
Harris, Jesse, 237
Harrison, Leland, 71
Harz Mountains, 210, 211, 323
Hastin, Jim, 173
Hearst, John R., 300
Heinkel, 128
Hemmons, P.D., 182, 183
Hentsche, Police Capt., 282
Herzstark, Curt, 155
Hess, Rudolf, 331
Hessen-Kassel, Elisabetta, 157
Hessen-Kassel, Heinrich, 157
Hessen-Kassel, Moritz, 157
Hessen-Kassel, Otto, 157
Heydrich, Reinhard, 67, 185, 331
Hibbs, Ben, 301
Hickey, Doyle O., 258
High, Stanley, 301, 302
Higuera, Wencie, 243
Himmler, Heinrich L., 13-14, 15, 17, 18, 25, 57, 61-62, 86, 112, 113-114, 117, 128, 130, 182n, 185-186, 190, 204-205, 207, 215, 225-226, 229, 230, 263, 293-294, 329, 331, 338
  Marriage to Margarete Concerzowo, 14
  Mistress of, 14
  Suicide of, 329
Himmler, Burwitz, Gudrun, 14
Hindenburg, Paul von, 155
Hitler, Adolf, 2, 7, 8, 9, 10, 11, 14, 20, 43-44, 57, 63, 66, 73, 84, 85, 99, 113, 114, 117, 133, 138n, 155, 157, 185, 204, 205, 207, 208, 215, 238n, 263, 267n, 281, 293, 294, 324, 328, 331, 338
  Assassination attempt on, 152
  Suicide of, 328
Hitler Youth (*Hitlerjugend*), 20, 227, 238, 325, 331
Hodges, Counrtney H., 203, 209-210
Hodson, Stanley, 242-243
Hof, Germany, 319
Hoge, William, 206, 237
Hogg, Charles A., Sr., 304
Holocaust, 11
Holocaust Memorial Museum, U.S., 13
Homberg, Germany, 207
Homosexuals, persecution of, 29, 61, 80, 94, 188
Horn, Otto, 142
Höss, Rudolf, 18
Hotel zum Erbprinzen, 197
Hottelstedt, Germany, 251, 253, 255
Hoven, Waldemar, 33, 87, 91, 92, 92n, ***92***, 93, 94
Hoyt, James, 253, 255
Hrsel, Emil, 142
Hugo Boss, 128
Hull, Cordell, 71
Hungary, 42n, 207, 264
Hussein, Saddam, 340

I

I.G. Farben, 18, 73, 88
Innemann, Kvetoslav, 142
International Camp Committee, 251, 252
Iraq, 340
"Iron Curtin," 338
Irzyk, Albin F., 244
Israel, 58, 144, 146
Israel, David, 317
Italy, 7, 66, 80, 100, 104, 115, 121, 133, 151, 155-157, 174, 187
Izak, Ed V. 298, ***298***
Izydorczyk, Jan, 142

J

Jabotinsky Group, 221
Jabotinsky, Ze'ev, 221
Jackson, Henry, 298,299
Janson, Paul-Emile, 155
Japanese Empire (Japan), 66, 310
Jena, Germany, 196, 293
Jensen, Carl P. (aka **Carl Vaernet**), 95
Jewish Agency for Palestine, 122, 124
Jewish Army of Stateless and Palestinian Jews, 123
Jewish Telegraphic Agency, 78
Jews, 10-11, 61-62, 104, 105, 157, 188, 191-192, 196, 207, 212, 231, 263, 300, 304, 308-310, 312, 313, 314, 315, 316-318, 320, 325
  Extermination of, 63, 64-65, 66, 69, 70, 71, 75, 76, 78-79, 79, 80, 122
  Himmler's "attempts to save," 185, 207, 293-295
  Kristallnacht, 39
  Laws to restrict, 10, 39, 85
  Pogroms, 10, 39
Jodl, Alfred, 331
Jonastal, Germany, 212, 224
Jouhaux, Leon, 155

K

Kahn, Bernard, 311
Kaiserslautern, Germany, 206
Kaltenbrunner, Ernst, 185, 208, 331
Kammler, Hans, 118-119
Kampeck, Hermann, 27
Kapo(s), 17, 17n, 28, 41, 50, 119, 144, 201, 230
Kassel, Germany, 206, 207, 248
Katzen-Ellenbogen, Edwin, 96, 97-98, 99-103, ***101***, ***103***, 181n
Keffer, Frederic, 253-256, ***249***
Keitel, Wilhelm, 331
Kerr, E. Coe, Jr., 264
Kersten, Felix, 293-294
Kertesz, Imre, 144n
Kesselring, Albert, 214, 238, 266
Kestel, Josef, 30, 32-33

Kiel, Emil C., 334
Kiev, U.S.S.R., 64-65
King, George, 314
King, Myles A., 174
Kinnis, Arthur G., 158-161, 163, 167, 169, 173, 179-180, 181, 182, ***184***
Kjung, Nikolaj, 142
Klein, Rene, 150-151
Kloss, Andrea, 280-282, 287
Kloss, Erich, 280-282, 287, 288, 291
Koblenz, Germany, 203
Koch, Artwin, ***34***, ***35***, 36
Koch, Gisele, ***35***, 36
Koch, Gudrun, 36
Koch, Margerete Ilse, 25, ***26***, 27, 33, ***34***, ***35***, 36, 65, 91, 175, 292n, ***333***, ***336***
  Trial of, 330, 333-337
  Death of, 337n
Koch, Karl Otto, 24, 25, ***26***, 27, 30, 33, ***33***, ***34***, ***35***, 36, 48, 65-66, 69, 73, 175, 215
  Execution of, 216
Koch, Otto, 259, 262, 280-281
Kodak, 128
Kogon, Eugen, 40, 48, 49, 50, 90, 92, 103, 226, 232
Kohn, Murray, 224, 227, 338
Konzentrationslager (See Concentration camps)
Kook, Hillel (See **Bergson, Peter H.**)
Krakow, Poland, 128, 190
Krebs, Hans, 214
Kretschmer, Karl, 57
Kristallnacht, 39, 318
Krupp AG, 73-74, 128, 146-147, 147n
Kuhn, Harry, 142
Kunkel, John C., 298
Kuntz, Albert, 188
Kursk, battle of, 113, 115

L

Lamp shades, human-skin, 175-176, 292-293, 304, 337
Landsberg Prison, Germany, 20, 92n, 94n, 326
Lange, Herbert, 63
Lau, Yisrael M., 144, ***145***, 265
Laufer, David, 220, 221, 222
Laufer, Leo (aka **Shmuel Lieb**), 219-225, 239-240, 241, 273-274, ***274***
Lavi, Naftali, 144
Lee, John, 322-323
Leipzig, Germany, 89, 99, 120, 166, 171, 194, 195, 196, 271n, 321, 323
Leiserofef, Eric, 244
Leonding, Austria, 338
Levin, Meyer, 272
Lewis, Emanuel, 335-336, ***335***
Ležáky Czechoslovakia, 67n
L'Hopital, René, ***277***, 292
Liddell Hart, Basil H., 309, 310
Lidice, Czechoslovakia, 67n
Liszt, Franz, 20
Łódź , Poland, 195, 219, 220, 221-222, 223
London Agreement, 331
London, England, 179, 273
Long, Breckinridge, 70, 71, 127
Lorner, Georg, 128
Lübeck, Germany, 67, 329
Lubersac, Raoul de, 264
Lublin, Poland, 65, 73n
Luce, Claire B., 298, 300
Ludwigslust, Germany, 324-325
Lukehart, Richard C., 272
Lüneberg Heath, 329
Luther, Martin, 85
Luxembourg, 68, 235

M

McBride, Horace L., 209, 323
McCloy, John J., 186-187
Magdeburg, Germany, 137
Main River, 206
Mainz, Germany, 206
Manasco, Carter, 298, 300
Manchester, William, 74
Mandel, Georges, 154
Manring, Gordon M., 304
Mantler, Marshall J., 315
Marchant, Jeff, 158
Marie, André, 215
Marshall, George C., 193n, 272, 297, 308, 310, 314
Marseilles, France, 159
Masur, Norbert, 206
Maurer, Gerhard, 137
Medical experiments (at concentration camps), 81, 85-86, 86n, 87, 90-91, 92, 93-94, 94-95, 95-96, 188, 278-279, 285-286
  Doctors involved in, 87, 92, 93, 94, 95, 96
  "Special Treatment 14f13," 82-83
  T-4 euthanasia program, 63, 82
  War-crimes trials of Nazi doctors, 86n, 88n, 90, 92n, 94n
Mein Kampf, 8
Mendelssohn, Felix, 20, ***87***
Mendelssohn, le, Joseph, 95-96
Mennecke, Friedrich, 83
Merbach, Hans E., ***321***, 321-322
Merkers, Germany, 267-268
Merseberg, Germany, 196
Messerschmitt, 128
Metz, France, 209
Michel, Jean, 119, 133
Middleton, Troy H., 203, 205, 206, 210
Milgram, Stanley, 58-59
Mitchell, Pvt., 264
Möbius, Kurt, 57
Montgomery, Bernard, L., 329
Mordy, Capt., 279
Morgen, G. Konrad, 65-66
Morse, Gilman E., 248
Moselle (Mosel) River, 203, 206
Mott, James W., 298

Mrugowsky, Joachim, 87, 89, ***89***, 93, 94
Mühldorf, Germany, 323
Mühlhausen, Germany, 209
Müller, Heinrich, 192
Mullinex, Charles, 285-286
Munich, Germany, 157, 321
Murphy, Robert D., 270
Murrow, Edward R., 302
Musi, Jean-Marie, 208
Mussolini, Benito, 7, 157

N

Nadich, Judah, 315
National Buchenwald Memorial, 339
National Socialist German Workers Party, 20
Nazi(s), 7, 9, 10, 187, 189, 226, 293, 303, 313, 316, 327, 330, 338
Nazi Movement, 9
Nazi Party, 8
Nazi Persecution Relief Fund, 268n
Netherlands, 68, 179, 330, 331
Neumann, Alois, 142
Neurath, Konstantin Freiherr von, 331
Newman, Al, 258
Newton, Alfred, 164
Newton, Henry, 164
Nickols, Bruce, 243, 244
Niemöller, Martin, 323-324
Nietsche, Friedrich, 20
Norden bombsight, 187
Normandy, France, 161, 185, 206
Norway, 44, 63, 163n, 184, 330
Nostitz, Paul, 21
Nürnberg (Nuremberg) International War-crimes Tribunal, 62, 330-333
Nürnberg (Nuremberg) Laws, 10, 39, 85
Nurtman, Moishe, 145-146

O

OB West, 238
Obersalzburg, Germany, 338
Odom, Charles B., 279
Oflag III (POW camp), 206n
"Olga" Project, 224, 225
Olympic Games (1936), 8, 338
Olympic Stadium (Berlin), 338
Omaha Beach, Normandy, 329
Opel (subsidiary of General Motors), 128
Operations, military
  Argument, 120-121, 203
  Bagration, 151
  Barbarossa, 63
  Dragoon, 185
  Fortitude, 140, 140n
  Gitter, 152
  Husky, 115
  Hydra, 116-117
  Jericho, 186
  Lumberjack, 203
  Market Garden, 185
  Mission 132, 165-166
  Nordwind, 190, 217
  Overlord, 133-134, 161
  Paperclip, 111n
  Plunder, 207
  Torch, 80
  Varsity, 207
  Wacht-am-Rhein, 189-190
Oranienburg, Germany, 205
Orenstein, Salek, 144, 170-171, 201-202, 233-234
Organization Todt, 68
Oslo, University of, 184
Ott, Charles H., 292
Oulins, France, 159

P

Paderborn, Germany, 338
Palestine, 72, 221
Pantanella, Italy, 186
Papen, Franz von, 331
Paris, France, 159, 160, 161, 185
Patterson, Frank, 159
Patton, George S. Jr., 140, 130n, 140n, 203, 205, 206, 209, 210, 213, 235-236, 267-271, ***269***, 273, 275, 277-282, 315, 316
Paul, Marcel, 142
Paulus, Friedrich von, 78, 104, 170, 215
Paxton, Steve, 173
Pearl Harbor, attack on, 66
Peenemünde (See Army Research Center Peenemünde)
Pehle, John W., 186
Pierce, Marie A., 99
Piotrkow, Poland, 265
Pister, Hermann Franz Josef, 67-68, 67n, 68-69, ***68***, 83, 147, 178, 183, 198, 208n, 214, 215-216, 229-230, 233, 248, 250, ***337***
Plauen, Germany, 319
Plaza, Heinrich, 94
Philipp of Hesse, ***156***, 157
Pilsen, Czechoslovakia, 321
Pohl, Oswald, 15, ***15***, 16, 74n, 128, 132-133, 137, 146-147, 185, 207
Poland, 43, 44, 57, 63, 68, 69, 70, 157, 183, 185, 186, 188, 189, 190, 191, 192, 193, 207, 217, 221, 222, 330, 331
Poller, Walter, 91
Poznan, Poland, 223
Prague, Czechoslovakia, 232
Priest, Warren, 282, 305
Prokhorovka, U.S.S.R., 113
Puccini, Giacomo, 155
Pulitzer, Joseph III, 300, 301
Putsch, 14

Q

Quandt, Harald, 328
Quirk, James T., 302

R

Radios, clandestine, at Buchenwald, 139, 207, 234-236
Raeder, Erich, 331
Raible, Erna, ***35***
Railroads, German, 191, 192, 195-196, 232-234, 339
Rancy, Jacques, 38
Rappaport, Mel, 267, 316
Red Cross, 125, 141, 162, 181n, 182, 195-196, 208
"Red Triangle," 235-236, 252, 254, 268n
Regen River, 320
Regensburg, Germany, 120
Reich Transport Ministry, 192
Reid, Richard, 302
Remagen, Germany, 203
Reparations (to former prisoners), 268n
Réthore, Col., 275, 276
Reynaud, Paul, 154
Rhine River, 203, 206, 207
Ribbentrop, Joachim von, 44, 331
Richards, James P., 298
Richey Program, 317
Riegal, Pete, 196
Riegner, Gerhardt, 70-71, 78
Rjukan, Norway, 163
Romana, Princess Mafalda, 155, ***156***, 157, 174,
  Children **Enrico, Maurizio, Ottone**, ***156***, 157
  Daughter **Elisabetta**, 157
  Husband **Prince Phillip of Hesse**, ***156***, 157
Romania, 42n
Rommel, Erwin, 152
Roosevelt Administration, 69, 79, 80, 81, 300
Roosevelt, Eleanor, 126
Roosevelt, Franklin Delano, 71, 79, 80, 81, 104, 122-123, 125, 126, 127, 148, 194, 267
Rose, Billy, 123, 126
Rose, Gerhard, 87
Rosenberg, Alfred E., 85, 331
Rosenfeld, Martin, 321-322
Rosner, Andrew, 227-228, 238-239, 337-338
Rostock, Paul, 87
Roth, Otto, 139, 142, 251-252
Rötz, Germany, 320
Royal Air Force (RAF), 69
Royal Canadian Air Force (RCAF), 179
Rudolph, Arthur, 111
Rush, Ralph G., 243-244

S

Sagan, Poland, 183
Salat, Solomon, 325-326
Salt, Frank, 172
Saltenstall, Leverette W., 298
Sauckel, Ernst Friedrich Christoph "Fritz," 19, 29, 73, 74, ***280***, 281, 331
Sauckel Werk, Fritz, 109
Scandinavia, 42n
Schacht, Hjalmer, 155, 331
Schaffer, Fritz, 336
Schellenberg, Walter, 208, 294
Schiedlausky, Gerhard, 87, 95, 101-102
Schiller, Friedrich, 20, 197
Schindler, Oscar, 128
Schirach, Baldur von, 20, 331
Schirmer, Henrietta H., 262
Schmidt, Hans H.T., 216, ***216***
Schmidt, William R., 209
Schmuhl, Lorenz, 292
Schneider, Albert, 246-247
Schroeder, Oskar, 87
Schulte, Eduard, 70
Schumann, Clara, 20
Schumann, Robert, 20
Schuschnigg, Kurt von, 323
Schuster, Franz, 142
Schwalbe V, 217
Schweinfurt, Germany, 120
Scotland, 316
Sears, Hayden A., ***245***, 246
Second Reich, 3
Selb, Germany, 319
Serbia-Bosnia-Herzogovina, 340
Seyss-Inquart, Arthur, 331
SHAEF, 268, 294, 315
Shapiro, William, 218, 320
Shepard, Lt., 196
Short, Dewey, 298, 300
Shoskes, Henry, 69
Shulman, Herman, 124-125
Sicherheitsdienst (SD), 185, 227, 316
Sicily, 115
Siemens, 128
Silverman, Samuel S., 71
Simakov, Nikolai, 142
Sitte, Kurt, 37
Slave laborers, 11, 13, 33, 40, 44-45, 52, 61, 73-74, 76, 77, 81, 111-113, 116, 118-120, 121, 122, 128-129, 136-139, 140, 143, 147, 149-151, 165, 179, 197, 205, 212, 315
Smirnov, Ivan, 142
Snodgrass, Harry, 304
SOE (Special Operations Executive). 163-164, 163n, 163n
Sofia, Bulgaria, 157
Sommer, Martin, ***29***, 30, 32
Sonderbauvorhaben III (aka S-III), 212, 213, 240
Soudan, Eugene, 215
Southgate, Maurice, 164
Soviet forces, 190, 193, 204, 207, 209, 263, 293, 294, 326
  Liberation of Auschwitz, 190
  Soviet POWs killed at Buchenwald, 294-295
Soyfer, Jura, 155
Spain, 159
Speer, Albert, 39, 74, 113, 117, 118, 121, 129
Spitz, Vivien, 90, 103n
SS (*Schutzstaffel*), 13, 14, 193, 230, 231, 235, 243, 249, 250, 252, 254, 256, 257, 292, 294, 301, 323, 324, 325-326, 338
  SS-Führerschule, 16-17
  SS-Leibstandarte Adolf Hitler (LAH), 15

SS-Oberführer, 67n
SS Sonderlager Hinzert, 67-68, ***68***
SS-Totenkopfverbande (SSTV), 15, 16, 20-21, 42, 43
SS-Verfügungstruppe (SS-VT), 15
Stalag Luft III, 183
Stalin, Josef, 44, 194, 213n
Stalingrad, U.S.S.R., 215
Stanley, Jack F., 196-197
Stauffenberg, Klaus von, 152, 155
Steyr, Germany, 120
Stieve, Hermann, 86
Stone, Walker, 300-301
Strasbourg, France, 187-188
Strasbourg, University of, 188
Strauss, Richard, 20
Streicher, Julius, 331
Stumpfegger, Ludwig, 332
Sturmabteilung or SA (See Brown Shirts)
Stuttgart, Germany, 120
Sue, Norman, 272
Sulzberger, Arthur, 122
Supek, Rudi, 142
Sweden, 186, 294
Switzerland, 186, 208, 294

T

Taillez, Jean, 146, 172
Task Force Baum, 206n
Tattooed skin (See also Lampshades), ***38***, 337
Taylor, Telford, 96
Tenenbaum, Edward A., 254
Thälmann, Ernst, 155
Thiel, Walter, 116n
Thielbeck (ship), 325
Third Reich, 9, 11, 37, 43, 66, 73, 79, 80, 82, 88, 129, 162, 185, 215, 225, 226, 229, 263, 268, 293, 323, 328, 331, 332, 338
Thomas, Elbert D., 298
Thomason, R. Ewing, 298
Thuringia, 18, 19, 20, 21, 117, 211, 232, 305
Thyssen, Friedrich "Fritz," 155
Tiefurt Palace, 19
Torture, 188, 300, 303, 337
Trautloft, Hannes, 183
Treaty of Locarno, 43
Treaty of Versailles, 8, 43, 105,
Tripartite Gold Commission, 268n
Troistedt, Germany, 259, 262
Truman, Harry S., 267
Typhus, 88-89, 90-91. 223, 242, 278-279, 283, 291, 293

U

United Nations, 80, 124-125, 125n
United Nations Displaced Persons Branch, 330
United Nations War Crimes Commission, 189, 302
U.S.S.R. (Soviet Union), 44, 63, 190, 193, 294, 330, 331, 338
United States, 66, 70, 71, 78-79, 99, 107, 125, 127, 148, 247, 309, 314, 318, 327, 331
Congressmen visit camps, 279, 298-300, ***299***
Editors and publishers visit Buchenwald, 280, 300-302, ***301***
Indifference to Nazi war crimes, 247, 307, 327
United States Army commands and units
Twelfth Army Group, 203, 209, 210, 293, 329
First Army, 203, 209-210
Third Army, 203, 209, 210, 235-236, 254, 256n, 259, 267, 270, 281, 292, 302
VIII Corps, 203, 205, 206
XII Corps, 203, 205, 206, 268, 271
XX Corps, 206
82nd Airborne Division, 324-325
101st Airborne Division, 326
2nd Armored Division, 267
4th Armored Division, 205, 206, 209, 235, 237, 240, 244-247, 254, 272
6th Armored Division, 205, 206-207, 209, 235, 248-249, 253, 256, 275, 285, 304, 305, 316, 323
8th Armored Division, 323, 324
9th Armored Division, 203
10th Armored Division, 205
11th Armored Division, 205, 321
12th Armored Division, 205, 326
1st Infantry Division, 326, 331
2nd Infantry Division, 323
3rd Infantry Division, 258, 323
4th Infantry Division, 324
5th Infantry Division, 205, 304
26th Infantry Division, 205, 326
42nd Infantry Division, 324
45th Infantry Division, 311, 322, 324
36th Infantry Division, 326
63rd Infantry Division, 326
65th Infantry Division, 205
69th Infantry Division, 323
71st Infantry Division, 325
76th Infantry Division, 205, 209
80th Infantry Division, 205, 209, 259, 262-263, 264, 266, 323
83rd Infantry Division, 323
84th Infantry Division, 323
86th Infantry Division, 323
87th Infantry Division, 205, 209, 304
89th Infantry Division, 205, 209, 237-238, 243-244, 248, 337-338
90th Infantry Division, 205, 323
94th Infantry Division, 205
95th Infantry Division, 323
97th Infantry Division, 323
99th Infantry Division, 323
103rd Infantry Division, 326
104th Infantry Division, 258, 323
120th Medical Evacuation Hospital, 282-285, 297, 298
121st 120th Medical Evacuation Hospital, 284
Eighth Air Force, 69, 120-121, 196
401st Bombardment Group, 165

464th Bombardment Group, 186
487th Bombardment Group, 196-197
613th Bomb Squadron, 165
615th Bomb Squadron, 171
837th Bomb Squadron, 198
Utah Beach, Normandy, 206, 209

V

V-1 rocket, 107, 107n, 117, 148, 165, 205, 207n, 277
V-2 rocket, 107-108, 111, 112-113, ***112***, 113, 114, 117, 118, 120, 121, 137, 150, 165, 178-179, 205, 207, 277
Vatican, 157
Victor Emmanuel III, 155
Victor, Paul Heinz, 28
Vilna, Lithuania, 70
Vinnichenko, Yakov, 193
Volkswagen, 128
Vorys, John M., 298
Vosges Mountains, France, 187-188, 190

W

Wachsmut, Heinz,213
Waffen-SS, 15, 42, 42n
Hygenic Institute of, 89
Wagenen, James H. van, 246-247
Wagner, Erich, 36-37, ***37***, 87
Wagner, Mitiek, 243
Wagner, Richard, 20, 85
Wajchendler, Chaim, 233
Waldeck und Pyrmont, Erbprinz Josias, 65, 248, 332, ***333***
Walker, Walton H., 203, 205, 206, 210, 268, 271, 277
Walther, Armin, 139, 234
Wannsee Conference, 66
Ward, Harry, 253-255
War-Crimes tribunals, 330-333
War Refugee Board, 186, 189
Warsaw, Poland, 70, 75
Washington, D.C., 273, 298, 300, 315
Waters, John K., 206n
"We Will Never Die" pageant, 126-127, 313
Wehrmacht (German Army), 16, 43, 77, 212
Weimar, Germany, 1-7, ***1***, 10, 16, 19-21, 23, 25, 33, 54, 66, 84, 106, 109, 117, 120, 131, 153, 170, 171, 174, 176, 178, 179, 195, 209, 211, 216, 217, 227, 232, 233, 235, 251, 254, 259-263, ***260***, 267, 275, 277, 279, 280-282, 283, 287, 288, 291, 293, 303, 304-305, 321, 322, 338
Bombing of, 196-199, ***199***, 201-202, ***201***
Capture of, 259-263, ***260***, ***261***
Citizens visit Buchenwald, 279, 280-282, 287-291, ***288***, ***289***, ***290***
Occupation of, 227
Weimar Republic, 10
Weismann, Leon, 138
Weizmann, Chaim, 122, 124
Welles, Sumner, 71-72, 79
Werber, Jacob "Jack," 30, 32, 47, 109, 131, 143-144, 146, 175-176, 215-216, 233
Werl, Germany, 323
Werner, Claire, 213
Werra River, 210
Wertz, Lt., 197
Wesel, Germany, 207
Weser River, 210
West Wall ("Siegfried Line"), 209
Wewelsburg Castle, 338
Wherry, Kenneth S., 298
Whitney, Carl, 335-336, ***335***
"Why We Fight" (film), 318
Widerman, Moishe (and family), 75, 76-77
Widerman, Robert Max (aka Robert Clary), 75-78, ***75***, 194-195, 197, 200, ***200***, 250-251, 252, 256-257
Wiechart, Ernst, 155
Wiesbaden, Germany, 206
Wiesel, Eliezer ("Elie"), 144, 144n, 252, ***278***, 239
Wilder, Krulik, 234
Wilhelm Gustloff-Werk II (See Gustloff-Werk II)
Williams, William E., 284
Wilson, Woodrow, 99
Winkeln, 29
Wise, Rabbi Stephen S., 69, 71-72, 78-79, 80-81, 122, 123, 124,125, 126, 127
Wodzislaw, Poland, 190-191
Wolsyn, Poland, 223
Wood, Eric F., 292
Woodside, J.P., 264
World Jewish Congress, 70, 71, 78, 293
Worms, Germany, 206

X-Y-Z

Yalta Conference, 194, 203
Yeo-Thomas, Forest, 255
Zenkl, Petr, 98, 155
Zimbargo, Philip G., 59-60
Zionist Organization of America, 126
Zyklon-B, 88, 189
Zylberberg, Perec, 201, 234